INTERNATIONAL & COMPARATIVE PHYSICAL EDUCATION AND SPORT

(Edited, with essays by)
Earle F. Zeigler
Ph.D., LL.D., D.Sc., FAAKPE
The University of Western Ontario
Canada

T0380755

Trafford Publishing
2009

Printed in Victoria, BC, Canada.

ISBN: 978-1-4269-0643-5 (sc)
ISBN: 978-1-4269-0645-9 (eb)

*Our mission is to efficiently provide the world's finest, most comprehensive book publishing
service, enabling every author to experience success. To find out how to publish your book, your
way, and have it available worldwide, visit us online at www.trafford.com*

Trafford rev. 11/17/09

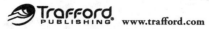 www.trafford.com

North America & international
toll-free: 1 888 232 4444 (USA & Canada)
phone: 250 383 6864 ♦ fax: 812 355 4082

Dedication

To the memory of
DOROTHY AINSWORTH,
LYNN VENDIEN,
WILLIAM JOHNSON,
and **RAYMOND CISZEK.**

These dedicated professionals, working within the AAHPERD understood how truly important it is for the "allied professions" to understand and promote the international and comparative aspects of physical activity education and educational sport worldwide

Foreword

Darwin Semotiuk
Past-President, ISCPES
Canada

It is with great pleasure that I have the opportunity to provide some comments on Earle Zeigler and this important scholarly contribution to the area of comparative and international sport and physical education. Indeed, the compilation of important works in Earle Zeigler's **International and Comparative Physical Education and Sport** is long overdue, and a most welcome addition to the body of published materials in this exciting and increasingly relevant field of study. Most would not know that Earle Zeigler is one of the real pioneers in championing the cause of this field of study both within the profession and the discipline. In this book, he has assembled some of the more significant articles that happened to have been produced during his nearly seven decades of professional service and scholarship. What is most remarkable here is that this volume has been produced in the year that Earle Zeigler will be celebrating his 90th birthday. What a story and what a wonderful statement on the unselfish loyalty and dedication this fine human being has shown to his profession and colleagues over this span of time!!! Thank-you Earle Zeigler.......we are in your debt.

As Past-President of the International Society for Comparative Physical Education and Sport (ISCPES), I would like to provide some thoughts on this organization, its past, present and future. ISCPES is basically a volunteer organization that has operated and continues to operate on a very constrained budget. The Society will be celebrating its 31th anniversary on December 29th 2009, having been founded at the First International Seminar on Comparative Physical Education and Sport held at the Wingate Institute of Physical Education in Israel in 1978. It is a research and educational organization. The Society has as its central mission..........'to promote, stimulate and encourage research and scholarly activity in comparative and international physical education and sport'. These broad objectives are realized through academic meetings which are held every two (2) years, through the publication of a newsletter, a scholarly journal (*International Sports Studies*) and Conference Proceedings and through facilitating collaborative research projects and professional international networking. The Biennial Conference has been hosted throughout the world: Israel, Canada, the United States, Germany, Hong Kong, England, the Czech Republic, Japan, Belgium, Australia, Venezuela, Cuba and most recently in Macau, China.

Over the years, the Society has been blessed with exceptional leadership and voluntary participation from its members. Time, energy, commitment and professional contribution are linked to the following names who have had impact on the Society and its activities – Vendien, Simri,

Howell, Bennett, Pooley, Haag, Broom, Zeigler, Fu, Hardman, Krotee, Chandler, Reekie, and Clumpner. The list can go on.........

If one were to compile a report card on ISCPES, I can conclude that, overall, it has been a pretty successful organization. Its Conferences have been well attended and productive. Its publications have made, and continue to make, solid contributions in the global academic community. Indeed, this positive impression and international reputation can be directly linked to the people who have made things happen. The challenge before ISCPES is to become even better in all areas. Hence, I would ask each of you to give consideration to responding to the challenge personally.

What does the future hold? Clearly there are a number of issues and directions that require the attention of the Society. These include:

- Increasing the number of members along with improving their participation and involvement
- Taking the Society's publications up a notch
- Expanding existing international networking and collaborative research opportunities
- Becoming more effective and efficient in using computer/communication technologies and the internet
- Developing new strategies for transition and succession planning – the Society need to engage young, active and capable scholars
- ISCPES needs to become more entrepreneurial, creative and commercial in managing its affairs
- The Society needs to broaden its focus and reach to include countries in Africa, the Caribbean, South America, South-East Asia, Eastern Europe and the Middle East, and finally,
- The Society needs to become more proactive in dealing with important issues before the global community.
- Today, we are living in a new world where the term globalization has continued, and will continue, to take on new meaning. With the click of a mouse, information can be transmitted to the far reaches of the globe, We are all being invited to become 'citizens of the world'. Through this publication, Earle Zeigler has extended this invitation to each of us and our profession. Indeed, I believe the following words say it all.

"..............there is no greater service than that of the man or woman who sows the seed of the right idea in the right places."

Darwin M. Semotiuk, PhD,
The University of Western Ontario,
London, Ontario, Canada, May, 2009

Conceptual Index

PREFACE

Earle F. Zeigler
Canada

The idea of editing and authoring a book on the important topic of comparative physical (activity) education and (educational) sport has been in my mind for years. The ongoing interest of my good friend and colleague at the University of Western Ontario, Darwin Semotiuk (immediate past president of the ISCPES) in the work of the Society kept its ongoing role close to my mind's eye. Hence, when I learned that Anthony Church (Laurentian University) had received the go-ahead to organize an ISCPES conference in June of 2009, I decided that now was the time to follow through with the idea of organizing such a volume.

After due consideration, I decided to divide the body of the text into five parts as follows:

Part One: Historical Orientation: An Emerging
              Post Modern Age
Part Two: Comparative Physical Education
              and Sport: In Retrospect
Part Three: How to Develop the Body of Knowledge
              About Comparative Physical Education
              and Sport
Part Four: A Descriptive Research Format
              and Exploratory Studies
Part Five: Looking to the Future in Physical Activity
              Education and Sport

After explaining how I became interested in the international and comparative aspects of the field in the Introduction, I then discussed several aspects of the history of our work through the efforts of it pioneers in the AAHPERD, ICHPERSD, and ISCPES. I urged all professional educators related to the field to "spread the word" at all levels about the immediate objectives and long-range aims of our evolving quasi-profession/quasi-discipline. I recommended that we should rededicate ourselves right now to become sufficiently motivated to lead the field of physical (activity) education and (educational) sport to reach its potential both at home and abroad to help provide a brighter future for all people everywhere.

In Part One: Historical Orientation: An Emerging Post Modern Age, I began with an effort to set the stage historically for what was to follow. I inquired whether humans in earlier times enjoyed to any degree what we today might define as "quality living." In this vein, I asked, also, to what extent these humans had an opportunity for "freely chosen, beneficial activity…" In the next selection, after enumerating the significant developments that have transformed our lives, I considered to what extent we were ready to enter a postmodern age.

In Part Two: Comparative Physical Education and Sport: In Retrospect, I turned for direct assistance to the earlier work of three colleagues: Brian T. P. Mutimer (Canada), William Johnson (Illinois) and Ken Hardman (England). The first two papers by Mutimer and Johnson were written almost 40 years ago, but each has valuable information orienting us to the subject. The third and fourth selections in this section are by Ken Hardman from the end of the 20th century and the early 21st century. These excellent papers are unique and provide direct insight into the present situation in relation to the topic at hand.

In Part Three: Developing a Body of Knowledge About Comparative Physical Education and Sport, I ask a direct question in Selection #7: "What Should We Do About What We Don't Know?" Of course, this question can be asked of the entire field itself, not just the international and comparative area. Simply put, there is no body of knowledge about the subject in the form of ordered generalizations available in any form for the professional practitioner. I seek to explain how this basic problem can be overcome by the field and by those people primarily interested in the international and comparative aspects of it.

In Part Four: A Descriptive Research Format, Recommended Research, and Exploratory Studies, I turned to the work of several colleagues first: Eric Broom (England and Canada) and Donald Morrison (Canada). In "An Approach to Research in Comparative Physical Education and Sport, Broom completed an outstanding doctoral study employing Bereday's comparative (method) technique of broad descriptive research. At about the same time (the 1970s), Donald Morrison carried out a fine study at the University of Alberta (with guidance from Max Howell and Al Affleck) in which he very carefully delineated a number of factors and relationships to be considered in comparative research related to physical education and sport.

Next there are three exploratory studies by the author/editor using the comparative research technique. One (Sel. #10) is titled Professional Preparation in Physical Education in the United States and Canada (1960-1985): A Comparative Analysis. The second (Sel. #11) looks at "Cross-Cultural Comparison and International Relations in the Mid-1980s. Finally, Selection #12 titled "Assessment of the International Scene in Physical Activity Education and Educational Sport in 1994" concludes Part Four.

In Part Five: Looking to the Future in Physical Activity Education and Sport, in Sel. #13, I seek to answer the question as to "How the Profession of Sport and Physical Education Might Provide Experiences Basic to Peace."

This includes specific program recommendations for the field of physical education and sport.

In Sel. #14, we (Darwin Semotiuk and I), who worked with a committee on the subject, offer for consideration "A Proposed Creed and Code of Ethics Because of troublesome developments in the area of sport, I then decided to include a selection (#15) titled "The Sport Management Profession in the 21st Century." Finally, in Sel. #16, I confront all of us interested in the international and comparative aspects of our work in the ISCPES by asking the question: "The 21st Century: What Should We Do Now?" In doing so, I seek to explain what "we should avoid" and "what we should do" as we face the professional task ahead.

In conclusion, I want to thank those friends and colleagues who permitted me to use their valuable contributions. I know that I speak for them when I urge all who may read these words to "take up the torch" and move it much further along that we were able to do.

Earle F. Zeigler
British Columbia, Canada
2010

Introduction

The International Society for
Comparative Physical Education and Sport

Earle F. Zeigler
Canada

Writing and assembling a book about the international and comparative aspects of physical education and sport was very interesting for me. It made me recall how I got interested in that aspect of our field in the first place.

After a move in 1949 from Yale University to the University of Western Ontario in Canada, I was anxious to keep up my contact with the American scene as well as learn about the Canadian one. I was able to do this through my ongoing membership starting in 1943 in the American Association for Health, Physical Education, and Recreation, as well as through an affiliation with the former College Physical Education Association (an organization for men now merged with the NAKPEHE).

At an AAHPER Convention in 1952, I attended the annual international relations session. There Dorothy Ainsworth of Smith College, a founder and stalwart in this aspect of our work, noted my interest at that time. Hence, in 1952 I was invited to write the "International Scene Column" in AAHPER's professional journal *(JOPER)*. Other people I remember from those days for their contributions include Lynn Vendien (UMass), Bill Johnson (Illinois), Leona Holbrook (Utah), and Ray Ciszek (AAHPER).

I have retained my interest in this highly important aspect of our field ever since. In 1971, with contributions from Max Howell and Marianna Trekell, a work titled *Research in the History, Philosophy, and International Aspects of Physical Education and Sport: Bibliographies and Techniques* (Champaign, IL: Stipes) was published. Our hope was to stimulate solid scholarly endeavor in the international and comparative aspects of the field. As I consider what has happened since, I can only ask: "What indeed has happened in the past 39 years?" The only conclusion one can come to is this: somehow a relatively small number of us in the profession who understand the need for cross-cultural understanding and knowledge carried on under the aegis of several professional associations (the AAHPERD and the ISCPES. However. at present we must become more aggressive and creative in this direction.

Literally "we don't know what we don't know" about the scholarly and professional development of physical activity education and educational sport worldwide. However, we do know that we have *a professional obligation* to promote world brotherhood and peace through the production of pure and applied knowledge about possible values inherent in such activity at all educational levels. Such promotion extends naturally and automatically to the area of international and comparative physical education and sport. We need more people like those stalwarts who have served our Society so ably since its inception. For example, past president Eric Broom (Canada) comes to mind as an excellent example, as does John Pooley (England; then the USA). In addition, Ken Hardman (England) has made a unique contribution to the Society *and* to the literature through his assessment of scholarship in this aspect of the field. And "aficionados" will remember the solid contribution of Frank Fu [Hong Kong] along the way...)

The International Council for Health, Physical Education, and Recreation (ICHPER–SD), with Dong Ja Yang (President), Yoshiro Hatano (Secretary-General), and Bill Stier (SUNY, Brockport) have also been working very hard to improve this situation, but it is definitely an uphill struggle. I must tip my hat too to the earlier dedicated efforts over the years by Carl Troester of AAHPERD. Finally, Julian Stein's devotion to the development of the excellent *Journal of the ICHPER* of AAHPERD was a most significant contribution as well.)

Our own ISCPES journal, begun with verve by Uri Simi, and the *International Journal of Physical Education* (published originally as *Gymnasion)* promoted so well by ICHPER past president, Herbert Haag for many years, deserve strong commendation. Nevertheless, in this era of satellite communication, we should be seeing increased–not less–general and specialized knowledge about other lands on the part of all citizens in the countries served. (Here in North America what we see and hear mostly on television is "news and views of conflicts and disasters.")

Another way to improve the situation is to make certain that fine undergraduate and graduate professional courses are available where we work at both the undergraduate and graduate levels for *both* professional and general education students. This is going to be unusually difficult what with the steadily developing trend in universities toward "*kinesiology and exercise science*" and "*sport management*", a move that appears to automatically downgrade programs that prepare young professionals to serve as physical activity educators and coaches in educational institutions. Well-taught *professional* programs related to international and comparative physical education and sport–with curricula including fine laboratory experiences–can do much to motivate young people to find a life purpose in this profession and subsequently raise the level of world understanding and involvement.

We should be urging all people to give some thought to the desirability (even the necessity) of joining those of their colleagues who are striving to "spread the word" at all levels about the immediate objectives and long-range aims of our evolving quasi-profession/quasi-discipline. This struggle to promote greater opportunity for people of all ages and conditions to become involved in purposeful, developmental physical activity should grow in the 21st century and on into the indefinite future. It should be coupled with greater individual freedom and improved social values and norms.

The International Society for Comparative Physical Education and Sport (ISCPES) was established in December 1978 to promote and strengthen the specialized area of international and comparative study in physical education and sport. Thirty years later, despite the vigorous effort of outgoing ISCPES president, Darwin Semotiuk (U. of Western Ontario), Roy Clumpner Western Washington University), Scott Martyn (Univ. of Windsor). and Rosa de D'Amico (Venezuela), we appreciate that there is still abysmal ignorance in North America, for example, and seemingly elsewhere about this field. This statement does indeed appear to be true both on this continent and in the rest of the world. With the recent election of Walter Ho of Macau as new president of ISCPES, we trust that he and his associates will continue the effort to move the Society ahead in both "professional" and "scholarly" ways.

> Note: I recognize the danger of "naming names" as I have been doing above. Through my ignorance I'm sure I have omitted some people who should have been mentioned. Please excuse me for any such omission and rest assured it was not by intent!

Viewed in perspective, we in this field are most fortunate. We now know that fine programs of physical activity can not only help people live their lives more fully, but that people will also live longer if they are involved regularly. Our task is to convince ever more people to become more than mere observers, to rise to active–and even creative levels–in this great struggle for a "better tomorrow" for all people in the world. We need to produce more "professional missionaries" to help us reach our ultimate goal!

This, then, is how we in comparative and international sport and physical education should "look to the future"" and thereby become secure in the knowledge that we have indeed done our part. However, as is the case with worthwhile but truly difficult tasks, such improvement will not come easily or soon–certainly not in the lifetimes of those reading these words. It can only come eventually through the ongoing efforts of a sufficient number of professional educators making quality decisions generation after generation.

We need to rededicate ourselves right now to become sufficiently motivated to lead the field of physical (activity) education and (educational) sport to reach its potential both at home and abroad. We have it within our grasp to help provide a brighter future for all people everywhere.

Earle F. Zeigler
British Columbia, Canada
2010

Part One

Selection #1
International Perspective on "Quality of Life":
Genes, Memes, and Physical Activity

Earle F. Zeigler
Canada

Two historical questions have important implications for the area of international and comparative physical education and sport:

1. Did humans in earlier times, equipped with their coalescing genes and evolving memes, enjoy to any significant degree what discerning people today might define as "quality living?" (Memes are sets of "cultural instructions" passed on from one generation to the next; see below, also.)

2. Did earlier humans have an opportunity for freely chosen, beneficial activity in sport, exercise, play, and dance of sufficient quality and quantity to contribute to the quality of life (as viewed by us today)? The phrasing of these questions–whether humans in earlier societies enjoyed quality living, including fine types of developmental physical activity–is no presumptuous. It reminds one of the comedian whose stock question in response to his foil who challenged the truth of the zany experiences his friend typically reported: "Vas you dare, Sharlie?"

What makes a question about the quality of life in earlier times doubly difficult is whether humans can be both judge and jury in such a debate. On what basis can we decide whether any *social* progress has indeed been made such that would permit resolution of such a concept as "quality living." There has been progression, of course, but on what basis can we assume that change is indeed progress? It may be acceptable as a *human* criterion of progress to say that we are coming closer to approximating the type of accomplishments that we think humans should have achieved both individually and socially.

However, Simpson (1949) believes it is shortsighted to assume automatically that such is "the only criterion of progress and that it has a general validity in evolution." He concludes, therefore, that human progress is actually relative and not general, and "does not warrant a choice of the line of humans' ancestry as <u>the</u> central line of evolution as a whole." Yet, he does concede "that man is, on the whole but not in every single respect, the pinnacle so far of evolutionary progress" *on this Earth* (pp. 240-262).

A Conception of History (Nevins)

Of course, we should also understand initially that a number of different "approaches" to the historical analysis of human history have been taken by scholars (e.g., "x number" of great civilizations, "great man" theory). The one that I adopted after reflection early on in my writing is what I identify as a pragmatic approach. Allan Nevins' broad conception of history (1962) seemed to offer that possibility in the best possible way when he stated:

Although when we use the word "history" we instinctively think of the past, this is an error, for history is actually a bridge connecting the past with the present, and pointing the road to the future. This conception of history as a lantern carried by the side of man, moving forward with every step taken, is of course far ampler than the concept of a mere interesting tale to be told, a vivid scene to be described, or a group of picturesque characters to be delineated (p. 14).

The "Tragic Sense" of Life (Muller)

Proceeding from this conception with the topic at hand, I realized immediately that any assessment of the quality of life in prerecorded history must be a dubious evaluation at best. However, I was intrigued by the work of Herbert Muller who has written so insightfully about the struggle for freedom in human history. I was impressed, also, by his belief that recorded history has displayed a "tragic sense" of life. Whereas the philosopher Hobbes (1588-1679) stated in his *De Homine* that very early humans existed in an anarchically individualistic state of nature in which life was "solitary, poor, nasty, brutish, and short," Muller (1961) argued in rebuttal that it "might have been poor and short enough, but that it was never solitary or simply brutish" (p. 6). Accordingly, Muller's approach to history (1952) is "in the spirit of the great tragic poets, a spirit of reverence and or irony, and is based on the assumption that the tragic sense of life is not only the profoundest but the most pertinent for an understanding of both past and present" (p. vii).

Muller's rationalization for his "tragic" view is simply that the drama of human history has been characterized by high tragedy in the Aristotelian sense. As he states, "All the mighty civilizations of the past have fallen, because of tragic flaws; as we are enthralled by any Golden Age we must always add that it did not last, it did not do" (p. vii). This brings to mind the possibility that the 20th century of the modern era could turn out to be the Golden Age of the United States. This may be true because so many misgivings are developing about our blind optimism concerning history's malleability and compatibility in keeping with American ideals. As Heilbroner (1960) explained in his "future as history" concept, America's still-prevalent belief in a personal "deity of history" may be short lived in the 21st century. Arguing that technological, political, and economic forces are "bringing about a closing of our historic future," he emphasized the need to search for a greatly improved "common denominator of values" (p. 178). However, all of this could be an oversimplification, because even the concept of civilization is literally a relative newcomer on the world scene.

Arnold Toynbee (1947) came to a quite simple conclusion about it all is his monumental A study of history—that humankind must return to the one true God from whom it has gradually but steadily fallen away. There is a faint possibility that Toynbee may turn out to be right, but we on this Earth should not put all of our eggs in that one basket. We had best try to use our heads as intelligently and wisely as possible as we get on with striving to make the world as effective and efficient—and as replete with good, as opposed to evil, as we possibly can.

Here we can well be guided by the pact that Goethe's Faust made with the Devil. As a German student and instructor originally, I recall the essence of the pact struck by Faust with the then-presumed purveyor of the world's evil. It was as follows: If ever the time were to come when Faust was tempted to feel completely fulfilled and not bored by the power, wealth, and honor that the horned one had bestowed upon him, then the Devil would have won, and accordingly would take him away to a "much warmer climate." Eventually, by conforming to the terms of the agreement, Faust is saved by the ministrations of the author (Johann Wolfgang von Goethe). However, we today can never forget for a moment that previous civilizations were not somehow saved miraculously—not one made it! "Man errs, but strive he must," said Goethe, and we as world citizens today dare not forget that dictum.

The "Adventure" of Civilization

In retrospect, the adventure of civilization began to make some headway because of now-identifiable forms of early striving which embodied elements of great creativity (e.g., the invention of the wheel, the harnessing of fire). The subsequent development in technology, very slowly but steadily, offered humans some surplus of material goods over and above that needed for daily living. For example, the early harnessing of nature created the irrigation systems of Sumeria and Egypt, and these accomplishments led to the establishment of the first cities. Here material surpluses were collected, managed, and sometimes squandered. Nevertheless, necessary early accounting methods were created that were subsequently expanded in a way that introduced writing to the human scene. As we now know, the development of this form of communication in time helped humans expand their self-consciousness and to evolve gradually and steadily in all aspects of culture. For better or worse, however, the result of this social and material progress has created a mixed agenda characterized by good and evil down to the present.

As Muller (1952) concluded, "the adventure of civilization is necessarily inclusive" (p. 53). By that he meant that evil will probably always be with humankind to some degree, but it is civilization that sets the standards and accordingly works to eradicate at least the worst forms of such evil. Racial prejudice, for example, must be overcome. For better or worse, there are now more than six billion people on earth, and that number appears to be growing faster than the national debt of the USA! These earth creatures are black-, yellow- or brown-, and white-skinned, but we now know from genetic research that basically there is an "overwhelming oneness" in all humankind that we dare not forget (Huxley, 1967).

As various world evils are overcome, or at least held in check, scientific and accompanying technological development will be called upon increasingly to meet the demands of the exploding population. Gainful work and a reasonable amount of leisure will be required for further development. Unfortunately, the necessary leisure required for the many aspects of a broad, societal culture to develop fully, as well as for an individual to grow and develop similarly within it, has come slowly. The average person in the world is far from a full realization of such benefits. Why "the good life" for all has been so slow in arriving is not an easy question to answer. Of course, we might argue that times do change slowly, and that the possibility of increased leisure has really come quite rapidly once humans began to achieve a degree of control of their environment.

Of course, there have been so many wars throughout history, and there has been very little if any let-up in this regard down to the present. Sadly, nothing is so devastating to a country's economy. In retrospect, also, in the Middle Ages of the Western world the power of the Church had to be weakened to permit the separation of church and state. This development, coupled with the rising humanism of the Renaissance in the latter stages of that era, was basic to the rise of a middle class. Finally, the beginnings of the natural sciences had to be consolidated into real gains before advancing technology could lead the West into the Industrial Revolution (i.e., Toffler's "Second Wave").

Recommended Approaches for Improving Life's Quality

Csikszentmihalyi (1993), seeking to help humans "free themselves of the dead hand of the past," has proposed selected "approaches to life that will improve its quality and lead to joyful involvement." However, he stresses that humans are now confronted with a "memes versus genes" dilemma. "Meme" is the term introduced in the 1970s by the British biologist, Richard Dawkins, who coined the noun from the Greek term mimesis to describe a set of "cultural instructions" passed on by example from one generation to another. A gene is, of course, the basic physical unit of heredity about which we are hearing increasingly.

Csikszentmihalyi is fearful that humans' previous "adaptive successes"—the very ones that have helped people survive down to the present—need to be re-assessed in the light of present conditions lest they destroy our future. He is referring here to (1) the organization of the brain, (2) the emergence of a primitive self, (3) the genetic instructions that helped us survive through past millennia, and (4) the competition with other people that is the result of the selective forces on which evolution is based. In addition, he is also concerned about a further danger—"the threat of the artifacts we have created to make our lives more comfortable" (p. 119). The problem here is that these "permanent patterns of matter or information produced by an act of human intentionality" (p. 120), although new on the humans' evolutionary stage, can over time assume lives of their own, so to speak. For example, the results of a few "mimetic parasites," such as the mind-altering drugs, alcohol and tobacco, have been literally devastating to a number of societies or segments thereof.

Arguing that our unique heritage "brings with it an awesome responsibility" because we are at the "cutting edge" of evolution, he affirms that now we "can either direct our life energy toward achieving growth and harmony or waste the potentials we have inherited, adding to the sway of chaos and destruction" (pp. 3-4). Csikszentmihalyi is basically searching for ways that could "integrate the growth and liberation of the self with that of society as a whole" (p. 5). Essentially, he is recommending that we diligently seek what he calls "flow experiences" which are characterized by,

(1)   clear goals with instant feedback;
(2)   opportunities for acting decisively in situations where personal skills are suited to given challenges;
(3)   actions taken merging with awareness to facilitate concentration
(4)   resulting concentration on the task at hand such that there is complete psycho-physical involvement;
(5)   a sense of potential control prevailing;
(6)   a loss of self-consciousness involving transcendence of ego boundaries occurring as the person experiences a sense

of growth and of being part of some greater
entity;

(7)   a sense of time altered so as to seem to pass
        faster; and

(8)   an experience that becomes autotelic, and
        thus creating the feeling that it is worth
        doing for its own sake (pp. 178- 179).

He theorizes further that, even though intense flow experiences are
relatively rare in everyday life, such experiences should indeed be
increasingly possible in the play, work, study, or religious ritual of humans,
IF AND ONLY IF the conditions outlined above are present.

Zeldin (1994), in his highly interesting book, *An intimate history of
humanity*, both complements and supplements the work of Csikszentmihalyi
by offering what he calls a "new vision of the past." He urges humankind to
revisit the various individual feelings and personal relationships evidenced
throughout history. In the process he recommends that individuals "form a
fresh view both of their own personal history and of humanity's whole record
of cruelty, misunderstanding, and joy" (p. vii). This revised vision of the past
can be gradually achieved as the 21st century develops, Zeldin affirms, also–
agreeing with our conference theme-setter (Csikszentmihalyi)–by deliberate
efforts to reverse, through considered re-examination now and in the future,
the unpleasant and unrewarding experiences of distant generations in the
past. Because of this urgent need to remove the past's "dead hand," Zeldin is
telling us starkly and simply that "those who don't learn from past
experiences are doomed to repeat them!"

Zeldin stresses, also, the urgent need for society to:

(1)   help people revive their hopes as they search for their
        roots,
(2)   acquire immunity to loneliness,
(3)   invent new forms of love,
(4)   give respect instead of seeking power,
(5)   learn how to serve as intermediaries between
        people,
(6)   free themselves from fears,
(7)   develop rewarding friendships,
(8)   survive today's nuclear family crisis, and
(9)   choose a purposeful way of life.

He sees these as some of the ways in which we can turn future achievement
of now often hidden aspirations into "flow experiences."

Interestingly, Lenk (1994), from a social-philosophical perspective, also envisions the need for "value changes" in what he calls the "achieving society." He asks the question, "Is life more about work or more about pleasure?" He answers by suggesting that societal conditions may increasingly be such that people will require additional opportunities for "creative achievement and active involvement." Proceeding from an "achievement theme" he developed previously, Lenk affirms also that "we are in need of a new positive 'culture' of achievement and a humanized creative achievement principle" (pp. 92-93).

The Fundamental Importance of Individual Freedom

The delineation by Csikszentmihalyi of the contribution that "flow experiences" can make in people's' lives, as well as Zeldin's call for a new "vision of the past" as we move into the future, would require substantive individual freedom within a positively permissive society. As we look back to earlier eras, therefore, the vital missing link in most people's lives as they sought to fulfill their purposes was the absence of the necessary individual freedom. The definition of freedom I will use here is the relatively neutral, objective one accepted by Muller (1961, p. xiii) in his *Freedom in the ancient world*: "The condition of being able to choose and to carry out purposes." This means that the individual is neither hampered by external constraints nor coerced to do other than he or she wills. It assumes the ability, coupled with a positive desire, to make a conscious choice between known alternatives.

Human Evolution

Admittedly, permitting a conscious choice between alternatives will permit the presence of "population pockets" where there is a demand to give creationism co-equal status with the teaching of a Darwinian long-range approach to human evolution in the schools. As humans we, who tend to think we are "the greatest," may be excused from wondering occasionally why the Creator took such a long and laborious route with so many odd variations of flora and fauna to get to this point of "present greatness." For literally hundreds of thousands of years, the forebears of present-day humans struggled on chipping flints and making their tools. As they used their brains and their hands, both that proved to be an enormous biological advantage, it now seems apparent that in their primitive self-consciousness they were not living only for the moment like their contemporaries, the apes.

The power that these advantages provided humans, an aid combined with technological advancement, somehow nevertheless only offered minimal levels of freedom. As mentioned above, the early development of language as a means of communication was vitally important. This distanced sub humans even more from the apes as cultural evolution became much faster than biological evolution. In a sense, culture brought with it "good news" and "bad news." The bad news was that humans were to a large degree trapped in a world that they themselves created. Fixed habits and beliefs are strong inhibitors of change, growth, and of what might be called progress. The good news is that change did occur, albeit very slowly, and growth did take place.

To most people such change and growth did represent true progress. For example, prehistoric humans interbred, and in this way broadened their genetic base. This lends credence to the present-day argument introduced above that humans today—brown or yellow, black, and white—are indeed one race. This fact helps us to appreciate the development of worldwide cultural evolution. Unfortunately, however, progress has never been a straight-line affair. In the final analysis, this must be the answer for those of us who idealistically thought that the world would be in quite good shape by the year 2000! It may also provide solace to those of who wonder (1) why education finds it so difficult to get sufficient funding; (2) why professors in so many countries must often assume a "Rodney Dangerfield complex"; and (3) why physical education/kinesiology, despite evidence mounting daily as to the value of developmental physical activity, so often finds itself in dire straits within the domain of education and in the eyes of the public.

Physical Culture Down Through the Ages

Lest we in the profession presently blame ourselves too much for our profession's perennial plight, we should keep in mind the words of Thomas Woody (1949) who produced perhaps the most scholarly work extant about physical education in the ancient world. "Turn where one will," Woody explains, "it is impossible to find physical culture adequately presented in books dealing with the general history of education" (p. vii). (To this I hastily add the opinion: or anywhere else for that matter!)

We might ask, "Why is this so?" I believe the answer is that, throughout recorded history down, supposedly learned people have simply not understood either planned or playful physical activity's potential for improving the quality of life, for providing flow experiences, if you will. We might therefore argue that the highest aim of the profession of physical (activity) education and (educational) sport could well be the ordered assembly of the scientific and scholarly principles and generalizations that underlie such developmental physical activity.

It is a safe assumption that the values and norms of a culture have a profound influence on the way people carry out their daily functions. Accordingly, we are now in a position to inquire as to how value determinations have influenced developmental physical activity historically in those activities that we now call exercise, sport, dance, and play. History has told us clearly that physical activity has been a basic part of the fundamental pattern of living of every creature of any type that has ever lived on Earth. Yet Woody (1949) tells us further that "lip-service has been paid increasingly to the dictum 'a sound mind in a sound body,' ever since western Europe began to revive the educational concepts of the Graeco-Roman world." As he avers, "there is still a lack of balance between physical and mental culture" (p. vii).

Most interestingly, the answer to our plight may well rest in Woody's words that relate to the early "wisdom" of a Greek named Plato who left the world with a mixed message on the topic of the human body. The mind-body dualism that he has evidently created led indirectly to the Roman "sound mind in a sound body" dictum of Seneca. Further, this denial of the "wholeness" of the human organism has carried through down to the 20th century. And as the world moves on in the 21st century, I believe that the field of physical education/kinesiology [or whatever silly name appeared this week!] must strongly build on the "unified organism" concept provided for us by the related discipline of psychology, along with the continuing research of its applied psychologists.

Writing at the turn of the 21st century, I sought to leave behind a challenge to the next generation of scholars and professional practitioners that those of us in this generation were not able to meet. The challenge is for them to devise the necessary ways and means of informing the American public about the principles of developmental physical activity–of physical education and kinesiology, if you will–upon which the field's professional practice can now be based logically.

Physical Education's 13 Principal Principles

On December 28, 1951, speaking at the general session of the former College Physical Education Association in Chicago, Illinois, the eminent Arthur H. Steinhaus of George Williams College, Chicago, with "many misgivings," offered what he called the four "principal principles" of physical education to the profession (1952). He explained that the term "principal principles can and does mean the most important or chief fundamental theories, ideas, or generalizations" (p. 5).

Steinhaus' effort in 1951 preceded the analytic summary carried out in "The Contributions of Physical Activity to Human Well-Being," a supplement to the *Research Quarterly* in May, 1960. There, as explained by Ray Weiss, a joint effort was made by scholars in the allied professions to present evidence that physical activity can indeed contribute to wellbeing of humans. These scholarly professionals were stating to the best of their knowledge what we felt that *really* knew, and what we felt that we were very close to knowing at that time.

As we in physical education/kinesiology move along in the 21st century, we can affirm that our steadily growing body of knowledge has provided our profession with a much more substantive knowledge base than that which existed at the middle of the present century. With similar misgivings to those mentioned by Professor Steinhaus, we can now affirm with reasonable assurance that our "principal principles" have increased in number to thirteen! It is perhaps pointless to attempt to determine precisely to what extent this increase can be attributed more to the efforts of the profession's natural science scholars than to those of the more recently added social science and humanities scholars, not to forget the important contributions emanating from our allied professions and related disciplines. That there is some overlap in these principles will be obvious as they are read, but this increase in the number of principal principles suggested points to the wisdom of continually searching for evidence wherever it is to be found.

The following, then, are the principles or generalizations that under gird our professional practice t the beginning of the 21st century. Steinhaus' four principles have now been merged with nine others to make a total of thirteen. Many of you in this room have made a greater or lesser contribution to what has now become the "knowledge heritage" being "passed on"—as our AAKPE seal states—to recent Academy inductees and their colleagues for further investigation and development:

Principle I: The "REVERSIBILITY Principle"

The first principle affirms that circulo-respiratory (often called cardio-vascular) conditioning is inherently reversible in the human body.

(A male, for example, typically reaches his peak at age 19 and goes downhill gradually thereafter until eventual death. This means that a person must achieve and maintain at least an "irreducible level" of such conditioning to live normally.)

Principle II: The "OVERLOAD Principle"

The principle here is that a muscle or muscle group must be taxed beyond that to which it is accustomed, or it won't develop; in fact, it will probably retrogress.

(Thus, the individual must maintain reasonable muscular strength in his/her body to carry out life's normal duties and responsibilities and to protect the body from deterioration.)

Principle III: The "FLEXIBILITY Principle"

This principle states that the human must regularly put his or her various joints through the range of motion for which they are intended.

(Inactive joints become increasingly inflexible until immobility sets in. If inflexibility is a sign of old age, the evidence shows that most people are becoming old about age 27! A person must not neglect maintenance of bodily flexibility.)

Principle IV: The "BONE DENSITY Principle"

The evidence explains that developmental physical activity throughout life preserves the density of a human's bones.

(The density of the human's bones after maturity is not fixed or permanent, and the decline after age 35 may be more rapid than is the case with fat and muscle. After prolonged inactivity, adequate calcium in an individual's diet and weight-bearing physical activity is essential for the preservation of bones. Prevention of bone loss is much more effective than later efforts to repair any bone damage incurred.)

Principle V: The "GRAVITY Principle"

This principle explains that maintaining muscle-group strength throughout one's life, while standing or sitting, helps a person fight against the force of gravity that is working continually to break down a body's structure.

(Maintaining muscle group strength and tonus, along with the best possible structural alignment of one's bones through the development of a proper "body consciousness," will help the individual to fight off gravity's potentially devastating effects as long as possible.)

Principle VI: The "RELAXATION Principle"

Principle VI states that the skill of relaxation is one that people should acquire in today's increasingly complex world.

(Oddly enough, people often need to be taught how to relax in today's typically stressful environment. Part of any "total fitness" package should, therefore, be the development of an understanding as to how an individual can avoid chronic or abnormal fatigue in a social and physical environment that is often overly taxing.)

Principle VII: The "AESTHETIC Principle"

This principle explains that a person has either an innate or a culturally determined need to "look good" to himself/herself and to others.

(Socrates may have decried "growing old without appreciating the beauty of which the body is capable." This is a "need": to make a good appearance to one's family, friends, and those who one meets daily at work or during leisure. Billions of dollars are spent annually by people striving to "make themselves look like something they are not" naturally. Why do people do this? Quite probably, they go through these "body rituals" both to please themselves and because of various social pressures. Thus, if a person is physically active, while following the above six principles, one's bodily appearance can be preserved normally, naturally, and inexpensively.)

Principle VIII: The "INTEGRATION Principle"

Principle VIII asserts that developmental physical activity provides an opportunity for the individual to get "fully involved" as a vital living organism.

(So many of life's activities challenge a person only fractionally in that only part of his or her sensory equipment and even less of the individual's motor mechanism are involved. By their very nature, physical activities in exercise, sport, play, and expressive movement demand full attention from the organism—often in the face of opposition—and therefore involve complete psycho-physical integration.)

Principle IX: The "INTEGRITY Principle"

The integrity principle states that a completely integrated psycho-physical activity should correspond ETHICALLY with the avowed ideals and standards of society.

(The integrity principle goes hand in hand with desirable integration of the human's various aspects (so-called unity of body and mind in the organism explained in Principle VIII immediately above). Fair play, honesty, and concern for others should be uppermost in an individual's pattern of developmental physical activity.)

Principle X: The "PRIORITY OF THE PERSON Principle"

Principle X affirms that any physical activity in sport, play, and exercise that is sponsored through public or private agencies should be conducted in such a way that the welfare of the individual comes first.

(Situations arise daily in all aspects of social living where this principle, one that stresses the sanctity of the individual, is often forgotten. In a democratic society, a man or woman, or boy or girl, should never be forced or encouraged to take part in some type of developmental physical activity where this principle is negated because of the desire of others to win. The individual's personal growth and development is more important than the reputation of any sport organization in which he or she may take part. Sport should serve as a "social servant.")

Principle XI: The "LIVE LIFE TO ITS FULLEST Principle"

This principle asserts that, unless a person moves his or her body with reasonable vigor according to principles I-VI above, it will not serve that individual best throughout life.

(Human movement is what distinguishes the individual from the rock on the ground. Regular, reasonably strenuous physical activity helps a person to meet the normal daily tasks and the unexpected sudden demands that may be required live life fully and to protect oneself from harm.)

Principle XII: The "FUN AND PLEASURE Principle"

Principle XII states that the human is normally a "seeker of fun and pleasure," and that a great deal of the opportunity for such enjoyment is achieved by full, active bodily movement.

(The opportunity for such fun and pleasure will be missing from a person's life if he or she does not maintain at least an "irreducible minimum" level of physical fitness.)

Principle XIII: The "LONGEVITY Principle"

This final principle affirms that regular developmental physical activity throughout life can help a person live longer.

(The statistical evidence is mounting that demonstrates the wisdom of maintaining an active lifestyle throughout life. Succinctly put, all things being equal, a physically active person who is physically active will live longer!)

Flow Experiences and "The Good Life"

These 13 "principal principles" represent what we believe we know about wisdom of keeping these generalizations about planned physical activity in mind throughout life. The key task for the field of physical activity education and kinesiology is to help people of all ages, whether they are "accelerated, normal, or 'special population'," to actually implement this knowledge daily into their lives. If it is possible at present for some people to deliberately plan for and then include such flow experiences in their life patterns, and thereby to improve their quality of life, it is accordingly reasonable to assume (to hope?) that many more people will have the opportunity (i.e., the freedom) to do so in the future). However, before this will happen, those presently unconvinced must be convinced of the possibility and desirability of adding such experiences to their lives. This leads inevitably to the perennial question in education as to the knowledge, competencies, character, and personality traits for which we should educate in the years ahead.

Such choices will inevitably depend on the values and norms of the culture in which people live. As we appreciate, values are the major social forces that help to determine the direction a culture will take at any given moment. Such values as social values, educational values, scientific values, and artistic values make up the highest level of the social system in a culture. It can, therefore, be argued that these values represent the "ideal general character" (e.g., rule of law, social-structured facilitation of individual achievement, equality of opportunity). As we understand further, overall culture in itself serves a pattern-maintenance function as a society relates to the functional problems it faces. In this connection pattern-maintenance and integration are internal problems, whereas adaptation and goal-attainment are external (Johnson, 1994, 1969).

In addition, the values that people hold for themselves in a society at a given time have a direct relationship to how we conceive the nature of the human being. There have been a number of attempts to define such nature on a rough historical time scale. For example, Morris (1956) offered a fivefold chronological series of definitions as to how to conceive the human being, including analyses in the following order:

(1) rational animal,

(2) spiritual being,

(3) receptacle of knowledge,

(4) mind that can be trained by exercise, and

(5) problem-solving organism.

In the mid-1960s, Berelson and Steiner (1964) traced six images for humankind throughout recorded history, but more from the standpoint of behavioral science. They identified them as follows:

(1) philosophical image,

(2) Christian image,

(3) political image,

(4) economic image,

(5) psychoanalytic image, and

(6) behavioral-science image.

Whatever one conceives to be his or her basic nature (e.g., problem-solving organism with a behavioral science image), as this person matures we can reasonably expect that considerable thought will be given as to what constitutes "the good life." As we know people from all levels of society have been offering advice on this topic since time immemorial. Csikszentmihalyi has recommended that we search for approaches to living–that is, flow experiences–that "improve its quality and lead to joyful involvement." In so doing, "the growth and liberation of the self" will be combined "with that of society as a whole" (p. 5).

Kateb's Delineation of "The Good Life"

To help us answer the question about ways to improve the quality of life, as well as how this might be accomplished joyfully, I return to the possibilities for "Utopia and the Good Life" outlined by George Kateb (1965, pp. 454-473). He recommended a progression of possibilities or definitions of the good life as:

(1) laissez faire,
(2) the greatest amount of pleasure,
(3) play,
(4) craft,
(5) political action, and
(6) the life of the mind.

His conclusion was that the life of the mind offers the greatest potential in the world as we know it now or as we may know it in the future.

As we put these possibilities in historical perspective, it is immediately obvious that only a very small percentage of people throughout recorded history have had sufficient freedom and wherewithal to choose and carry out those purposes they might have chosen initially. For example, laissez faire (No. 1 above), the greatest amount of pleasure (2), and play (3) could only be chosen (i.e., were available) as life patterns by a minute percentage of earlier humans in any search for flow experiences.

If by craft (4) is meant pursuit of an art or manual skill, then the number of those people for whom such was possible and who were probably involved in the development and use of craft in the past for survival and/or recreation rises significantly. Undoubtedly, depending on their freedom to pursue such endeavor, flow experiences could well have been one outcome of this involvement. Number 5, political action as a possible pursuit in the search for a good life, presents a significantly lesser opportunity, numerically speaking, for flow experiences because of the station in life inherited, not to mention the freedom, temperament, and constitutional vigor required for such involvement.

Kateb's final possibility as an approach to a search for the good life was titled "the life of the mind." He felt that "the man (sic) possessed of the higher faculties in their perfection is the model for utopia and already exists outside it . . ." (p. 472). This is an interesting conclusion that might be foreseen, of course, from a university scholar. Also, it can be argued that pursuit of the so-named "life of the mind" should increasingly be part and parcel of the life of each person in enlightened societies of the future.

Flow Experiences Via a Transcending Multiple

In conclusion, I believe that men and women, now and in the future, can increase their exposure to flow experiences by combining all of Kateb's approaches into one viable, multiple, all-encompassing approach. At least five of these six approaches to the good life are directly or indirectly related to the role that developmental physical activity in sport, exercise, and dance can play in a society generally, as well as in the lives of people specifically (Zeigler, 1979, p. 12).

Fine educational experience has been related historically to the mastery of various subject matters. Accordingly–and I believe mistakenly–we do not typically understand so-called formal education to fully encompass *all* of the changes that take place in individuals based on their total life experience. Because of this truncated outlook, somehow the movement experience, the quality human motor performance experience aspect of education, of recreation, of all life–these *flow* experiences of a unified organism, if you will–has been slighted historically down to the present. Huxley (1964, p. 31) called it the disregard for the "education of the non-verbal humanities," of the "psycho-physical instrument of an evolving amphibian." This is the historical reality faced by the profession in 2008 of the Common Era.

Notes

1.   Sincere appreciation is expressed to the many scientists and scholars, both within our field and in related disciplines and allied professions, whose efforts have made the statement of these principles possible at the close of the 20th century.

2.   Steinhaus' original principles are included in the 13 principal principles formulated above. Note, however, that his "principle of integration and integrity" has been divided in two so as to create two separate principles.

References

Berelson, B. & Steiner, G.A. (1964). *Human behavior: An inventory of scientific findings*. NY: HarcourtBrace.

Contributions of physical activity to human well-being. (May 1960) *Research Quarterly*, 31, 2 (Part II): 261-375.

Csikszentmihalyi, M. (1993). *The evolving self*. NY: HarperCollins.

Heilbroner, R.L. (1960). *The future as history*. NY: Harper & Row.

Hobbes, T. *De Homine*.

Huxley, A. (1964). *Tomorrow and tomorrow and tomorrow*. NY: New American Library.

Huxley, J. (January 1967). The crisis in man's destiny. *Playboy*, 93-94, 212-217.

Johnson, H.M. (1969). The relevance of the theory of action to historians. *Social Science Quarterly*, 21, 2:46-58)

Johnson, H.M. (1994). Modern organizations in the Parsonsian theory of action. In A. Farazmand, *Modern organizations:Administrative theory in contemporary society* (pp. 57 et ff.). Westport, CT: Praeger.

Kateb, G. (Spring 1965) Utopia and the good life. *Daedalus*, 94: 454-473.

Lenk, H. (1994). Value changes and the achieving society: A social-philosophical perspective. In *Organisation for Economic Co-operation and Development, OECD societies in transition* (pp. 81-94).

Morris, V.C. (1956). Physical education and the philosophy of education. *JOPHER*, 27, 3: 21-22, 30-31.

Muller, H.J. (1954). *The uses of the past*. NY: Mentor Books.

Muller, H.J. (1961*). Freedom in the ancient world*. NY: Harper & Bros.

Nevins, A. (1963). *The gateway to history*. Garden City, NY: Doubleday & Co.)

Simpson, G. (1949). *The meaning of evolution*. New Haven & London: Yale University Press.

Steinhaus, A.H. (1952). Principal principles of physical education. In *Proceedings of the College Physical Education Association.* Washington, DC: AAHPER, pp. 5-11.

Woody, T. (1949). *Life and education in early societies*. NY: Macmillan.

Zeigler, E.F. (1979) Sport and physical activity's role in the behavioral science image of man and women. In E. F. Zeigler, *Issues in North American sport and physical education*. Washington, DC: AAHPER.

Zeigler, E.F. (1989). *An introduction to sport and physical education philosophy*. Carmel, IN: Benchmark.

Zeigler, E.F. (1994). Physical education's 13 "principal principles,"*JOPERD*, 65, 7: 4-5.

Zeldin, T. (1994). *An intimate history of humanity*. NY: HarperCollins.

Selection #2
An Emerging Postmodern Age Confronts
Comparative Physical Education & Sport

Earle F. Zeigler
Canada

We who are dedicated to promoting development in the area of comparative physical education and sport need to fully comprehend what an emerging postmodern age holds in store for us. North Americans, for example, may well find that their unique position in the history of the world's development will in all probability change radically in the 21st century as well. All indications point to the position that the years ahead are really going to be difficult ones for the world's citizens wherever they may be located.

Maintaining world peace is undoubtedly the most threatening problem facing civilization. The United States, as the leading nuclear power at present, has taken upon itself one approach to the ongoing, massive problem of maintaining large-scale peace. (And they have repeatedly gone to war to preserve it!) Of course, a variety of countries, both large and small, may or may not have nuclear arms capability as well. That is what is so worrisome.

Additionally, all of the world will be having increasingly severe ecological problems, not to mention the ebbs and flows of an energy crisis. Generally, also, there is a worldwide nutritional problem, as well as an ongoing situation where the rising expectations of the underdeveloped nations, including their staggering debt will somehow have to repay. (This said, keep in mind that the so-called developed nations typically have enormous debts too.) These are just a few of the major concerns looming on the horizon.

Indeed, although it is seemingly truer of the United States than Canada, history is going against American in several ways. This means that their previous optimism must be tempered to shake them loose from delusions they have somehow acquired. For example, despite the presence of the United Nations, the United States has persisted in envisioning itself--as the world superpower--as almost being endowed by the Creator to make a variety of crucial political decisions. Such decisions, often to act unilaterally with the hoped-for, but belated sanction of the United Nations, have resulted in United States-led incursions in the Middle East in the two wars and into Somalia for very different reasons. And there are other similar situations that are now "history" (e.g., Cuba, Afghanistan, the former Yugoslavia, Rwanda, Sudan, Haiti, respectively, not to mention additional suspected incursions).

Nevertheless, there is reason to expect selected U.S. retrenchment brought on by its excessive world involvement and enormous debt. Of course, any such retrenchment would inevitably lead to a decline in the economic and military influence of the United States. With the way international affairs are now developing, therefore, who can argue logically looking to the future that the present uneasy balance of power is a healthy situation? Norman Cousins appeared to have sounded just the right note more than a generation ago when he stated: "the most important factor in the complex equation of the future is the way the human mind responds to crisis" (1974, pp. 6-7). The world culture as we know it must indeed respond adequately to the many challenges with which it is being confronted. The societies and nations must individually and collectively respond positively, intelligently, and strongly if humanity as we have known it is to survive.

Significant Developments Have "Transformed Our Lives"

In this discussion of national and international developments, undertaken with an eye to achieving some historical perspective, we should also keep in mind the specific developments in the last quarter of the 20th century. For example, Naisbitt (1982) outlined the "ten new directions that are transforming our lives" that were followed subsequently by "megatrends" concerning women's evolving role in societal structure (Aburdene & Naisbitt, 1992). The original "ten directions" were as follows:

(1) understanding the concepts "information society" and the "Internet,"
(2) moving to "high tech/high touch,"
(3) comprehending the shift to world economy,
(4) seeing the need to shift to long-term thinking about ecology,
5) moving toward organizational decentralization,
(6) adapting to the trend toward self-help,
(7) participating in the ongoing discussion of the wisdom of participatory democracy as opposed to representative democracy,
8) getting involved in the shift toward networking,
9) reviewing the "north-south" orientation, and
(10) viewing of decisions as "multiple option" instead of "either/or."

The ever-increasing, lifelong involvement of women in the workplace, politics, sports, organized religion, and social activism occasioned a subsequent listing referred to above. Together they helped us to understand that a new world order has descended upon us as we began life in the 21st century.

Shortly after Naisbitt's first set of Megatrends appeared, a second list of 10 issues facing *political* leaders was highlighted as "Ten events that shook the world between 1984 and 1994" (*Utne Reader*, 1994, pp. 58-74). Consider the following:

(1) the fall of communism and the continuing rise of nationalism,

(2) the environmental crisis and the Green movement,

(3) the AIDS epidemic and the "gay response,"

(4) the continuing wars and the peace movement,

(5) the gender war,

(6) the religious and racial tension,

(7) the concept of "West meets East" and resultant implications,

(8) the "Baby Boomers" came of age and "Generation X" has started to worry and complain because of declining expectation levels,

(9) the whole idea of "globalism" and international markets, and

10) the computer revolution and the specter of Internet.

The World Has Three Major Trading Blocks

The listing of the above developments is interesting, but it is also disturbing. A search for a full understanding of it may possibly help us to cope with such change. Actually the world's "economic manageability" may have been simplified to a degree by its division into three major trading blocs: (1) the Pacific Rim (dominated by Japan?), (2) the European Community very heavily influenced by Germany, and (3) North America dominated by the United States of America. While this appears to be true to some observers, interestingly perhaps something even more fundamental has occurred. Succinctly put, world politics seems to be "entering a new phase in which the fundamental source of conflict will be neither ideological nor economic." In the place of these, Samuel P. Huntington, of Harvard's Institute for Strategic Studies, believes that now the major conflicts in the world will actually be clashes between different groups of civilizations espousing fundamentally different cultures (*The New York Times*, June 6, 1993, E19).

These clashes, Huntington states, represent a distinct shift away from viewing the world as being composed of first, second, and third worlds as was the case during the Cold War. Huntington is arguing instead that in the 21st century the world will return to a pattern of development evident several hundred years ago in which civilizations will actually rise and fall. (Interestingly, this is exactly what the late Arnold Toynbee postulated in his earlier famous theory of historical development.)

For example, with the dissolution of the Union of Soviet Socialist Republics (USSR), Russia and the remaining communist regimes face complicated social issues as they seek to convert to more of a capitalistic economic system. Russia is understandably concerned when surrounding "new nations" contain fractious multi-national populations (with some looking to a union with "the West). Additionally, a number of other multinational countries have either dissolved as "entities," or are showing signs of potential breakups (e.g., Yugoslavia, China, Canada, certain African countries). Further, the evidence points to the strong possibility that the developing nations are becoming ever poorer and more destitute with burgeoning populations and widespread starvation setting in.

Further, Western Europe is facing a demographic time bomb even more than the United States. This has happened because of the influx of refugees from African and Islamic countries, not to mention refugees from countries of the former Soviet Union. It appears further that the European Community will be inclined to appease Islam's demands. However, the multinational nature of the European Community will tend to bring on economic protectionism to insulate its economy against the rising costs of prevailing socialist legislation.

Still further, there is some evidence that Radical Islam, along with Communist China, may well become increasingly aggressive toward the Western culture of Europe and North America. At present, Islam gives evidence of replacing Marxism as the world's main ideology of confrontation. For example, Islam is dedicated to regaining control of Jerusalem and to force Israel to give up control of land occupied earlier to provide a buffer zone against Arab aggressors. Further, China has been arming certain Arab and African nations. (Question: How can we in the West be too critical in this regard when we recall that in the past [and present?] the U.S.A. has also selectively armed countries when such support was deemed in its interest?)

As Hong Kong is gradually absorbed into Communist China, further political problems seem inevitable in the Far East as well. Although North Korea is facing agricultural problems, there is the possibility (probability?) of the building of nuclear bombs there. (Further, there is the ever-present fear worldwide that small nations and terrorists will somehow get nuclear weapons too.) A growing Japanese assertiveness in Asian and world affairs also seems inevitable because of its typically very strong financial position. Concurrently, the flow of foreign capital from Japan into North America has slowed down somewhat because Japan is being confronted with its own financial crisis caused by inflated real estate and market values. There would obviously be a strong reaction to any fall in living standards in this tightly knit society. Interestingly, still further, the famed Japanese work ethic has become somewhat tarnished by the growing attraction of leisure opportunities.

The situation in Africa has become increasingly grim because the countries south of the Sahara Desert (that is, the dividing line between black Africa and the Arab world) experienced extremely bad economic performance in the past two decades). This social influence has brought to a halt much of the continental effort leading to political liberalization while at the same time exacerbating traditional ethnic rivalries. This economic problem has accordingly forced governmental cutbacks in many of the countries because of the pressures brought to bear by the financial institutions of the Western world that have been underwriting much of the development. The poor are therefore getting poorer, and health (AIDs!) and educational standards have typically deteriorated even lower than they were previously.

The Impact of Negative Social Forces Has Increased.

Shifting the focus of this discussion from the problems of an unsettled "Global Village" back to the problem of "living the good life" in the 21st century in North America, we are finding that the human recreational experience will have to be earned typically within a society whose very structure has been modified. For example, (1) the concept of the traditional family structure has been challenged strongly by a variety of social forces (e.g., economics, divorce rate); (2) many single people are finding that they must work longer hours; and (3) many families need more than one breadwinner just to make ends meet. Additionally, the idea of a steady surplus economy may have vanished, temporarily we hope, in the presence of a substantive drive to reduce a budgetary deficit by introducing major cutbacks in so-called nonessentials.

The Problems of Megalopolis Living Have Not Yet Been Solved

Additionally, many of the same difficulties associated with megalopolis living in the 1960s still prevail and are even increasing (e.g., declining infrastructure, rising crime rates, transportation gridlocks, overcrowded schools). Interestingly, in the same year–1967!–Prime Minister Lester Pearson asked Canadians to improve "the quality of Canadian life" just as Canada celebrated her 100th anniversary as a confederation. And still today, despite all of Canada's current identity problems, she can take some pride in the fact that Canada has on occasion been proclaimed as the best place on earth to live (with the United States not very far behind). Nevertheless, we cannot escape the fact that the workweek is not getting shorter. Further, Michael's prediction about four different types of leisure class still seems a distant dream for the large majority of people.

Still further, the situation has developed in such a way that the presently maturing generation, so-called Generation X, is finding that fewer good-paying jobs are available and the average annual income is declining (especially if we keep a steadily rising cost of living in mind). What caused this to happen? This is not a simple question to answer. For one thing, despite the rosy picture envisioned a generation ago, one in which we were supposedly entering a new stage for humankind, we are unable today to cope adequately with the multitude of problems that has developed. This situation is true whether inner city, suburbia, exurbia, or small-town living are concerned. Transportation jams and gridlock, for example, are occurring daily as public transportation struggles to meet rising demand for economical transport within the framework of developing megalopolises. In addition, gasoline prices are vacillating, but they are also "going through the roof."

Certainly, megalopolis living trends have not abated and will probably not do so in the predictable future. More and more families, where that unit is still present, need two breadwinners just to survive adequately. Interest rates, although minor cuts are implemented when economic slowdowns occur, remain quite high. This prohibits or discourages many people from home ownership. Pollution of air and water continues despite efforts of many to change the present course of development. High-wage industries seem to be "heading south" in search of regions where lower wages can be paid. Also, all sorts of crime are still present in our society, a goodly portion of it seemingly brought about by unemployment and rising debt at all levels from the individual to the federal government. The rise in youth crime is especially disturbing. In this respect, it is fortunate in North America that municipal, private-agency, and public recreation has received continuing financial support from the increasingly burdened taxpayer. Even here, however, there has been a definite trend toward user fees for many services.

What Character Do We Seek for People?

Still further, functioning in a world that is steadily becoming a "Global Village," we need to think more seriously than ever before about the character and traits that we seek to develop in people. The so-called developed nations can only continue to lead or strive for the proverbial good life if children and young people develop the right attitudes (psychologically speaking) toward (1) education, (2) work, (3) use of leisure, (4) participation in government, (5) various types of consumption, and (6) concern for world stability and peace. Make no mistake about it. If we truly desire "the good life," education for the creative and constructive use of leisure–as a significant part of ongoing general education–should have a unique role to play from here on into the indeterminate future.

What are called the Old World countries all seem to have a "character." It is almost something that they take for granted. However, it is questionable whether there is anything that can be termed "character" in North America (i.e., in the United States, in Canada). Americans were regarded as heterogeneous and individualistic as a "people" earlier, as opposed to Canadians. But the Canadian culture–whatever that may be today (!)–has "progressed" strongly in recent decades toward multiculturalism--not to mention the "nation notion" of many living in French-speaking Quebec, of course--as people arrived from many different lands. (Of course, Canada arose from two distinct cultures, the English and the French.) Still further, Canada has not been able to resolve its problem with indigenous "First Nations."

In mid-20th century, Commager (1966), the noted historian, enumerated what he believed were some common denominators in American (i.e., U.S.A.) character. These, he said, were:

(1) carelessness;
(2) openhandedness, generosity, and hospitality;
(3) self-indulgence;
(4) sentimentality, and even romanticism;
(5) gregariousness;
(6) materialism;
(7) confidence and self-confidence;
(8) complacency, bordering occasionally on arrogance;
(9) cultivation of the competitive spirit;
(10) indifference to, and exasperation with laws, rules, and regulations;
(11) equalitarianism; and
(12) resourcefulness (pp. 246-254).

How may Canadian character be described as opposed to what Commager stated above for Americans? To help us do this, a generation ago, Lipset (1973) made a perceptive comparison between the two countries. After stating that they probably resemble each other more than any other two countries in the world, he asserted that there seemed to be a rather "consistent pattern of differences between them" (p. 4). He found that certain "special differences" did exist and are as follows:

> Varying origins in their political systems and national identities, varying religious traditions, and varying frontier experiences. In general terms, the value orientations of Canada stem from a counterrevolutionary past, a need to differentiate itself from the United States, the influence of Monarchical institutions, a dominant Anglican religious tradition, and a less individualistic and more governmentally controlled expansion of the Canadian than of the American frontier (p. 5).

What Happened to the Original Enlightenment Ideal?

The achievement of "the good life" for a majority of citizens in the developed nations, a good life that involves a creative and constructive use of leisure as a key part of general education, necessarily implies that a certain type of progress has occurred in society. However, we should understand that the chief criterion of progress has undergone a subtle but decisive change since the founding of the United States republic. This development, for example, has had a definite influence on Canada and Mexico as well. Such change has been at once a cause and a reflection of the current disenchantment of some with what others regard as technologic progress. Recall that the late 18th century was a time of political revolution when monarchies, aristocracies, and the ecclesiastical structure were being criticized on a number of fronts in the Western world. Additionally, the factory system was undergoing significant change at that time. Such industrial development with its greatly improved machinery "coincided with the formulation and diffusion of the modern Enlightenment idea of history as a record of progress. . . ." (Marx, 1990, p. 5).

Thus, this "new scientific knowledge and accompanying technological power was expected to make possible a comprehensive improvement in all of the conditions of life--social, political, moral, and intellectual as well as material." This idea did indeed take hold slowly and eventually "became the fulcrum of the dominant American world view" (Marx, p. 5). By 1850, however, with the rapid growth of the United States especially, the idea of progress was already being "dissociated" from the Enlightenment vision of political and social liberation.

Technology and Life Improvement.

By the turn of the twentieth century, "the technocratic idea of progress [had become] a belief in the sufficiency of scientific and technological innovation as the basis for general progress" (Marx, p. 9). This came to mean that, if scientific-based technologies continued to develop in an unconstrained manner, there would be an automatic improvement in all other aspects of life! What happened, inasmuch as this theory became coupled with onrushing, unbridled capitalism, was that the ideal envisioned by Thomas Jefferson in the United States was turned upside down (so to speak). Instead of social progress, guided by such values as justice, freedom, and self-fulfillment for all people, rich or poor, these goals of vital interest in a democracy were neglected in a burgeoning society dominated by supposedly more important instrumental values (i.e., useful or practical ones for advancing a capitalistic system).

So the fundamental question still today is, "which type of values will win out in the long run?" In North America, for example, it seems that a gradually prevailing concept of cultural relativism was increasingly discredited as the 1990s witnessed a sharp clash between (1) those who uphold so-called Western cultural values and (2) those who by their presence are dividing the West along a multitude of ethnic and racial lines. This is occasioning strong efforts by disparate groups to promote fundamentalist religions and sects. These groups are composed either those that have been present historically or by those groups that have recently been imported. These factions are characterized typically by a decisive right/wrong morality.

Postmodernism as an Influence

The orientation and review of selected world, European, North American, regional, and local developments occurring in the final quarter of the 20th century might seem a bit out of place to some who read this book. It may be asked whether this has a relationship to the value system in place in North America. My response to this question is a resounding "Yes." The affirmative answer is correct, also. if we listen to the voices of those in the minority within philosophy who are seeking to practice their profession, or promote their discipline as if it had some connection to the world as it exists. I am referring here, for example to a philosopher like Richard Rorty (1997). He, as a so-called Neo-pragmatist, exhorts the presently "doomed Left" in North America to join the fray again. Their presumed shame should not be "heightened" by a mistaken belief that only those who agree with the Marxist position that capitalism must be eradicated are "true Lefts." Rorty seems truly concerned that philosophy once again become characterized as a "search for wisdom," a search that seeks conscientiously and capably to answer the myriad of questions looming before humankind all over the world.

While most philosophers have been "elsewhere engaged," what has been termed postmodernism has become a substantive factor in intellectual circles. I must confess up front that I have personally been grumbling about– and seeking to grapple with–the term "postmodern" for years. Somehow it has now become as bad (i.e., misunderstood or garbled) as existentialism, pragmatism, idealism, etc.). I confess, also, that I have now acquired a small library on the topic. At any rate, I recently read *Crossing the Postmodern Divide* by Albert Borgman (Chicago, 1992). I was so pleased to find something like this assessment of the situation. I say this because, repeatedly, I have encountered what I would characterize as gobbledygook describing what has been termed "civilization's plight." By that I mean that what I encountered typically was technical jargon, almost seemingly deliberate obfuscation by people seemingly trying to "fool the public" on this topic. As I see it, if it is worth saying, it should be said carefully and understandably. If not, one cannot help but think that the writer is a somewhat confused person.

At any rate, in my opinion this effort by Borgman is solid, down-to-earth, and comprehensible up to the final two pages. Then he veers to Roman Catholicism as the answer to the plight of moderns. It is his right, of course, to state his personal opinion after describing the current situation so accurately. However, if he could have brought himself to it, or if he had thought it might be possible, it could have been more useful if he had spelled out several alternatives, possibly other desirable directions for humankind to consider in the 21st century.

Is this modern epoch or era concluding? An epoch approaches closure when many of the fundamental convictions of its advocates are negated by a substantive minority of the populace. It can be argued that indeed the world is moving into a new epoch as the proponents of postmodernism have been affirming over recent decades. Within such a milieu there are strong indications that all professions are going to have great difficulty crossing this so-called, postmodern gap (chasm, divide, whatever!). Scholars argue that many in democracies, under girded by the various rights recommended (e.g., individual freedom, privacy), have come to believe that they require a supportive "liberal consensus" within their respective societies.

Post-modernists now form a substantive minority that supports a more humanistic, pragmatic, liberal consensus in society. Within such a milieu there are strong indications that present-day society is going to have difficulty crossing the "designated," postmodern divide. Traditionalists in democratically oriented political systems may not like everything they see in front of them today, but as they look in other directions they flinch even more. After reviewing where society has been, and where it is now, two basic questions need answering. Where is society heading? And. most importantly, where should it be heading?

Some argue that Nietzsche's philosophy of being, knowledge, and morality supports the basic dichotomy espoused by the philosophy of being in the post-modernistic position. I can understand at once, therefore, why it meets with opposition under girded by traditional theocentric religions or sects (i.e., in the final analysis, it is God "who calls the shots."). It can be argued, also, that many in democracies bolstered by the various rights being propounded (e.g., individual freedom, privacy) have come to believe–as stated above–that they require a supportive "liberal consensus." However, conservative, essentialist elements functioning in such political systems feel that the deeper foundation justifying this claim of a requisite, liberal consensus has been never been fully rationalized--keeping their more authoritative orientations in mind, of course. The foundation supporting the more humanistic, pragmatic, liberal consensus, as I understand it, is what has been called postmodernism by some.

Postmodernists subscribe largely to a humanistic, anthropocentric belief as opposed to the traditional theocentric position. They would subscribe, therefore, I think, to what Berelson and Steiner in the mid-1960s postulated as a behavioral science image of man and woman. This view characterized the human as a creature continuously adapting reality to his or her own ends (1964).

Thus, the authority of theological positions, dogmas, ideologies, and some "scientific infallibilism" is denied strongly. A moderate postmodernist--holding a position I feel able to subscribe to once I am able to bring it all into focus--would at least listen to what the "authority" had written or said before criticizing or rejecting it. A strong postmodernist goes his or her own way by early, almost automatic, rejection of tradition. Then this person presumably relies on a personal interpretation and subsequent diagnosis to muster the authority to challenge any or all icons or "lesser gods" extant in society.

If the above is reasonably accurate, it would seem that a postmodernist might well feel more comfortable by seeking to achieve personal goals through a modified or semi-postmodernistic position as opposed to the traditional stifling position of essentialist theological realists or idealists. A more pragmatic "value-is-that-which-is proven-through-experience" orientation leaves the future open-ended.

Whatever your personal orientation may be, you will be faced with decisions of varying complexity that must be made every day for the rest of your life. Read on. . . .

Part Two:

Selection #3
In Retrospect #1: A Review
of Comparative Physical Education

Brian T.P. Mutimer
St. Francis Xavier University
Canada

Note: This comprehensive article
was written by Dr. Mutimer in 1969-70.)

Introduction

Why offer a course in comparative physical education? What *is* comparative physical education? These are among the first questions that a prospective teacher of the subject must answer, and they provide an excellent starting point for a general discussion.

There are a number of valid reasons for offering a course on the subject. The one most often quoted is the pragmatic one. By knowing other people's successes and failures, we will be able to improve our own system. For some, however, the answer is rather like that of the mountain climber when asked why he climbs the mountain: because it's there! In other words the mere fact that there are other people working in the same field is stimulus enough for some practitioners to want to know (1) what *they* are doing, (2) how *they* are doing it, and (3) why *they* are doing it-and so on. The "global village" is a fact. Thus, many people feel that it behooves us all to know each other, and what better way than looking at one's own field on a world-wide basis? The present writer feels that while it is the pragmatic reason, the desire to acquire knowledge to be used in bettering one's own system, that is most often used to defend comparative study, in fact very rarely do people apply the lessons they have learned from others. Some of the reasons for this failure will be discussed below

.

The question-"What is comparative physical education?"-is simple and straightforward. The answer, unfortunately, is not. At first sight there is no problem, "comparative" is self explanatory and every physical educator knows what "physical education" is. This is true, of course, but it is a sad fact that very few physical educationalists would agree on a definition, although there would be a lot of common ground. If this disparity between definitions is true within a country, and it is submitted that it is true, then how much more will opinions differ between countries? Even on the broadest of definitions, it may be difficult to get agreement. Is physical education part of education, so that comparative physical education becomes part of comparative education, or is it a discipline in its own right? On the other hand, can one speak of comparative education as being a discipline, or is it simply part of, say, comparative sociology, psychology, philosophy, or "whatever"?

The reader may well take an instant position as he reads these rhetorical questions, but he may rest assured that sound as his reasoning is, definite as his opinions are, and obvious as his stance may be, there are others who will take equally self-evident, definite, and sound positions that are quite different.

Why give a course in comparative physical education? What is comparative physical education? It is the purpose of this paper to discuss these and other related questions in the hope that both the reader and the writer will be enabled to come to a position based on some thought and consideration of the problem involved.

Defining Comparative Physical Education

Comparative education is at least as old as Plato who borrowed from Sparta and Egypt for his educational system as outlined in *The Republic*. There is little doubt that in a sense there has been comparative education for as long as there has been man. It is even possible that comparative *physical* education pre-dates comparative education, in that it is likely that members of one group or tribe who found a good way of teaching their youngsters the art of hunting would find themselves imitated by their near neighbours.

In its modern sense, however, comparative physical education is a young off-spring of a young parent:

> The starting point of comparative education as a
> field of study is often associated with the
> appearance in 1817 of Marc Antoine Jullien's
> Esquisse et vues préliminaires d'un ouvrage sur
> l'éducation comparée.[1]

If accurate, this makes comparative education some one hundred and fifty years old. Dr. Dorothy Ainsworth, world physical education leader, and many-times president of the International Council for Health, Physical Education, and Recreation and the International Association of Physical Education and Sports for Girls and Women, suggests that comparative *physical education* has existed for only about one third of that time:

> Previously, (i.e. earlier than fifty years before 1968,
> when the article was written" only a few

organizations such as the YMCA and YWCA have been concerned with these fields.[2]

The 150 years of comparative education have seen many books, articles and texts of various natures published, but the number of publications devoted to comparative physical education is severely limited. In fact, apart from ICHPER and UNESCO, nobody seems to have written anything of note until Vendien and Nixon produced their work in 1968[3]. Of course, many of the publications on comparative education contain some information on comparative physical education. However, this simply serves to underline the fact that the latter is normally considered as part of the former, not as a field of study in its own right. It is also true that there have been many articles and some books written on physical education within a particular country or area, but these have not been on a comparative basis.

For years the battle has raged over the question: "What is physical education?" Many physical educators, struggling for academic equality with their peers, have stubbornly insisted that it is a discipline, an academic field of study. Borrowing frantically from many disciplines, physical educators have striven for respectability. However, they have only succeeded in producing many sub-groups, each of which moves further away from the traditional concept of physical education–and also further away from each other! So today people are graduating from physical education departments, schools, and colleges with bachelors, masters, and Ph.D. degrees whose academic background is often far removed from anything that remotely resembles physical education. Theses are being written for, and accepted by physical education units, that are well researched, scholarly, and almost completely unrelated to the field of physical education. This is the case in some North American universities especially where there is not only difficulty in deciding what name should be" given to physical education, but also in what is covered by the term "physical education."

There seems to be little wonder that, if there are problems in defining physical education-and there are probably as many definitions as there are physical educators-that there must be problems also in defining *comparative* physical education. If the members of the profession in any one country cannot agree upon their own area of study, how much worse must it be to define the accepted limits in more than one country? For instance, does physical education include recreation, sport, and research? Is it restricted to what goes on in the schools, or are the activities of community clubs and organizations to be included? Where does professional preparation and teacher training fit in? Are both professional and amateur forms of sport included in the title "Physical Education"? These and related questions are not only of fundamental importance to the physical educator, but also need to be answered by the "comparativist" before he or she can begin scholarly work.

In one sense, no social science-and that includes comparative physical education-can exist by itself. It is impossible, other than for purely practical reasons, to disassociate one social science from another. Each one needs every other one and, in a sense, all social sciences are part of one whole. This inter-relationship will be discussed in detail later, but for the moment the point is made that the outlines of comparative physical education are necessarily fuzzy.

Is Comparative Physical Education a Discipline?

Can comparative physical education be considered a discipline? If one defines a discipline as an area of study with its own body of knowledge and with its own methodology, then there seems to be no doubt that, at present, comparative physical education cannot be considered a discipline. One could concede that there is a distinct body of knowledge available and that there is a methodology and also accompanying research techniques peculiarly suited to this body of knowledge. However, such knowledge is borrowed from other social sciences. When the number of works on the subject is as limited as it is, it becomes apparent that the body of knowledge has yet to be extracted from other such bodies. Therefore, comparative physical education is not a discipline in the terms of the definition.

There are, of course, two aspects to comparative physical education: the "academic" and the applied aspects of study of whatever it is that said to be. By "academic" the writer means the library and classroom work, and by "applied", that portion of the work that is intended for use. This would include for instance, the study of the programmes of the newly emerged nations in order to assist an emerging nation to benefit from past successes and failures in setting up its own programme. It might mean studies of a particular problem throughout all those societies that have experienced it, in order to try and make the best possible decision for one country. Canada is almost always able to use the U.S.A. for such comparisons, for whatever problems Canada suffers, it seems that the States have gone through them ten to twenty years before. It does not follow that Canada can accept answers because they have worked in the U.S., nor can she simply drop them because they have failed in the States. She can, however, look at the reasons for failure and/or success and see if those reasons apply equally to her and make her decision accordingly.

Another aspect of the "applied" side of comparative physical education is that which might be termed experimental. It is conceivable that pilot projects could be set up based upon study of other countries. Thus, if it could be shown that under these sets of circumstances it has been found that this condition can flourish, a pilot project could be set up to try to validate the theoretical construct.

These possibilities all contribute to the concept of comparative physical education as a discipline, but they are only possibilities and need to become actualities before any claims to discipline status can be seriously entertained. It is my opinion that physical education is in danger of losing its claim to discipline-status because of the way in which members of the profession are trying to carve off little pieces and associate them with other disciplines. Such a process will eventually lead to physical education no longer having a body of knowledge that it can call its own. If this does happen, *comparative* physical education will also cease to function as a separate area of study. Up to now, comparative physical education has tended to cover the full gamut of physical activity with the emphasis on the physical activity that is carried on in the educational systems, whereas "physical education" is coming to mean just that part of physical activity that is conducted in the school systems. To help clarify the situation, the following might be considered as working definitions of the more common terms:

a. *Physical Activity*: This is the generic term covering all forms of human movement, and may, therefore, include sport, games, physical education, recreation, work, etc.

b. *Play*: Any activity that is carried on for the intrinsic rewards of the activity itself.

c. *Games*: Those play activities in which there is an element of competition; that are bounded by limits of time and space and governed by rules that are not fixed, in that they may be changed as the game progresses, and are supplied by the participants.

d. *Sport*: Those physical activities in which the element of competition is present; that are bounded by limits of time and space, and in which the participants agree beforehand to abide by a fixed set of rules which are externally supplied.

e. *Work*: Any activity carried on for an extrinsic reward.

f. *Recreation:* Any activity carried on for the purpose of restoring homeostasis.

g. *Physical Education*: Those physical activities carried on in the schools and other institutions for "educational" purposes.

h. *Education*: The process in which a deliberate attempt is made to change a person either physically, mentally or emotionally other than by drugs, surgery, etc.

i. *Comparative Education*: The process of examining two or more educational systems in order to compare likenesses and dissimilarities,

j. *Comparative Physical Education*: The process of examining the physical activities carried on in two or more societies, cultures, countries or areas for purposes of comparing likenesses and dissimilarities.

Note: It can readily be seen that these definitions are not mutually exclusive, and that there is, in fact, a good deal of overlapping.

Is Comparative Physical Education a Sub-discipline?

If it is agreed that physical education, as a form of comparative studies, is not a discipline, it is most natural then to consider it as part of comparative education (i.e., a sub-discipline of the larger field). However, this raises the obvious question of whether one can consider comparative education to be a discipline. To be sure, people in the field of comparative education consider it to be a discipline and speak of it in that context. Edmund J. King, for instance, when speaking of the purpose of comparative education uses the term "our discipline,"[3] but in this article he points out that there is a danger that other people will state "that comparative education not merely does not belong to the constructive social sciences, but does not even belong to the genuine academic disciplines."[4] Later King suggests that the esteem in which comparative education is held, is low:

Even the academic planners setting up new universities or research departments leave most of us out of account in their growing departments of "Comparative Studies" or "Area Studies". How many of them really consider our work on a par with that of economists, sociologists, and the like? We have a body of knowledge; we have out tools of enquiry; we have a conspectus of the world and its problems focused on education, which is mankind's most remarkable activity. Some of us, in our personal capacities, are actually brought into planning. But what about Comparative Education itself, and all its parts? In public esteem, if the truth be told, we are not of the stature of Jullien, Cousin, Mann, Mathew Arnold or Sadler. We are 'just one more course' in teachers' colleges. This is no comment by me, but the judgment of many contemporaries.[5]

Howell and his co-authors also tread warily on this question of the status of comparative education:

> Comparative education has long been a field of academic study. That is not to say that it is a discipline in its own right, but it is considered as an essential and academic study, and also a most popular one. Comparativists like Edmund King, George Bereday, and A. D. C. Peterson in recent years (sic) have done much to place the subject in an academic framework and increase its respectability...

> Comparative education is too broad a field, and individual disciplines will benefit by intensified study of their subject. Thus we will see in the future, in all probability, a growth of fields such as comparative sociology, comparative educational psychology and so on. Physical education is one of these that will develop comparativists.[6]

It will be seen that in the opinion of these experts, comparative physical education is a part of comparative education and the latter is not a discipline.

R. Freeman Butts reinforces this viewpoint when he says:

> Some of my colleagues are now even going so far as to claim that there really is no such identifiable field of study as comparative education or international education; they claim that each is merely a particular dimension of one or more of the separate and already well-established social science disciplines in education. Just as education has no disciplinary integrity of its own as a field of study, I have heard it argued, so comparative and international education have no integrity of their own among the other educational specialties that DO have a disciplinary base, such as the history of education, philosophy of education, sociology of education, economics of education, and the like...

> Some of my colleagues argue, for example, that the only legitimate disciplinary studies of education derive from the well recognized fields of anthropology, sociology, economics, political science, history, philosophy, and psychology. These, apparently, are the modern seven liberal arts and sciences. Since comparative and international education are not

disciplines in themselves, all that can be known or need to be known about them can come through the study of one or more of the magic seven.[7]

Is Comparative Physical Education a Sub-sub-discipline

There would seem to be little doubt that one could argue for comparative sociology being a discipline that would naturally include education and thus physical education. Whatever reasonable criteria are laid down, it would seem that this broad area of study would manage to comply with them. It seems, also, therefore, that comparative physical education can certainly (1) claim to be part of the discipline of comparative sociology, and (2) can assert its place as a section of comparative education, with less chance of substantiating a claim for that branch of knowledge to be considered a discipline and may even be able to call itself a discipline.

Whatever its name and status, comparative physical education needs to be defined. It is basically the study of different systems of physical education in order that they may be examined for similarities and differences. To be executed well, this requires an eclectic approach. At the moment the most popular method of studying different systems is what one might term the social-science method, whereby the investigator "searches for repetitive patterns and regularities in social relationships,"[8] But "comparative education was traditionally considered an offshoot of the discipline of history,"[9] which meant that an historical approach was most often used in the past.[10]

The historical approach meant not only writing about past events, but also identifying antecedent factors and forces that had influenced education in form, policy, and practice, and that determined the development and present status of the educational system. Naturally, consideration was given also to the philosophical, nationalistic and melioristic factors involved in the educational process. Ulich, Kandel, and Hans, for instance, wrote their treatises this way. They reconstructed the past, by narrating past events and by interpreting those events in terms of the antecedent forces that helped shape them and then abstracted certain problems or generalizations from the current situation that they felt could be seen in the past.[10] A study of this type has, of course, obvious merit, but equally, it is limited in scope and fails to offer anything like a complete picture. If this brief comment seems to reject out of hand a valid and worthwhile method of investigation, let it be said that this is not the intention, but that in a short paper a more detailed exposition is neither possible nor warranted.

What can we say of the present methods in comparative education? They are those of social science in general and utilize what may be termed the scientific method. The ultimate purpose of any science is prediction and control. The social scientist attempts to establish universal laws by

54

formulating explicit hypotheses and then testing them. He tries to replicate situations in order to confirm or refute the data available. The instruments that he uses are also subject to replication. Thus, the social scientist (1) observes social phenomena, or in our case, educational phenomena; (2) formulates hypotheses; and (3) tests them in order to try to establish some laws. In the field of comparative education, such laws will be of the type that say: "When one state of affairs exists, then another state will necessarily exist; or when one state (or condition) is changed, then another will necessarily change too."

A social-science approach to comparative investigation in physical education may be termed a functional approach in that the emphasis is on the function of the phenomenon studied rather than its structure. Thus, one might be examining sport in two different countries and looking at it from the point of view of the purpose that it serves in the culture (e.g., as an expression of nationalism, as a form of military training, as an expression of the underlying tenets of the culture, as a form of catharsis, and so on. This way of looking at sport is completely distinct from that which is concerned with, for instance, the methods of financing sport within a society. Let it be said, however, that neither method is complete by itself, but only uses different emphases in order to arrive at the truth.

Let us also examine the idea of the "truth". The point was made that comparative physical education is part of comparative education, which in turn is part of the social sciences. Even more, all of these are part of the particular culture and cannot be divorced from it. To isolate any part of the culture without a concomitant examination of the society as a whole may result in the analysis of variables that are not relevant; yet, they may be "true". For instance, it may be true that there are more baseball players in the United States of America than there are in Canada, but such a statement tells us nothing about relative populations, status of differing sports, facilities, the national psyche or, in fact, anything other than that there are more baseball players in one country than another. The statement is true, but it tells us nothing of any real importance.

This short discussion has attempted to make the following points:

    a. Comparative physical education may or may not be a discipline.

    b. The research methodology and accompanying techniques of comparative physical education are that of the social sciences.

    c. Comparative physical education cannot be discussed separately from the rest of the culture.

Any discussion of it must be made from the broad base of that culture.

In the final analysis, it does not matter whether that this field of study called comparative physical education can be called a discipline, or whether its academic status is high, or whether its methodology is its own or borrowed. It does matter, however, that whether it is a discipline, and if as such it is accepted by its sister disciplines, it will (1) attract good–caliber people, and (2) members of other disciplines will be the more likely to aid, confer with, and accept aid from those who are engaged in the study of comparative physical education. It is important, also, that the broad research methodology (e.g., descriptive) and techniques employed (e.g., comparative), wherever they came from, be viewed as being sufficiently stringent by members of other professions. In addition, it does matter because, as has been stated, discussion of physical education is meaningless unless it is in the context of the total culture. In addition, to use this kind of broad-based view, it is necessary to incorporate the work of all social scientists and especially those involved in comparative studies.

Comparative physical education is in a particularly vulnerable position. *[Ed. Note: And this is still true some 40 years after Mutimer expressed this opinion.].* It is, by definition, closely allied to the field of physical education, which is–in the Western world at any rate–still struggling to get away from the "drill" concept and to become accepted as an academic discipline. Further, it is linked with comparative education. Still further, as King explains, comparative education is also involved in the same struggle. Finally, the point was made that few publications of any note have been written on the subject, which implies that there are few scholars of any magnitude working in the area. This, of course, means that there is that much more difficulty in attaining any semblance of disciplinary status. The fact should be noted that there are only a few scholars working in comparative physical education does not necessarily detract from the standards held by those few. It does mean that the work output, however high the caliber, will be limited in quantity relative to what probably is needed.

The result, therefore, is an area of study in which few are working, in which the boundaries are ill defined, and which is not held in high esteem. Despite all this, comparative physical education is a worthwhile area of study. In fact, as far as the field of physical education is concerned, it can be argued that it is a vital study.

Rationale for Comparative Physical Education

Why bother with this area of investigation in the first place? This is a natural question to follow: "Why bother with it at all?" There has to be a reason for whatever man does, for he is a rational creature. The fact that there are comparative studies being carried out in physical education means that some people have answered, to their own satisfaction, the question of why such studies should be undertaken. There is, in all disciplines, a rising tide of interest in comparative work, and this appears to be as true of physical education as any other area. For example, Nixon states:

> In recent years, a tremendous wave of interest has developed concerning the international aspects of physical education. Professional magazines abound with articles written by American physical educators who have visited other countries, and who then want to share their observations with their colleagues.

Among the reasons given by various authors are: (1) to improve international relations, (2) the fact that modern technology has made the world so small that it is imperative to know one's neighbours, (3) the simple desire to know, (4) to learn from others, (5) to teach others, (6) to improve oneself, and so on. Thus, in this discussion, a more detailed look will be at those reasons that this writer considers most important.[11]

International Relations

The English language is full of clichés. Some examples of this are "to know is to love", "the grass is always greener the other side of the hill", "the fear of the unknown", and others. They convey the twin ideas that, if only one can get to know one's neighbours, one will no longer fear them and will be able to live in peace with them; that there is a tendency to exaggerate when knowledge is incomplete. There are comparativists who feel that within the basic concept of "knowing one's neighbours" there lies ample justification for comparative studies.

There is much to be said for this point of view. It seems to be axiomatic that fear is a driving force often leading to war and that this fear can be lessened by learning that the "enemy" is, after all, human. He, too, has hopes and dreams and fears, weaknesses as well as strengths, and a desire to live in peace. In fact, he and she are very much like oneself.

Imitation is the sincerest form of flattery. When one country, or one group within that country, borrows an idea from another there is typically a strengthening of the amicable ties between them. The borrower has stepped outside his own parochialism and found something good in another's way of life. The borrowee, if one might coin a term, cannot help but feel flattered by the fact that someone has thought enough of his ideas to borrow from them. It may spur the borrower to further efforts in order to maintain the supremacy that is acknowledged tacitly when his methods are copied. In addition, in some cases, it may cause him to try to stop the other's use of them, but in a field like physical education this is unlikely.

Even if there were to be no copying, no borrowing and no exchange of practice, the mere fact of knowing more about a people is sufficient to lessen tension, to soften antipathy, and to make relations better. Simply to realize that the other person has the same, or similar problems as oneself, and that he too is looking for answers to them, is enough to enable one to see the other person in a different, and better, light.

Vendien and Nixon put it this way:

As educators today consider the one-world concept, comparative education in all fields has reached significant heights. Increased knowledge and understanding is the only reasonable approach to peaceful existence. Cross-cultural studies serve to:

(1) supply information and interpretive material about health, physical education and recreation around the world that is specially designed for graduate courses in comparative physical education;
(2) do much to develop talent in constructive leadership;
(3) stretch one's intellectual capacity by supplying information about the aspirations, ideas and experiences of others;
(4) aid in assessing and improving one's own educational system as a result of insights and perspectives gained through comparative analysis; and
(5) promote international professional collaboration*, especially at research levels.

Comparative studies in health, physical education and recreation, as in other disciplines, give more insight into a way of life in another land. Although studies in this field and other educational areas have little or no effect upon the power politics of the world or decision making at the top levels, they become one more facet of international understanding.[12]

The Global Village

It is a fact that modern methods of transportation and of communication have turned the world into a "global village". It is patently absurd to continue to live as if people in other countries did not exist. They are there; communication is not only possible; it is easy. It seems obvious that one should take advantage of the situation to get to know all the inhabitants of the "village" and share problems and solutions. The whole idea relates to that of improving international relations and, in fact, cannot really be separated from it. In addition, it is contained within the idea of a liberally educated person.

It is becoming increasingly obvious that any one nation's problems are the world's problems. For example, the population growth of India and China is not solely the concern of the Indians and the Chinese, but that of everyone. Not only do the conditions caused by such population growth pose grave threats to world peace, the sheer proliferation of humans on this planet threatens the very existence of humans. Thinking of a war as "local" no longer makes sense. Any war anywhere now involves everybody everywhere. Modern technology has made barriers between people purely artificial. Nobody on this earth is more than minutes away from destruction by someone else.

While the problems of physical education are, perhaps, of less magnitude than war or famine, they belong to the world and should be looked at from a world-wide viewpoint. This should be done without losing sight of the fact that, while the basic problems in every society may be similar, there are still great differences.

Once more, the point has to be made that there is need for a thorough grounding in the background knowledge and information. The first thing that is required is the facts, which is what makes the reports emanating from the International Council on Health, Physical Education, Recreation, and Dance, for instance, so valuable. The facts and opinions, while indispensable, are only a beginning, however. The first stage must be the collection of the facts, of course, but these facts should be interpreted in the light of all the influences that surround the phenomenon under, review. Anything less than may lead to wrong conclusions being drawn, even though the facts are accurate.[13]

There was, perhaps, a tendency in the days before the global village, to think that anything foreign was inapplicable to one's homeland. It was strange, or interesting, perhaps, but of no use outside its own country. Maybe there has been a swing in the other direction and now the mode of thinking is that the world is a small place, people are just people, wherever they happen to live and anything that is right in one part of the world is necessarily right in another. Not everyone thinks this way, to be sure. For instance, dominant nations have always tended to force their own ideas on those they dominate and have failed to see the good in other peoples' practices, and they still do.

The author hopes that this paper will help to show the fallacy in thinking that one's own problems are unique, as well as the fallacy in thinking that one's own problems are *not* unique.

The "Desire to Know" Syndrome

The "because it's there" syndrome is a major factor in human life. This is the force that drives men to climb mountains, to seek the answer to the riddle of the universe, and also to the mystery of the microorganism. The mere fact that there are other people elsewhere who are facing the same problems and, perhaps, answering them in a different way, is enough for some men to want to investigate, examine and learn. Perhaps this is the most honest and the most human reason behind comparative studies. It covers those who would reply that they undertake such work because they enjoy it, and those who would say that someone has to do it. The urge to know, to understand and, to empathise is one of the major factors in lifting man from the level of the beasts.

As Bereday says:

> The foremost justification for comparative education as for other comparative studies is intellectual. Men study foreign educational systems simply because they want to know, because men must forever stir in quest of enlightenment. Just as it is a travesty of informed living to use an automobile without knowing the principle upon which it is based, it is a mockery of pedagogy to study child-rearing practices without being aware of their endless variations, not only in historical time but also in geographical perspective. *Knowledge for its own sake is the sole ground upon which comparative education needs to make a stand in order to merit inclusion among other academic fields*[13]

(**Note**: The emphasis above is the present writer's.)

Bereday stresses further that comparative education is far from being esoteric, and that it contributes both to pedagogy and the field of the social sciences.

Learning from Others

The idea that perhaps by studying what other people are doing we can learn from their successes and mistakes, and thereby improve out own system, is a pious and humble thought. It is the reason most often put forward as the rationale for undertaking comparative work. Is it a valid reason? How often has one system been modified by knowledge of another?

It seems likely that the main time when other people's ideas are incorporated into a system is the period when the system is being first instituted. We then get a man like Ryerson in Canada, for example, who set out to determine what was being done elsewhere in the world and to bring back the best features for his, as yet, untried system. Another major opportunity for borrowing from others is when there is a drastic change in a system perhaps for political reasons, or because of a sudden change in the economic structure of a country. The election of the Communist Party under the leadership of Tito in Yugoslavia might serve as an example of both a political and an economic change. The political move led to borrowing from the U.S.S.R. in educational matters. In addition, the change from a purely agricultural to a predominantly industrial economy led to a great need for trained personnel. This, in turn, meant that the educational system had to be completely revised.

Occasionally, it may be that a need for some change is felt in, or in addition to, a system. Then work in other countries may be examined to assist the change. One example might be the varying awards schemes, such as the "Duke of Edinburgh" awards in Canada, or the various fitness awards-schemes that are rife in the United States. There were precedents for this type of incentive and doubtlessly they were borne in mind when the newer schemes were inaugurated.

If it is true that changes are made only because of a felt need, then changes will not normally be made because of a comparative study. However, comparative studies will be commissioned when a change is to be made. If this is true, then the rationale that comparative studies should be undertaken in the hope of reforming one's own system is faulty. It may be that the results of an existing study would be used by someone contemplating a change, but it seems more likely that he or she would investigate the particular aspect personally, if only because the viewpoint obtained would not necessarily be the same as that of the study's investigator. Furthermore, it is unlikely that the study would have been made at just the time when it was needed, unless it were commissioned. So, it may well be that the most a comparative study is likely to do is provide a head-start for someone who wishes to make a change. This, in itself, is a good reason for undertaking comparative studies, but it is not the same as providing a stimulus for change.

John E. Nixon reinforced this view of the role of comparative physical education studies, when he said:

> it can be contended that very few comparative education studies have fundamentally influenced governmental policy in education so as to effect significant change.[14]

Missionary Zeal

The obverse of the desire to improve oneself by acquiring knowledge of others is the desire to improve others because of a belief that one has something better to offer. This missionary zeal is often good, but sometimes tragic. The mass importation of a system, be it religious, educational, or anything else, rarely meets with success because it does not take into consideration the "soil" into which the "transplant" is to be placed. This problem will be discussed at greater length below. For the moment, however, it should be noted that this is one driving force behind comparative studies.

Often, of course, the missionary zealot bypasses the comparative study. For some the intent is to study the system so that differences from that of the investigator (in whose eyes "different" is synonymous with "inferior") are seen and changes (improvements) may be made to bring it up to the standard of the investigator. For others this is a wasteful step, and all that needs to be done is to move in the new system, lock, stock, and barrel. In addition, if any parts of the old happen to fit, that is fine; if they do not, well that is simply unfortunate. In recent times the British have been, perhaps, the worst culprits–or the best exponents, depending upon one's viewpoint–of this type of "improvement", although it seems likely that the Americans will soon surpass them.

Apologists for the method will point to India, Australia, and Canada to show that the graft can take and produce good results, but in fact where the transplanted system has worked it has worked among people who are, to all intents and purposes, British. This is true even in India where the native peoples who have adopted and thrived on the British system have also adopted much of the British culture. However, most of the people have not adopted the system, nor have they felt any benefit for it. In Australia and Canada, of course, the educational system, the outlook on sports, and the whole culture was transplanted from the homeland and has, over the years, developed into something quite distinct from that which existed, or exists, in Britain. These countries, then, are not examples of missionary zeal, but of a people taking their culture with them wherever they went.

Unfortunately, in many cases people with a mission have felt it their duty to play down physical activity, sports, games, and similar "devilish pursuits". Missionaries in the accepted sense of the word have traveled the world sowing seeds of guilt and making happy people cover their bodies, refrain from play and take their pleasures like medicine. The fact that in most cases this dastardly deed has been perpetrated for the highest motives only makes it that much worse.

Liberal Education

No one can be considered truly educated who lives in ignorance of his fellow man. If this is true in general how much more is it true in the narrower sense of one's own profession? In other words, can one be a good physical educator if one does not know what is going on in the world of physical education? Or, perhaps, would one not be a better physical educator if one kept abreast of happenings across the world? The answer seems to be so obvious as to require nothing further to be said. Surely, the chances of change, of improvement, of borrowing are greater at the individual level than at any other level? Surely no one would disagree that the more one knows about one's subject, even if much of that knowledge is not immediately applicable, the better?

Perhaps the aim of all education is to know oneself. Bereday states that "one studies foreign education not solely to know foreign peoples, but also–and perhaps most of all–to know oneself."[15] He says that understanding oneself and understanding others are the necessary pre-requisites to making comparisons.

Edmund King, the dean of comparativists puts it another way:

> If people look at themselves and their work in a
> wider context than usual, they not merely
> contribute more to their children and their country
> but will gain even more themselves.[15]

The foregoing are very wide categories, which, despite their width, are probably not all-inclusive. Let us look at some of the reasons given by individual writers for the study of comparative physical education. Vendien and Nixon, for instance, suggest that:

> in the light of cross-cultural studies it is possible to
> re-evaluate one's own educational system and
> determine what is best for meeting the goals of
> one's own society.[16]

The authors say further that the major basic assumptions underlying the development of comparative physical education materials are:

1. All students are enlightened by exposure to other
   cultural concepts and social systems. The
   comparative approach is educative in providing
   information about the unknown, in clarifying aims
   and practices taken for granted but little understood
   in one's own culture, in stimulating insights regarding
   program improvements, and in encouraging
   international professional collaboration.

2. The comparative education approach involves the
   hypothesis that:

(a) Any education system or part thereof is partially
    patterned by the traditional values and practices in
    the culture.
(b) Any educational system within a former colonial
    country is more strongly patterned by the cultural

traditions of the colonial power than by its own traditions, these foreign traditions usually being dysfunctional but in many ways permanently influential.

(c) Any educational system in a developing nation is subject to the danger of a sustained colonial pattern or a hastily copied Western pattern. Rationale and results should be examined and then adjusted, or changed according to conscious choice.

(d) Any educational system in a so-called developed nation is subject to the danger of assumed excellence - thus obsolescence becomes a possibility. Again, the rationale and results should be examined and then adjusted or changed according to conscious choice.

3. Any program of health, physical education, and recreation is part of the total education system, and as such has responsibilities both to the total system and to its specific portion of it.[17]

Howell and his co-authors stress the learning-from-others approach when they state that "we have so much to learn from other countries today."[18] They list, also, a number of features of other countries and then say:

These are all vital issues that should be developed and debated and understood, for it is possible they might profitably be introduced into our own culture.[19]

In support of their contention, the authors quote Edward T. Hall as saying that "the implicit purpose of our work is to be useful in the improvement of school systems - and therefore in the transformation of human society."[20]

Kandel in the introduction to his classic *Comparative Education* lists twenty problems that he considers to have cross-cultural significance and then states:

The chief value of a comparative approach to such problems lies in an analysis of the causes which have produced them, in comparison of the differences between the various systems and the reasons underlying them, and, finally, in a study of the solutions attempted...

The study of foreign systems of education means a critical approach and a challenge to one's own philosophy and, therefore, a clearer analysis of the background and basis underlying the educational system of one's own nation. It means, further, the development of a new attitude and a new point of view which may be derived from a knowledge of the reasons for establishing systems of education and of the methods of conducting them.[21]

Moehlman offers a slightly different slant on the reasons for carrying out comparative studies. Although he is advocating knowledge of others in order to understand them, his stress is slightly different:

Through a sympathetic study of a foreign educational system, one gains a window through which the scholar may become acquainted with the national character and aspirations of another people. The next generation is being shaped by today's schools and colleges. The study of the motivation, the goals, and the techniques of a system of educations is an important step toward understanding both this generation and the next. Achievement of such understanding is a firm step toward survival.[22]

He, in turn, uses two quotations which he feels justify the study of comparative education: "To know thyself, compare thyself to others" (Tacitus) and "Those who forget their past are condemned to repeat it" (Santayana).[23]

Social Institutions Influencing Comparative Physical Education

The one point on which there is complete agreement by all writers on comparative education is that it is essential to understand the whole society of which the educational system is but a part. Different writers say it in different ways, but the message is the same and it comes across loud and clear. Keeping, for the moment, to physical education comparativists one sees that Howell *et al.* say that, "a study of sport and physical education in the U.S.S.R., for example, cannot be done without a study of its geography, its topography, its culture and its history."[24] Vendien and Nixon say that the comparative education approach involves the hypothesis that: "any education system or part thereof is partially patterned by the traditional values and practices in the culture."[25]

Cramer and Browne, in writing about the influences on systems of education include (1) the sense of national unity, (2) the general economic situation, (3) fundamental beliefs and traditions, (4) the status of progressive educational thought, (5) language problems, (6) political background, and (7) attitude towards international cooperation in their discussion.[26] Similarly Nicholas Hans lists the following factors:

1. Natural factors: racial, linguistic, geographic, and economic.

2. Religious factors: Catholic, Anglican, Puritan [Hans was writing about England, the U.S., the U.S.S.R. and France].

3. Secular factors: Humanism, socialism, nationalism, democracy.[27]

The Report on the Expert Meeting, held from March 11-16, 1963 and published by UNESCO contained a statement echoing this position:

> "...it has always been realized by comparative
> educationists how strongly education is influenced
> by the economic, social structure, religious,
> political and other sectors of a social context,..."[28]

Other beliefs are available, but enough has been written to make the point that education, and physical education for that matter, is merely one facet of a country and cannot be adequately understood unless every other facet is known and understood. Obviously there are some factors that have a greater effect on education than others, and thus more attention paid to them in any study of the educational system. Some of the more obvious examples will be examined below in this paper.

A Definition of "Culture"

A number of words or terms in current use that are very difficult to define. Of these, "culture" is one of the most difficult. As is the case with many an important and oft-used term, it has changed its meaning with the years, but it has usually included the idea of the products of learned behaviour (i.e., the language, clothing, food habits, spiritual and moral values, institutions, and material culture, or technology.[29] Kluckhohn and Kelly's definition seems adequate for our purposes:

> A culture is an historically created system of
> explicit and implicit designs for living, which tends
> to be shared by all or specially designated
> members of a group at a specified point in time.[30]

One could quibble at the emphasis on the "specified point in time" in relation to comparative studies, because it is the dynamic aspect of a culture that interests us most. Obviously, however, any study is conducted at a specific point in time. In addition, it seems unnecessary to belabour the point that culture and education are inextricably mixed. In certain senses they are one, since education is simply the means whereby the culture is passed from generation to generation.

A Definition of History

If it is impossible to extract education from the rest of the culture, and it is (!) other than for academic purposes, it is equally impossible to consider history, culture, philosophy, etc. as separate factors in a civilization. It should be borne in mind constantly that any discussion, such as this, which attempts to look at one facet of the lives of a group of people is a purely academic exercise–and a rather sterile one at that. However, the scope of the subject is so great that, in order to attain a little order and some cohesion, it becomes necessary to create these artificial areas and look at them separately.

It is not the intention to define every term used in this paper, but if it were then one could spend as many pages writing about definitions of history, of which there are historians. It should be enough to say that "history" in this context is regarded as the story of culture. Thus if we could envisage history as a living, growing organism that could be sliced laterally at any given level at will–and that which would be exposed at the time of the slice would be a culture at a certain point in time.

All that is intended is to point out that, to understand the educational system and the part that physical education plays in any given culture at any given point, it is essential to know the history of that culture. For instance, one cannot understand the British preference for a "games philosophy" unless one knows something about the role of the Public School in British life. Another example is Yugoslavia's emphasis on military training that would be incomprehensible without some idea of the warlike nature of her immediate past. Similarly, the Communist Bloc countries' concentration on group activities would be puzzling unless one knew that there had been, within living memory, a revolution (whether bloody or peaceful) and that group activities were seen as a method of inculcating new ideals in the people.

One could continue, but the investigator hopes that the point has been made. If further clarification is needed one has only to look at the private schools in Canada (e.g., Upper Canada College), or the fact that squash racquets is played across the country, or that Swedish gymnastics is taught in the high schools–or even that there are such places as high schools. Seeing these things would not make sense to an outsider without knowledge of the conquest of New France by the British, the influence of the British garrisons, and the influx of ideas from the United States. To know is only the "first step towards understanding, and without understanding comparative physical education can never be more than an academic exercise.

Bruce L. Bennett, the excellent physical education historian stresses the need for the comparativist to study the history of the various countries being examined, and says:

May I suggest that the student of comparative
physical education needs both the *breadth* that
comes from a study of contemporary life in other
countries and the *depth* that can only come from a
study of the history of those countries.[31]

A Definition of Philosophy

Philosophy is another of the terms that may mean almost whatever
one wants it to mean. In the context of this paper, one could talk about the
philosophy that the individual brings to his work, be that person a teacher,
administrator, or civil servant. Thus limited, we would not have mentioned
the philosophies that motivate the many bodies and organizations that affect
education and physical education in any society.

However, let us take a quick look at philosophy in a broad sense. If one
examines the ontological and epistemological position adopted by the
majority of people in a country, then almost inevitably it will be seen that the
beliefs lie somewhere between spiritual monism and material monism,
which lead to rationalism on-the one hand and empiricism on the other.

If the former view is taken, it is axiomatic that the only route to
knowledge is by way of the intellect. Accordingly, it is a simple step to
believing that education must be *of* the intellect and *for* the intellect. In such
circumstances, the curriculum becomes overloaded with subjects that are
susceptible to learning through the intellect, such as mathematics, and less
stress is placed on the applied subjects, such as physical education.

If we were to adopt the philosophic position of empiricism, this would
mean that all knowledge is obtained through the senses. In holding such a
position, one is forced into concluding that education must be by experience
of the observable world. Thus, practical subjects are given importance, and
physical education is commonly included among them. In a society in which
spiritual monism is the prevails, we can expect that physical education will
suffer in status and can hope for little more than being considered a service
programme at best. If the dominating view is that of empiricism then
practical or applied subjects, including physical education, will be given
pride of place.

The question can then be asked as to what kind of person a believer in
each system thinks he is educating. For the rationalist, the intellect is the all-
important component, and the human is viewed as "a mind that happens to
be encased in a body" (as Plato argued). This dualistic concept is the result of
many influences. Asceticism and belief in the immortality of the soul, as well
as in rationalism have all aided in creating a "two-part man" with the
physical side debased. The empiricist often takes a much more holistic view
of man and will revere the body and see its natural impulses as good.

However, some empiricists see the body as a machine and view it as a complicated arrangement of materialistic attributes acting in accordance with physical laws. In this latter case, physical education, while it may attain a significant place in the curriculum, is used solely to produce physical results, with the emphasis on physical fitness, health, and concomitant cardio-vascular endurance.

The dualistic/holistic and rationalistic/empirical dichotomies are extreme positions that have influenced education and physical education since before Plato. The rationalistic-dualistic concept has dominated Western thought since that time, with a holistic concept gaining credence only on occasion (e.g., the period of Humanism associated with the Renaissance).

> [**Ed. Note:** This comprehensive essay was completed by Mutimer in 1970. In 1973, Prof. J. R. Fairs published what was to be a well-received paper pointing out Plato's "dualistic approach". See Fairs, J. R. (1973). The influence of Plato and Platonism on the development of physical education in Western culture. In E. F. Zeigler (Ed. & Au.), *A history of sport and physical education to 1900*, pp. 155-166 Champaign, IL: Stipes, 1975.]

The point made here is that, if the prevailing mode of thinking is dualistic, then physical education is likely to be downgraded. However, if the general philosophical viewpoint is holistic, then physical education will be given higher status in relation to intellectual subjects. If one is investigating the status of physical education in a culture and does not examine the current philosophical position, that person may not discover why the status is as it is.

Finally, the point bears repeating that philosophy is closely interwoven with everything that creates a national ethos: religion, politics, relations with neighbours, etc. ad infinitum. Of all these influences, religion is perhaps the most closely allied to philosophy.

The Importance of Religion

Knowledge of a country's religion is an indispensable part of knowing its views on physical education and sport. If one could know everything about two countries except for the physical education and sport program, and the two countries were identical in all else but religion, then one could make some very accurate guesses about the physical activities of the two countries. One might expect, for instance, that countries where the major religion is Christianity (e.g., Puritan, Lutheran or Calvinistic) would view sport and physical activities as necessary evils that should be relegated to the plane of physical training. The classical puritanical view has been that physical activity should be useful, not enjoyable. The Lord's Day Observance Acts, the view of dancing as potentially evil, and gambling as actually evil are relics of the age of strict Puritanism that are still with us. The degradation of the body and the exaltation of the soul and the intellect have led to many of the taboos in our society regarding the nude body, sex, biological functions, modes of dress, and so on.

In societies where the puritan (i.e., "puritan" with a small "p") influence has not existed, many of these attitudes are unknown. Where puritanical views of the body are held, physical education is almost bound to be regarded as something base, a necessary evil at best. In a non-puritan society one may get the kind of glorification of the physical that apparently was rife in Athens in the 5th Century. The foregoing is simply to show the kind of influence that religion may play. Puritanism is not restricted to the Puritanism of the Christian Church, but covers any religion or philosophy in which enjoyment, especially of a physical nature, is frowned upon. It goes without saying that there are sects within every religion that are more extreme than the rule, and that it is unlikely that the religious influence would be uniform across a country. The fact remains , however, that the more one knows of a specific religion, the more one will be able to understand the attitudes held towards physical education.

The Influence of Geography and Climate

J. R. Hildebrand stresses the importance of geography in forming sporting activities.[32] The view he expresses is perhaps one-sided, and it may be that when one writes for the *National Geographic* the writer does tend to stress geography; nevertheless his thesis is interesting. The influence that geography necessarily has on the sports in a country is obvious. For instance, one is unlikely to find mountain climbing a popular pastime in the middle of the Canadian prairies, or sailing in the middle of the desert, or surfing somewhere a thousand miles inland.

The mention of surfing inland may make the reader jump to attention and say that he knows of an inland surfing lake where the breakers are made to order. This is very true, and raises the point that geography may be losing its position to a degree to modern technology as a dominant factor in deciding what games will be played where. Let us take some obvious examples. Ice-hockey has now become possible in equatorial countries because of man's ability to make artificial ice. Man-made lakes have made inland aquatic sports a possibility, and snow-machines have enabled ski-jumps and runs to be put where none existed before, In fact, almost anything is possible given the necessary money. However, all of this is of very recent vintage, and there is no doubt that geography and climate have been great forces in determining historic national pastimes. This will undoubtedly continue indefinitely.

It is worth nothing that modern technology has been one other major form of influence in deciding which games are to be played. The ease with which travel is now possible has become remarkable. Games have been moved across frontiers in the past hundred years in a way that was not possible before. The spread of games by the British well exemplifies this trend and the ubiquity of soccer, for instance, epitomises the sporting "global village" that is a direct result of modern methods of travel. This is not to suggest that the transporting of games across national boundaries is a purely modern phenomenon. It is not. The example of the Japanese who have taken up baseball from their American conquerors doubtless had precedents going back to the Crusades and before. However, as in so many developments, the process has been increased and widened.

However, despite the inroads of 20th century "know-how", geography has been and still is a major factor in the games people play. There is little doubt that board games started in the southern parts of Asia, at least in part because of the heat, which made exertion unpleasant and because the sand made scratching a "board easy, while skiing and snow-shoeing, skating and walking on stilts–and even pole-vaulting were forms of adaptation made by humans to cope with the physical environment.

There is also little doubt that while air-conditioning, central-heating, covered stadiums, artificial lakes and snow wind etc. are all possible, for the majority of humankind they are far in the future. Geography and climate will continue to govern the sporting life, and the tendency will still be for "Mohamet to go to the mountain, rather than bringing the mountain to Mohamet."

The Influence of Neighbours

The first, and obvious, way in which one's neighbours can influence the games one plays is by adoption. If one wishes to meet one's neighbours in sporting combat, then both have to be playing the same game under the same rules. If they do not, there is a likelihood that sporting combat may rapidly turn to real combat. A classic example in North America is squash. The first squash that was played in Canada was the same as that played in England, whereas the Americans (using the name in its common, but loose sense) had their own form. Gradually the Canadians adopted the American game so that inter-national games could be played on equal terms. We now have the situation where every nation in the world where squash is played (an unconfirmed report places the number at 54) abides by the English rules, with two exceptions: Canada and the United States of America.

However, there are ways less obvious in which neighbours can affect the physical activities of a nation. For instance, if a country is faced with aggressive neighbours, one might reasonably expect a strong emphasis on those physical activities that are considered useful in war. A neighbour that is despised might lead to certain activities being eschewed simply because they are associated with the other group. In cases where the neighbour is highly regarded, one might find activities and methods imported wholesale even though they do not necessarily fit in with the general cultural pattern. If one were looking for examples of such a trend, Israel is a nation whose physical education is influenced by aggressive neighbours. A second example is the rejection of athletics by certain members of ancient Roman society because of the association with the Greeks. Finally, there is the introduction of ten-pin bowling into Britain because of her slavish desire to emulate the United States of America. The reader will undoubtedly think of other examples.

The influence of one's neighbours may take many other forms. The missionary zeal of her religious leaders could lead to a change in the attitudes towards physical education and sport. The decision by an American business firm to build a chain of health clubs, or bowling alleys, or ski-jumps across Canada would be one example of economics and one's neighbours having a decided influence. The art forms of one's neighbours can "invade" a country and cause a change in attitude to the body and thus a change in attitude towards physical activity. The avenues of influence are unlimited. Some methods of influencing one's neighbours are obvious and direct; others are subtle and easily missed. However, they are there, and a country like Canada is particularly susceptible to pressures to conform with her rich and populous neighbour.

One other "influence" worth mentioning is the lack (!) of influence. For instance, Britain has tended to develop her own forms of sport, games and physical education because of a lack of interest in her neighbours. Yet, this is not an all-pervasive characteristic. There have been influences, and it would be foolish to deny Ling, Gutsmuth, Jahn, Laban, etc. their rightful place in British physical education. Nevertheless, Britain's dominant position in world affairs, her national instinct for insularity, her belief that British is best, and her physical separation from the mainland of Europe have all contributed to the development of distinctly British forms of physical activity. It should perhaps be noted that this insularity is breaking down, and has been doing so for the past 50 or so years.

Again, all that is being attempted in this analysis is to show that understanding a country, its educational system, and its physical education and sport requires knowledge of all the factors that go to make the country what it is.

The Influence of Politics

Politics and sport is an area that has received and is receiving a great deal of attention from many experts. The ties between politics and other aspects of the culture, such as economics, nationalism, religion, neighbours, history and so on, are perhaps more obvious than in many other cases. The prestige that accrues to the government of a nation that is victorious in international sporting competition, both at home and abroad, has led to vast amounts of money being spent on sports by countries determined to prove their superiority to the newly emerging nations who want to show that they have arrived.

The use of physical education as a tool for building national character is evident in modern communist countries as well as it could in ancient Sparta. The identification of a people with its national team has been seen over and again and has led to riots expressing disappointment and riots of victory, in its extreme forms. In many countries sport and physical education are controlled by the political authority. Thus, funds are channeled into various aspects depending upon the goals of the particular party in power. Thus we may get a concentration of moneys in mass-participation, as in Sweden and Great Britain, or more emphasis placed on the elite, international caliber athlete who will bring fame to the country, as would seem to be the purpose in Canada now. It may be that, physical activity is used as a means of making better citizens, as in Yugoslavia, or as "opium for the masses" as in ancient Rome and the U.S.A. of today.

In any case, politics and politicians have great and obvious influence en physical education within the school system, recreation, and sport. The mere fact of designating areas as national parks and supplying facilities and amenities can be a decisive factor in the recreational habits of a nation. The decision to host the Olympic Games is a political move with far-reaching results. The question of whether to build gymnasia or science laboratories, or even whether to build large or small gymnasia are as much political decisions as are import tariffs on sporting goods, or restrictions on touring teams. Practically every major decision in physical education, sport, and recreation has a political base. One might be hard pressed to understand such things as athletic-scholarships in the U.S., or the numbers of top athletes who happen to hold commissions in the armed forces in some East European countries, unless one knows something of the politics and the feelings of nationalism that either exist or that the government wants to exist.

The Influence of Economics

An order of priorities is a political answer to an economic question. One may wonder how an under-developed nation can afford to send a team to the Olympic Games. However, the politicians responsible probably feel that the nation cannot afford not to send a team and thereby spend money on training, housing and transporting that team; money which could have been used on the "starving millions".

The fact that there is need for an order of priorities is based on economics. Physical education, sport, and recreation programmes have to be subsidised adequately. As with everything else, the countries that can best afford them are the rich. One could argue that no country is rich enough to spend money on sports while there are desperately poor people. Obviously, those who control the purse strings do not think this way. Countries like the U.S.A. and the U.S.S.R. have their poor; yet, they spend vast sums on all forms of physical activity. Small nations with an even larger problem, relatively speaking, still spend large amounts of money on sport. One only has to think of Mexico to realize that this is true. Nevertheless, a political decision has to be tempered with the economic reality; there is simply a limit to what can be done. If one is to comprehend the data one has accumulated on physical education and sport within a society, one needs to know the status of the economic situation under consideration.

The foregoing was intended to do no more than point out the necessity for looking at all aspects of a society if one wishes to understand any one aspect. For comparative physical education to be meaningful, it is necessary to study the countries as wholes. To prevent false conclusions drawn from limited accurate data, total knowledge is needed. All of the factors mentioned in this section are linked with physical education and sport in one way or another. The writer hopes that the need to know something about each of them has been shown. However, this list is not exhaustive. Perusal of almost any text on comparative work in any discipline will suggest areas not included here. The intention has not been to provide an exhaustive list, but to highlight the need for a look at total societies when making comparisons.

Comparative Physical Education: Its Execution

Comparative physical education studies should take an eclectic, interdisciplinary, multidisciplinary approach. To be effective physical education comparativists must have good working relationships both with comparativists in other disciplines and experts in other disciplines. The whole society must be examined if a thorough understanding of the physical education, sport and recreation is to be obtained.

Assuming for the moment the acceptance of these premises, the question arises: "How does one go about doing this? Comparative physical education, it has been said, is a young area of study. To date it has developed no methodology of its own. However, comparative education has had rather longer in which to develop its methods of carrying out scholarly comparisons. It would seem reasonable, then, for comparativists in the field of physical education to borrow techniques from their counterparts in other disciplines.

If one is about to undertake a comparative study, it is because of one or more of the reasons discussed above, or for some reason that has been omitted from that list. In any case there must be a reason, a rationale behind the proposed work. To some extent the emphasis of the study and the methods used, will be determined by the reason for undertaking the study.

For instance, if the intent is to adapt one society's system by introducing reforms based on a second system, one should be more concerned with the practicalities of the system (i.e., costs, availability of materials, the need for instructors etc. than if one were investigating the two systems simply to know and understand them better. The former would require a much more detailed breakdown of certain factors than the second, and the comparative techniques used might differ considerably.

There is also the consideration of cost. Unless a survey is commissioned by government, there is likely to be a restriction on the amount of money that can be spent in acquiring the data. To take the extreme case, the student writing a paper for a course will normally be restricted to the materials in his university library, plus what he can borrow through inter-library loan. This could be combined with any other miscellaneous data that he or she may be able to garner from staff and other students. If there is sufficient time, the student might be able to obtain some information from the country's embassy. However, the person's time, and sources of information are limited.

Conversely, a government-sponsored survey could employ hundreds of investigators each working at a specific task and with the full co-operation of the country being studied. Over time such a survey force could present a very detailed, up-to-the-minute report that would get much closer to the truth of the situation than a study carried out by a student.

Most studies, of course, fall somewhere between these extremes, rather closer to that of the student than that of a "mass-invasion." Nigel Grant, for instance, apparently, spent time visiting the countries that he covers in *Society. Schools and Progress in Eastern Europe* and watched at work pupils, teachers, school directors, professors, lecturers, students and education officials.[33] He also gathered information from literature, documents and similar sources. Grant had a prepared formula to guide his investigations. In common with the other books in the Society, Schools and Progress series, Grant had to investigate the historical and institutional background, the administration, the school system, family influences, and background social forces. One can assume that Grant spent several months making his visits and collecting his data.

Let us assume further that an author such as Grant takes one month per country to gather the information he requires. Let us still further assume that the information he does accumulate is up to date. In this book, there are seven countries discussed. This would mean that the information received about the first country is already seven months old by the time that the last country is completed. Even supposing that he required only one more month

_____

33

in which to write up the material, and the publisher were able to get the book on the market in six more months, the information of one-seventh of the book is already 14 months out of date by the time that the reader gets it. In addition, this may well be a conservative estimate. It would seem more likely that some of the data obtained would be anywhere up to a year old by the time that the author first gets it. This observation is particularly true of data provided in figures (e.g., the number of students, teachers, or specialists in a school system. The best that one can usually hope for is that the figures were accurate at the end of the previous academic year.

It could be that the information obtained is correct to the last fourteen months is good enough in most cases. In a period of rapid expansion, however, one could get a picture that was very much out of focus. Let us suppose, for example, that the country being surveyed is in the process of building 50 new high schools complete with every modern facility. At the time the survey is made none of the 50 is ready to accept students; however, by the time that the book reaches the reader all the fifty schools are in full use.

This may be a bad example, Any investigator who is taking the time to write a book on the subject is going to discover the fact that 50 new schools are in the process of being built. However, it could happen. If the investigator should be working within strict guidelines and, if he does not know the language of the country, he could miss this important fact. Even if he should catch such errors, many smaller discrepancies could easily escape him, and the total result might be to date his work well before it is printed.

One way to lessen the chances of this kind of mishap is to have an expert from the country write the book, or part of the book. This is the approach used by Vendien and Nixon in *The World Today in Health. Physical Education and Recreation*.[34] They supplied their chosen experts with the format in which they wanted the article written. In theory, therefore, they could give all their contributors the same deadline and have all the articles written at more-or-less the same time. Thus, although the information is out of date by the time that it reaches the reader, it is all dated by the same amount of time and the comparisons drawn are still valid. It also has the advantage that, presumably, the expert would know about such things as unfinished "schools or projected changes that would alter the scene in any major way in the near future."

An approach such as that of Vendien and Nixon has obvious advantages, not the least of which is the intimate view of the system that no outsider could hope to attain. There are, however, equally obvious disadvantages. The first is the matter of translation into a common language (English, in this instance). The contributor might be able to write his article in English (or whatever language in which the book is to be published). However, even if the writer does, and even if he or she writes as well in

English as in the mother tongue, the materials used must be translated and "something" could well be lost in the process.

The next major drawback to the Vendien-Nixon approach is that of bias. Any writer, any investigator, any person involved in accumulating information has a bias automatically. However, if the same person is collecting the data in all the countries that are being surveyed, the bias will be uniform throughout (as in Nigel Grant's work). If, however, one uses many investigators, the problem of bias is compounded and may make comparisons between and among countries less meaningful than they would otherwise be.

One can guard against this to a certain extent, of course, by such means as selecting contributors who have the same type of job and then giving them a very detailed morphology (i.e., the study of the forms of things) to follow. However, the weaknesses are easy to see and require no elaboration. Nevertheless, as well-matched as the contributors may be, they are still unique human beings with different interests and competencies.

The first step in any comparative study is to collect the facts. Comparative physical education is not a science. However, it does provides information, and it follows the normal pattern of the sciences in that description precedes explanation. Today almost everything written in the area of comparative physical education is descriptive, which is natural and right in a young aspiring-discipline. This is a stage that comparative education went through, and we might expect that comparative physical education will follow in the same path with the hope that one day it will reach the point that comparative education has:

> Currently, comparative education is concentrating on unfolding the possibilities and potentialities for testing hypotheses, producing valid generalizations, and evolving predictive methodologies as a basis for sound decision-making and policy formulation in education. Less importance is now attached to the search for what Holmes[35] calls "antecedent causes"

However, now we are still in the process of *collecting* data; so, it is here that reports like those issued by ICHPER are invaluable.[36] The writer does not know how well the information contained in the three reports was validated. If one can assume that the information is reliable, however, we have here an excellent beginning to cross-cultural surveys and studies. The idea of up-dating these reports is also noteworthy and necessary.

Essential as this kind of information is, it is, nevertheless, only the first step. The ICHPER reports actually contain two steps: the presentation of data and the classification of that data. The next stage is to interpret the data and to see them in the total context. The ICHPER reports demonstrate another research technique of descriptive method of research: the questionnaire. These questionnaires, samples of which are given in the reports, were sent out to "key individuals in each country." Of course. this allows great scope for bias.

How then is the physical education comparativist to obtain his data? The major possibilities are (1) questionnaire, such as those used by ICHPER; (2) individual visiting and interviewing, such as that undertaken by Howell and Van Vliet[37] and Grant[38]; (3) recruiting contributors to write about their own countries, as was done by Vendien and Nixon[39]; (4) by sending in a team of trained investigators, which has yet to be done in this field; (5) having people in the particular countries administer questionnaires as Kenyon did[40]; or (6) by simply relying upon the sources of information that are at hand wherever the investigator happens to be.

There are, of course, innumerable combinations and permutations of these basic techniques. For instance one might send a team of investigators armed with a questionnaire, or visit the countries and then supplement this first-hand knowledge with information from publications available in one's own country, as Howell and Van Vliet did. Naturally, if physical education, as a field of comparative study, wishes to be taken seriously and wishes to do a good job, then all the techniques, safeguards, and "know-how" of other disciplines must be employed. For instance, sampling techniques must be sophisticated, questionnaires must be rigorously designed, and results must be checked carefully.

If we accept Nixon's interpretation of what a comparative study should involve, such studies in physical education are very limited. He suggests that comparative studies involve four major steps:

(1) juxtaposition, or the systematic arrangement of data from two or more countries about common topics;
(2) establishment of the criterion upon which a valid comparison can be made between countries about each topic being analyzed;
(3) creation of a hypothesis from the outcomes of steps 1 and 2 which can be tested through the comparisons; and
(4) processing the technical comparison involving simultaneous analysis among several countries.[41]

Nixon then elaborates this theme. It is worthwhile looking at what he has to say, since he is one of the few writers who is primarily concerned with physical education. His statements are based on those of Bereday, in particular, a leading scholar in comparative education:

Bereday describes modern, cross-cultural, analytical methodology borne of time–tested experience by him and pioneer colleagues. There are two major simultaneous procedural steps: (1) juxtaposition, and (2) comparison. In essence, this methodology begins with (1) a defining statement or central theme which will be the basis for subsequent comparison, and is followed by (2) the thorough, systematic collection and reporting of relevant data from two or more countries simultaneously; and (3) a summarizing statement in hypothesis form that reflects the exacting nature of the comparative analysis being undertaken. In the juxtaposition step, a preliminary "matching" of relevant data from two or more countries is made to prepare them for comparison. First, an appropriate category system with the prerequisite categories, must be created by the investigator. This is required for the systematic inclusion of data to be compared. Second, the investigator studiously analyzes the comparative data in his search for an emerging hypothesis (or hypotheses). The hypothesis must be stated in terms relevant to the characteristics of the data so that the hypothesis can then be subjected to rigorous testing.

The juxtaposition step determines the extent to which comparison is feasible. It is a procedure which seeks to establish a basic consistency. This procedure in itself does *not* directly generate conclusions; it lays the basis for hypothesis development, hypothesis testing, and for validation of generalizations.

Hypothesis development and testing is crucial to comparative methodology. The hypothesis is created by the investigator's intellectual abilities to "tease out" and propose a tentative explanation of * the data which have been placed in juxtaposition for intense comparison and analysis. When a hypothesis has been identified and carefully stated it then is subjected to test by means of subsequent comparison of similar categories of data to determine the extent to which it is accepted, rejected, or modified.

Bereday mentions two types of comparisons following juxtaposition. One he calls "balanced" comparison which means that a match, or a balance, of every type of data has been made from one country compared to similar data from all other countries in the study. This procedure starts with a comparison of each country with every other country by systematic rotation of the data. It terminates with comparison of results by fusion or synthesis. The second kind of comparison is titled "illustrative". Educational practices in different countries are selected at random to illustrate, or exemplify, comparative points found in the juxtaposition charts. Because illustrations (are specific instances which are not repeated from example to example the kinds of statements which can be made from such analysis are not capable of assuming the characteristics of generalizations.[42]

In conclusion, whatever form the investigator's methodology adopts, he or she must examine all the influences that were outlined above. This investigator should be fully conversant with (1) the importance of the body in the culture(s) and the view taken of it; (2) the place occupied by dance; and (3) the role of physical education, education, sport and recreation as well as the organizational structure of these four aspects of the culture. The researcher should know (1) how clubs, organizations and associations related to sport work, (2) what professional training is offered for teachers, coaches, administrators, and volunteers and (3) what methods these people use in the execution of their positions.

Further, this person should have detailed information of the curricula in all the educational institutions involved and know both their differences and similarities throughout the systems. Most important of all, the investigator must understand and empathise with the people under study. Without empathy the researcher will only learn the "what" and the "how" and never the "why".

Practically every book on comparative education includes a conceptual framework to be used in the analysis of a system of physical education, although the name or title may differ. Some authors will call their framework a morphology some a schema, and so on. It would be inappropriate in a paper of this length to repeat any of these frameworks here, but the reader is referred to Morrison[43], Bennett[44], Vendien and Nixon[45], Bereday[46], and Nixon47 for discussions and examples. Morrison in particular discusses the conceptual framework in some depth, while Bennett sets his schema out in simple outline which makes it easy to review. Examination of the various frameworks shows that there is little to chose between them. They all stress the idea of viewing the total society; their major difference is one of detail.

Problems Associated With Research in Comparative Physical Education

Some of the problems associated with research in comparative physical education have been mentioned above. Now they will be assembled so that the difficulties can be clearly seen. In addition, some mention will be made of completed work in the field. Further, some recommendations will be made for the future.

Previous Scholarship in the Field. John E. Nixon, co-author of one of the very few textbooks in the field, has this to say about the available literature:

> The *JOHPER* Journal, *The Physical Educator* journal, and other professional publications contain numerous reports of the experiences of American physical educators in various countries around the globe,...

80

The available American literature on comparative physical education consists largely of articles containing personal descriptions of people, programs, and facilities as observed by the American visitor, and occasionally some statements of personal reactions, or impressions. Textbooks on comparative physical education still are extremely scarce. Examples are the two Monographs on *Physical Education Around the World*, William Johnson, editor, published by Phi Epsilon Kappa Fraternity; and *The World Today in Health, Physical Education, and Recreation*, by Lynn Vendien and John Nixon. These publications cannot rightfully be considered to contain material that has resulted from rigorous comparative research. At best they are examples of the early phases of the descriptive stage of comparative research. Even so the material is not organized with the end in view of organizing it for the juxtaposition step and consequent analysis which is major step number two in comparative research.

A cursory review of recent articles in *JOHPER* and the *Research Quarterly* and the list of titles of masters and doctoral theses and dissertations in the Microcard Catalogues do not seem to contain any studies which can be classified as rigorous comparative physical education research.[48]

Nixon also makes the point that there are very few fully qualified comparative researchers in the United States.

Morrison, in his investigation, looks at the recent research in comparative physical education and is "forced" to mention articles, theses, books etc. that do not really come under the aegis of comparative physical education.[49] For example, he includes: Marina Yu's *The History of Physical Education in China and the Factors Which Have Influenced its Growth and Developmen*[50]; Barbara Osborne's *An Historical Study of Physical Education in Germany and Its Influence in the United States*[51]; and Calvert, Morgan and Sayer's book *Physical Education and Sport in the Soviet Union*.[52] While these studies may be excellent pieces of work, they can hardly be classified as *comparative* studies.

However, as well as the studies those mentioned above, Morrison is able to include some studies that might legitimately be called comparative works. Included among these are:

Publications by the Council for Cultural Cooperation of the Council of Europe: "Youth and Development Aid"; "Physical Education and Sport"; and "Training the Trainer".[53]

The publications had limited value when new and–now that they are six to seven years old–they must be considered as being of less worth. "Training the Trainer", in particular, received very lukewarm reviews when it was first published.

.

The Place of Sport in Education-A Comparative Study, a UNESCO publication provided a good starting point, but could not be said to have done much more than that. It was a short study covering some thirty countries and, obviously, could offer little in-depth analysis. In fact it was not the intention of the researchers to present such an analysis; the intention was simply to provoke discussion and give rise to further studies.[54]

The ICHPER Questionnaire Reports [55], [56], [57], by the time that the 1967-8 revisions were carried out, covered 80 plus countries. They provide a good, concise, factual summary (with the exception of the *Status of Teachers of Physical Education*) that is based on individual judgment. However, it is obvious that, in dealing with over eighty countries in about 120 pages, they cannot provide any great depth. There are other limitations. The questionnaires were sent to key people in the countries surveyed and, therefore, the answers suffer from the problems of questionnaires in general. These problems were not helped by the presence of an investigator. It seems possible that the questionnaires were sent to only one person in each country and, if this is so, the results may well not be as complete as they might be. Nevertheless, for all their faults, these reports arc very good source materials even though they should be used with caution. For instance, apparent similarities between systems may be misleading, in that the emphasis given to them may not be the same. They should always be used in conjunction with other sources in order to balance their limitations.

The World Today in Health, Physical Education, and Recreation[58] is the only text book on the subject of comparative physical education known to this writer, other than the two monographs edited by William Johnson.[59] Vendien and Nixon attempt (in 432 pages) to:

> describe selected aspects of health, physical education, and recreation in countries representative of various parts of the world. With reference to twenty-six countries, particular emphasis is accorded historical, philosophical, and cultural backgrounds and influences; programs and practices; basic knowledge, concepts and content; professional aspects; and problems and trends.[60]

The first and obvious point is that with such a wide scope the depth is limited. This is not so much a criticism as a statement of fact. Any work that attempts to look at twenty-six countries must lack depth. The fact that twenty-one people were involved in writing the book, albeit within the same format, means that there is, necessarily, a shift of focus and bias between each one.

On the other hand, having an acknowledged expert in each country contributing to the total, means that the article on each country is probably of a high caliber and the writer Is close to the problems, to the successes and the failures.

Of course, closeness to a set of circumstances is not always good. Sometimes it prevents one from getting an overall view and it may lead to a greater bias (either for or against) than that possessed by an outsider.

This text also suffers, as was mentioned above, from the fact that some of the articles had to be translated. Others were written in English by writers whose first language was not English. Finally, as Nixon, one of the co-authors himself says, the material in the book has not "resulted from rigorous comparative research."[61] Yet, despite its drawbacks, this is, in effect, "the only game in town", and as such it has one great merit: it exists!

It not only exists, but (1) it is comprehensive; (2) it does give a reasonable picture of what is happening in the world; it is more-or-less up to date, and (3) it does attempt to give some general background to the state of physical education, health, and recreation in each country with which it deals.

Comparative Physical Education and Sport by Howell, M.L. *et al.* would have been a useful contribution to the field had it ever been made public, but as it is not generally available and would, presumably, have been considerably revised before publication it is inappropriate to comment further.[62]

Physical Education and Recreation in Europe by Howell and Van Vliet is a useful publication, but is conciseness and is now five or more years out of date. It does draw some interesting comparisons between the European countries and Canada, however. The reader may consider it worthwhile looking at the recommendations made by these authors and to ascertain how much or how little, has been carried out on the lines that they suggested.[63]

Values Held for Physical Activity by Selected Urban Secondary School Students in Canada, Australia, England and the United States [hereinafter referred to as "Values"] by G. S. Kenyon is a comparative study of a different sort.[64] This study demands the serious attention of physical educators and comparativists, since it is a novel effort in that it attempts, albeit not in depth, to see what effects the physical education programmes of different countries are having on the youngsters. The questionnaire technique is used, with all the problems that that implies. Yet, it is an interesting study and the instrument does distinguish between extremes of attitude (i.e., strongly pro-physical activity, and strongly anti-physical activity.[65] "Values" is a comparative work in the true sense of the word and it opens up a vast new field of enquiry, although it cannot be considered much more than a trial effort. The rest of the work in the field consists, as has been said, of articles of a descriptive nature, which are quite useful, but of limited value; of aspects of books written in comparative education and of governmental publications which are mainly propaganda. All in all there is a wide open area for research here, but the problems are many.

Other Problems. To this point, the difficulties inherent in the field not having a set methodology in (1) translation; in sources of materials; (2) in the rapidity with which data become dated and in (3) the costs of conducting suitably rigorous examinations have been discussed, and illustrated (the latter to a degree only). However, the problems for the ordinary student who wishes to write a term paper are somewhat different.

Probably the first problem that one runs up against is the dearth of information. Often the information available is patchy, in that one may be able to find quite considerable data on some aspects and little or none on others. While this makes it difficult to get anything like a clear picture of one country, it makes it almost impossible to make comparisons, as the "patches" of data on the one country are unlikely to coincide with those on another (or others). Often the sources of information are suspect. Just how much faith can we place in a publication put out by a government, or a government agency, for consumption abroad?

Next, the lack of data often makes it impossible to check the figures one is able to find, so that bias is often difficult to detect. Bias is one of the most persistent and troublesome of the problems faced by the student. Articles written by an authority from the country studied may be heavily biased either in favour or against the subject being considered; visitors to the country may be equally heavily biased. Some want to show that their own system is superior, and others out to prove that everyone else is doing more and better than is being done in their native land.

Even when the data are as reported objectively as possible, there is the ever-present danger of different meanings being assigned to the same terminology. We have ample evidence of this happening within Canada, and even more so within the English-speaking countries (e.g., what is a "grammar" school, or a "Public" school?) How much worse is it, then, when trying to compare usage within two different languages and two different countries to say nothing of the many languages and countries as there are in the ICHPER reports.

The lack of an agreed-upon methodology means that the student is reviewing information that is in no way prepared for comparative *analysis*. In addition, the investigator is given little or no guidance as to the best methods of analyzing the data that he does have. This state of affairs can only improve; the recent surge in interest, the incorporation of courses in comparative education at the post-graduate level, and the general realization that we have a viable, valuable, and valid field of study are all combining to help the situation. It must be noted, however, that there is still a large number of physical educators who display a complete lack of interest in comparative studies. Of course, this does nothing to assist the growth of the field.

The neophyte is faced, also, with the problem of the selection of variables in order to facilitate comparative studies. The investigator will find little aid to help solve this problem in the literature, although a search among texts on comparative studies in other disciplines may help.

In discussions of comparative research, stress is always laid–as it has been in this paper–on examining physical education within a total social context. However, it is obvious that this is impractical at least to the degree that is preferable, and is particularly difficult for the term-paper writer. Grant that the writer of a short article should concentrate on the particular problem at hand, and grant further that the researcher's main concern should be to isolate those factors that bear immediately on the problem chosen for study. The particular problem will not only determine what factors are relevant, but also how relevant they are.

This does not mean that the ideal of looking at the problem within the full context of the society should be lost, but simply that it has to be tempered by the realities of the situation. Further, the student will have to delve into works of the social science to obtain the background material needed to approach the problem at hand. Working in another discipline, or disciplines, is always difficult and tedious, no matter how rewarding.

With relatively cheap and easy travel available, it is often possible for people interested in comparative education to visit the countries and inspect the various systems for themselves. Obviously, this can be a great benefit; yet there are grave dangers here too. The "guided tour" is unlikely to offer an accurate picture, and the length of time that the visitor is likely to have is limited. The sources of information still come from those who have a "vested interest" in giving the visitor a roseate view, and the problem of translation is still present.

When comparisons are made, it is easy to fall into the error of contrasting the theory of one country with the practice of another. Visiting the countries in question does not make this much less likely. While these defects are real, they should not deter the prospective visitor from touring as widely and as often as possible. However, should make him or her conscious of the dangers of oversimplifying and assuming that he "knows it all" just because he has spent a few weeks "on location."

Howell and Van Vliet [66] were wise in writing up their report for the Fitness and Amateur Sport Directorate. As well as the benefits of having a fairly extensive tour, in which they were able to see for themselves and talk with people who knew the systems well, they used sources of information available in Canada in order to corroborate and check the first-hand information that they had obtained.

Mention was made above of the fact that the investigator not only has to decide what are the relevant factors, but how relevant they are as well. In other words, the researcher must decide how much weight to place on those factors that are determined to be relevant. The problem is further confounded by the fact that not only may the same factors not be relevant in any two systems; yet, even those that are the same may have different weightings within each of the societies being studied. For instance, hypothetically one could have two countries in which there was a fairly even Protestant/Roman Catholic split. In one, this split may have had a great effect on sport and games, and in the other little or no effect. The student not only has to decide–among the many influences that are apparent–whether this religious split is of importance, but further how important it is in each of the two societies. It may well be that some form of factor analysis may have to be used to help determine "what and how much."

Conclusion

The problems discussed in the field of study known as comparative physical education are manifold. This paper has touched on a number of them as best possible in the space allotted for this undertaking. In this writer's opinion, one of the most pressing problems at present is that of research methodology and accompanying techniques. When one considers that questionnaires, opinion polls, personal observation, interviewing, content analysis, inventories, psychometric scoring and scaling methods, and sociometric and matrix techniques are all available and worthwhile methods for use in the study of comparative physical education (to name only those that come easily to mind!). it can be seen that some sound, recognized methods and techniques must be adopted soon. Otherwise, data will be collected that is useless for comparative purposes.

Comparative international and developmental studies are in an embryonic stage of growth at present, but there is a widening interest in these areas and increasing numbers of graduate students are being trained in them. There is a deficiency in theoretical, conceptual, and methodological preparation, but the chances seem good that this problem will be addressed and remedied.

In conclusion, one might remember these words of Oliver J. Caldwell:

> To understand any system of education one must understand the people who created it: their land, history, and culture. Since such understanding is hard to achieve, complete, truthful and perceptive descriptions of education in other lands are hard to find.[67]

References

[1]Kazamias, A.M. and B.G. Massialas, *Tradition and Change in Education*. Englewood Cliffs, N.J.: Prentice-Hall, 1965.

[2]Ainsworth, D.S. Foreword in *The World Today in Health, Physical Education and Recreation* (C. L. Vendien and J. E. Nixon, Eds.). Englewood Cliffs, NJ: Prentice Hall, 1968.

[3]King, Edmund J. The Purpose of Comparative Education. *Comparative Education*, Vol. 1, No. 3 (June, 1965), p. 147.

[4]*Ibid.*

[5]*Ibid*, p. 148.

[6]Howell, M. L., Van Vliet, M. L., and Vinge, D. L. Comparative Physical Education and Sport. Unpublished document, University of Alberta, 1966.

[7]Butts, R. F. Civilization as Historical Process: Meeting Ground for Comparative and International Education." In *Studies in International Education*. (Reprinted from *Comparative Education* Vol. 3, No: 3, 1967, Institute of International Studies, Teachers College, Columbia University. p. 155.)

[8]Kazamias and Massialas. *op. cit.*, p.5.

[9]*Ibid*, p.6.

[10]*Ibid*, p. 10.

[11]Nixon, J.E. "Comparative, International and Development Studies in Physical Education". *Gymnasion*, Vol. VII, No. 1 (Spring 1970).

[12]Vendien, C. L. and J .E. Nixon. *The World Today in Health. Physical Education and Recreation*. Englewood Cliffs, NJ: Prentice-Hall, 1968. p.6.

[13]Bereday, G .Z. F. *Comparative Method in Education*. NY: Holt, Rinehart and Winston, Inc., 1964. p.6.

[14]Nixon, J. E. Op. Cit.

[15]King, Edmund J. *World Perspectives in Education*. Indianapolis, IN: Bobbs Merrill, 1962.

[16]Vendien, C. L. and J. E. Nixon. *op. cit.*, p.5.

[17]*Ibid*, p.6.

[18]Howell, M. L., Van Vliet, M. L. and Vinge, D. L., *op. cit.*, p.2.

[19]*Loc. Cit.*

[20]Hall, Edward T. *The Silent Language*. Garden City, NY:

Doubleday, 1959.

[21]Kandel, I. L. *Comparative Education*. Boston, MA: Houghton Mifflin, 1933, pp. xix-xx.

[22]Moehlman, A.H. *Comparative Educational Systems*. NY: Center for Applied Research in Education, 1964, p.3.

[23]*loc. cit.*

[24]Howell, M. L. et al. *op. cit.*

[25]Vendien, C. L. & Nixon, J. E., [op.cit.], [1]p. 6.

[26]Cramer, J. F. & Browne, G. S. *Contemporary Education*. NY: Harcourt, Brace and World, 1965.

[27]Hans, N. *Comparative Education*. London: Routledge and Kegan Paul, 1951.

[28]Holmes, B. & Robinsohn, S. B.. *Relevant Data in Comparative Education*. Hamburg, Germany: UNESCO Institute for Education, 1963, p. 12.

[29]Adams, D. K. *Introduction to Education: A Comparative Analysis*. Belmont, CA: Wadsworth, 1966.

[30]Kluckhohn, C. and Kelly, W. H. The Concept of Culture. In *The Science of Man in the World Crisis*. (R. Linton, ed.). NY: Columbia University Press, 1945, pp 78-107.

[31]Bennett, B. L. A Historian Looks at Comparative Physical Education. *Gymnasion*, Vol. VII:1 (Spring, 1970), p.11.

[32]Hildebrand, J. R. The Geography of Games. *National Geographic Magazine,* Vol. XXXVI. No: 2 (Aug. 1919).

[33]Grant, N. *Society, Schools, and Progress in Eastern Europe*. Oxford: Pergamon Press, 1969.

[34]Vendien & Nixon, *op. cit.*

[35]Holmes, B. *Problems in Education: A Comparative Approach*. London: Routledge and Kegan Paul, 1965, pp. 20-21.

[36]*ICHPER Questionnaire Reports (Parts I, II, and III, 1967-8). Physical Education and Games in the Curriculum; Teacher Training for Physical Education; and Status of Teachers of Physical Education.* Washington, DC: AAHPERD.

[37]Howell, M. L. *et al., op. cit.*

[38]Grant, N., *op. cit.*

[39]Vendien C. L. and Nixon, J. E., *op. cit.*

[40]Kenyon, G.S. *Values Held for Physical Activity by Selected Urban Secondary School Students in Canada, Australia, England and the United States*. Washington, DC: U.S. Office of Education. 1968.

[41]Nixon, J. E., *op. cit.*

[42]*Ibid.*

[43]Morrison, D. H. *A Rationale for the Development of Comparative Physical Education*. M.A. thesis, University of Alberta. 1967.

[44]Bennett, B. L. A Historian Looks at Comparative Physical Education. *Gymnasion*, Vol. VII, No. 1 (Spring), 1970.

[45]Vendien, C. L. and Nixon, J. E., *op. cit.*

[46]Bereday, G. Z. F. *Comparative Method in Education*. NY:

_____

1

Holt, Rinehart and Winston, 1964.

[47] Nixon, J. E., *op. cit.*, p. 5 et ff.

[48] *Ibid.*

[49] Morrison, D. H., *op. cit.*

[50] Yu, M. *The History of Physical Education in China and the Factors which have Influenced its Growth and Development.* M.A. thesis, Texas Women's University, Denton, 1969. (

[51] Osborne, B. J. *An Historical Study of Physical Education in Germany and Its Influence in the United States.* M.A. thesis, Women's College of the University of North Carolina, Greensboro, 1961.

[52] Calvert, J. S., Morgan, R. E. and C. Sayer, *Physical Education and Sport in The Soviet Union.* University of Leeds Institute of Education, Leeds, England, 1961.

[53] Council for Cultural Cooperation of the Council of Europe, *Series III–Out-of-School Education: (1) Youth and Development Aid; (2) Physical Education and Sport; (3) Training the Trainer.* Strasbourg, France, 1963-4.

[54] UNESCO. *The Place of Sport in Education—A Comparative Study.* Paris: UNESCO Publications, 1956.

[55] ICHPER. *Physical Education and Games in the Curriculum.* Washington, DC, 1969.

[56] ICHPER. *Teacher Training for Physical Education.* Washington, DC, 1969.

[57] ICHPER. *Status of Teachers of Physical Education.* Washington, DC, 1969.

[58] Vendien, C. L. and J. E. Nixon, *op. cit.*

[59] Johnson, W. *Physical Education Around the World.* Monograph 1 (1966) and Monograph 2 (1968). Indianapolis: Phi Epsilon Kappa Fraternity.

[60] Vendien, C. L. and J. E. Nixon, *op. cit.*, p. v.

[61] Nixon, J. E., *op. cit.*, pp 7-8

[62] Howell, M. L., Van Vliet, M. L. and Vinge, D. L. *Comparative Physical Education and Sport.* Unpublished document. University of Alberta, Canada, 1966.

[63] Howell, M. L. and M. L. Van Vliet. *op. cit.*

[64] Kenyon, G. S. *Values Held for Physical Activity by Selected Urban Secondary School Students in Canada, Australia, England and the United States.* Washington, DC: U.S. Office of Education, 1968.

[65] Mutimer, B. T. P. *Attitudes Towards Physical Activity of Grade 12 Boys in Two London Secondary Schools.* M.A. thesis, The University of Western Ontario, 1969.

[66] Howell, M. L. and Van Vliet, M. L., *op. cit.*

[67] Caldwell, O. J. Foreword, *in Comparative Educational Systems* by A. H. Moehlman, *op. cit.*

Selection #4
International Physical Education and Sport

William Johnson
USA

Note: This was written by Dr. Johnson in 1971

Introduction

An aura of mystery, and some confusion, clouds the minds of many in our profession when the topic "Comparative Physical Education" Is brought up for discussion. Such a state can be quickly dispelled when it is pointed out that elements of comparative physical education exist as physical educators visit foreign lands and make comparisons between aspects of physical education and sport observed abroad and conditions prevalent at home. The description and analysis of similarities and differences of international physical education and sports form the bases for comparative physical education.

Probably the most important purpose of international education and physical education is the hope that it holds for world understanding and good will in an era of crisis. While international education represents the key to a peaceful and prosperous future for all of mankind, international physical education, including competitive games and sports, can and does foster a better relationship between peoples and nations. It was recently proposed that the nations of the world would be wise indeed if the custom of the early Greeks in their Panhellenic celebration at Olympia were adopted - before the festival, heralds journeyed throughout Greece announcing a sacred truce among all the people that visitors and contestants might go to and from Olympia unmolested. Would that, in 1972, the year of the Olympiad, all men might lay down their arms and as visitors and contestants proceed on to Munich.

A composite definition of comparative education which applies equally well to comparative physical education and sport is given by George F. Kneller, "Comparative Education," Encyclopedia of Educational Research, 1960. He views comparative education as an attempt to;

.., study education in different countries in the light of the historical development of pertinent educational theories and practices and in consideration of the social, cultural, and economic growth of those countries, so that by increasing one's understanding of such conditions and developments the general improvement of education may be stimulated everywhere. (Kneller, 1960, p. 316).

Historical Background

While international interest in physical education, encouraged by advances in transportation, has multiplied tremendously during the last decade, actually comparative physical education and sport studies are relatively old. A recent article by Don Anthony of England, in Gymnasion (ICHPER'S Official Magazine) entitled "Physical Education as an Aspect of Comparative Education" points out features of the historical development of this field of study:

> The term *vergleichung* (comparison) was used in attempts to demonstrate that the Greek and Roman systems of education were best. Their notion of comparative education was an analysis of the past and present in order to determine best.
>
> A few of the more prominent educational works included Rousseau's *Emile* in 1762 and its subsequent implementation of education and physical education ideals by J. B. Basedow and C. G. Saizman.
>
> Leopold von Berchtold. a wealthy German philanthropist, in 1789, formulated a four-hundred page questionnaire which had some pertinent queries on physical education that is currently valid.
>
> Professor Cesar Basset, in 1808, stressed the comparative approach. He discussed "The utility of making, in foreign countries, observations of their modes of Instruction." His methods included to observe, compare and then to present the facts.
>
> Marc–Antoine Julien (1775–1848) in 1817, wrote "Esquisse" which is now thought to be a landmark in the history of comparative studies. With regard to physical education Julien's Plan employed a number of pertinent questions under the heading "Physical Education and Gymnastics." (Anthony, 1966, pp. 2-3).

Probably the best known example of an event that provided a wealth of opportunities for comparative physical education and sport, in ancient times as well as today, is the Olympic Games. The early games were conducted every fourth year for 1170 years, from 776 B. C. until they were abolished by the Roman Emperor Theodosius in 394 A. D. Baron Pierre de Coubertin revived the old Olympic Games in 1896, at Athens, giving comparative physical education and sport another opportunity to continue its development.

Current Trends

In recent years, when the need for increased understanding among countries is so obvious, a number of important efforts to keep interest in international physical education alive have been carried on:

> The importance of the revived Olympic Games has already been stressed.
>
> Phi Epsilon Kappa's *The Physical Educator* has promoted a featured column regularly entitled "Elsewhere in the World."
>
> The American Association for Health, Physical Education and Recreation's *JOHPER.* included periodic articles in an "International Scene" column.
>
> The International Relations Council of the AAHPER and its affiliated organizations have conducted a number of worthwhile projects .such as:
>
> Books Project (professional books sent to overseas institutions of teacher education in physical education).
> Newsletter (for domestic and foreign consumption).
> Care Kits (games and equipment for overseas organizations).
> People-to-People (good will projects).
> Pen Pals (correspondence with new friends overseas).
> Teacher Exchanges; and many more similar activities.

At each National Convention of the American Association for Health, Physical Education and Recreation and at many of the State and District Conventions, meetings, speeches, films, slides, socials and meetings other program items are organized for educators and students from foreign lands and for the many ICHPER members now becoming interested in widening their horizons of understanding in this important area of physical education.

The International Council on Health, Physical Education and Recreation, commonly known as ICHPER, an affiliate of the World Confederation of Organizations of the Teaching Profession, has actively promoted comparative physical education as confirmed by the locations of a decade of yearly Congresses (Amsterdam, New Delhi, Stockholm, Rio de Janeiro, Paris, Addis Ababa, Seoul, Vancouver, Dublin, Ivory Coast and Sydney). ICHPER also promoted comparative physical education by conducting Questionnaire Reports in some 50 countries on the following:

> *Part 1 - Physical Education and Games in the Curriculum*, 1968.
>
> *Part 2 - Teacher Training for Physical Education*, 1968.
>
> *Part 3 - Status of Teachers of Physical Education*, 1968.

In addition to the above, ICHPER publishes a Newsletter and a journal entitled *Gymnasion* which contains many comparative physical education articles. (ICHPER, 1963, pp. 64-104) and (ICHPER, pp. 4-1;i). Phi Epsilon Kappa's monograph series - *Physical Education Around the World* - had its inception from the yearly theme of Rho Chapter, University of Illinois, then under the leadership of Dr. Earle Zeigler, Many international students were on campus, and they contributed greatly to the success of the yearly program.

Through the further encouragement of Dr. Zeigler, Dr. C. 0. Jackson (Editor of The Physical Education), and Dr. R. R. Schreiber (Executive-Secretary of Phi Epsilon Kappa), the monograph series was launched under the editorship of Dr. William Johnson. Four years later monographs number one, two, three and four have been published and distributed widely in this country and overseas.

During the last decade there has been a strong surge of interest in international physical education, sport study, and research. In the colleges and universities of the United States alone, at least fifty institutions are offering one or more courses in International or Comparative Physical Education and Sport. The Phi Epsilon Kappa monograph series attempts, in a small way, to provide background materials for such courses.

A total of thirty-two countries have now been included in the four issues with thirty-five co-authors uniting in this joint professional effort. The co-authors were offered considerable latitude in the development of their articles within the following suggested topical outline: 1. General background; 2. Historical background; 3. Kindergarten-elementary; 4. Secondary; 5. College-university; 6. Teacher education; and 7. Special characteristics, such as sports clubs, facilities, Olympic Games emphasis, etc.

- Monograph No. 1 covered Britain, Canada, Finland, Germany, Israel, Japan, New Zealand, Pakistan, Russia and South Africa

- Monograph No. 2 included Australia, Ghana, Hungary, Iran, Mexico, Netherlands, Norway and Thailand-

- Monograph No. 3 covered Austria, Brazil, Colombia, England, Canada, Ethiopia, Hong Kong-Singapore and Iraq

- Monograph No. 4 included The Republic of China, Ecuador, Korea, Lebanon, Somali, Spain and two articles on the United States.

A fifth monograph is being written by a number of co-authors and will be available early in 1971.

Many other organizations and foundations in the United States and in other countries of the world promote various types of comparative physical education, but in a short paper such as this it is impossible to include a comprehensive list.

Comparative Content

The scope of comparative education and physical education-sport is broad and varied. Comparative Education has become quite well-established in nearly all of the major institutions of higher education in the United States. In physical education and sports a number of leading colleges and universities are now introducing new courses or are including extensive units in established courses of instruction.

Specific examples of existing courses might best illustrate the similarities and variations found in this emerging area. One example of content in Comparative Education and six of Comparative Physical Education are presented herewith:

> Example 1. From Education has been selected the content as outlined by Dr. Walter Kaulfers, Professor of Education, University of Illinois in his Comparative Education Course for Advanced Graduate Students
>
> - Education 303:
>
> Comparative Education: the study of contemporary school systems, from one culture to another, in terms of; 1) structure, 2) philosophical foundations; 3) historical, economic and geographical background; •!) their needs and problems; and 5) how to solve the problems.
>
> Comparative Education is an interdisciplinary subject. The student needs some knowledge of: a) History and Philosophy; b) Psychology; c) Sociology; d) Religion; and e) Helpful to know the language. (Kaulfers, 1965, p. I).
>
> Example 2. The course content as outlined by Professor C. W. Morgan, Dean, School of Health and Physical Education, Ithaca College, New York in his Comparative Physical Education course:
>
> Part I. General Comparison of Physical Education in Europe and the United States.

Unit I	General Philosophy and Objectives
Unit II	Organization and Administration
Unit IH	Curricula and Activities (at all levels)
Unit IV	Teaching Methods and Techniques
Unit V	Testing and Evaluation
Unit VI	Research in Physical Education
Unit VII	Facilities and Equipment

Unit VIII	Health Education
Unit IX	Recreation
Unit X	Teacher Preparation (Morgan, 1964, p. 1)

Example 3. The course content outlined by Professor Ben W. Miller, University of California at Los Angeles (UCLA) for his course, P. E, 280G, Comparative Physical Education and Sports:

- The comparative study of physical education and sports will include an analysis of:

- The similarities and differences in the general way of life shared or avoided by members of different world regions and societies (nations)

- The major institutions by which men live.

- The guiding beliefs and conceptions concerning the origin, capabilities and destiny of man.

- The result and nature of their physical education and sports program.

- At least six or seven of the following world regions will be selected for intensive comparative study:

> Western Europe
> Russia and Eastern Europe
> East Asia
> Southeast Asia
> The Middle East
> North Africa
> Sub-Saharan Africa
> Latin America
> The Commonwealth
> North America

The systematic comparative study will include some of all of the following elements of physical education and sports depending on their relevance to the world regions studied:

> Aims, objectives and philosophy.
> Organizational, agency or institutional auspices.
> Major legislative, administrative and supervisory controls.
> Programs for different age-interest groups and their scientific foundations.
> Leadership status and leadership preparation,
> Professional organization.
> Instructional methodology.
> Relationship with health education and recreation.

Measurement and evaluation, facilities and research.
Current status and future trends of programs (Miller, 1968, p. 1).

Example 4. The course content of Professor Robert D, Hoffs Comparative Physical Education studies at Eastern Michigan University, Ypsilanti:

To study comparatively in-depth recreation, physical education, methods of teaching, athletic training techniques, and facilities and equipment in the Scandinavian countries.

To study in depth the Olympic Game participation of the Scandinavian Countries in the light of the spirit and history of the Olympic Games,

To provide the opportunity for serious in-depth study of Swedish and Danish gymnastics, a discipline uniquely available abroad.

To provide the opportunity for "cultural shock" by immersing the participating students to the greatest extent possible in the foreign culture.

To involve European colleagues of the Director in the lectures and practical work. (Hoff, 1967, p. 1).

Example 5. The content of Professor William Johnson's course in International Physical Education and Sport, P. E. 303, at the University of Illinois includes:

P. E. 303 is a comparative study of aspects of physical education and sport in a number of selected countries. Typically, the nations included will be Denmark, France, Germany, Great Britain, Sweden and the U. S. S.R. Others will be chosen according to student interest.

The objectives, program, methods, personnel, facilities and evaluations of kindergarten, elementary, secondary, college/university and teacher preparation programs in physical education are also studied.

Additional concepts for investigation in international physical education are found in Zeigler's "Persistent Problems of Physical Education and Sport" listed below:

Values (aims) in Physical, Health and Recreation Education.
The Influence of Politics, Nationalism, Economics and Religion.
Methods of Instruction.

Professional Preparation.
The Bole of Administration.
The Healthy Body.
Physical Education for Women.
Dance in Physical Education.
The Use of Leisure.
Amateur, Semi-professional and Professional Sport.
Progress in Physical, Health and Recreation Education
(Zeigler, 1968).

Example 6. Suggested areas to cover in comparative research projects according to Dr. Lynn Vendien, University of Massachusetts:

Facts about the country
General Education
Physical Education
Composition
Professional Preparation
Status of Physical Education Teachers
Professional Association, Publications, Conferences
Problems in Physical Education today
Trends in Physical Education today
Research in Physical Education today
 Evaluation of Programs
References

 Example 7. A study outline developed by Dr. John Lucas, Penn State University, suggests another approach of value for the area of comparative study and research:

Culture and Geography
Education - Past and Present
Sporting Heritage
Modern Physical Education
Country studied compared to America

From the above examples one might conclude that many similarities in comparative content exist at the present time in this emerging area of study. Differences found in content should give variety to this broad field.

Comparative Methodology

Methodology in Comparative Education. Comparative education has achieved a certain amount of recognition over a considerably longer period of time than has comparative physical education and sport. As one part of education, physical education gains much by a consideration of comparative education methods used successfully over the years. The mode of inquiry most frequently utilized in comparative education is a descriptive technique called cultural analysis, i.e., in what sense is the formal system of education an expression of the culture from which it arises?

Don Anthony's article ID the ICHPER magazine, *Gymnasion* , quotes from Sir Michael Sadler (an Englishman, and probably the modern founder of the study of comparative education) concerning method in this area:

> In studying foreign systems we should not forget that the things outside the schools matter even more than the things inside the schools, and govern and interpret the things inside. But is it not likely that if we have endeavored, m a sympathetic spirit to understand the real working of a foreign system of education, we shall in turn find ourselves better able to enter into the spirit and tradition of our own national education, more sensitive to its unwritten ideals, quicker to catch the signs which mark its growing or fading influence, readier to mark the dangers which threaten it and the subtle workings of hurtful change? The practical value of studying in a right spirit and with scholarly accuracy the working of foreign systems of education is that it will result in our being better fitted to understand our own. (Anthony, 1966, p. 5).

George F. Kneller discusses methodology at some length in his section on Comparative Education in the 1960 *Encyclopedia of Educational Research*:

> The extent to which comparison may be used as a reliable method of understanding and solving of education problems is somewhat uncertain. Historically, the assumption has been that comparative education could use the same methods as comparative anatomy, comparative religion, or comparative government. The problem centers on the nature of what is to be compared; on this matter there are at least two schools of thought.
>
> One school advocates a method derived from one particular foreign system, with comparison, if made, limited to one's own product. The other school judges that comparative education is not worthy of the name unless it deals with the comparing of educational systems.
>
> The method of comparing systems involves both the vertical and horizontal approaches. Both must correspond to the goal the individual sets for himself. The horizontal approach is the more challenging but also the more difficult. This method seeks to analyze educational systems in all their elements and aspects, both separately and collectively. The most characteristic vertical approach is the practice of examining educational systems one

by one. Here the comparison with other systems is apt to be incidental or secondary. (Kneller, 1960, pp. 317-21).

A concrete example of educational methodology has been outlined by Professor Walter Kaulfers, University of Illinois, in his Advanced Graduate Course, Education 303, Comparative Education:

Research Methods:

Scientific Survey: most common. Important: Need a common denominator when measuring or comparing school systems (minutes-hours of instruction, age, etc.).

Documentary Method - Use reliable documents such as: laws, decrees, reports of the ministry of education, rules and regulations. May refer to UNESCO reports.

Interview (generally used in place of questionnaire). Consider: objectivity, control, validate questions (triple check for understanding).

Direct Observations - Check lists or rating scales.

Analytical Method - Used internally when cannot check original material or sources. Example: studying textbooks or examining examinations.

Experimental Method:

Many times difficult because of language problem.

AAHPER fitness tests abroad - an example of an experimental study.

Methodology in Comparative Physical Education and Sport

For the most part, pioneer efforts in comparative physical education and sport have been almost entirely descriptive in nature with only incidental discriminatory analysis and comparisons. Recent efforts (e.g., Bereday) in this area have adopted a comparative approach including:

Descriptive stage (Cataloging purely pedagogical data).

Interpretation stage (An analysis of the pedagogical data).

Juxtaposition stage (Establish the framework of the comparison). (Establishing similarities and differences).

Comparison state (Alternating information concerning the countries studied - simultaneous comparison).

A study recently completed by Don Morrison at the University of Alberta, Edmonton, Canada, was directed by a graduate committee composed of an anthropologist, historian, sociologist and a comparative educator. The purpose of the study was to provide a rationale for the development of comparative studies of systems of physical education. A rather elaborate "Conceptual Framework For Analyzing A System of Physical Education" was formulated. It will be discussed at length in another article in this publication.) This framework could well be adapted for many studies of comparative physical education and sport. It provides a plan for identifying the component sub-systems of physical education and for assessing their structures and functions. It also provides for the identification of the factors in the ecological setting and socio cultural situation of the system that may interact with it. Its success depends on its ability to direct the researcher to many of the factors which are relevant for understanding physical education and sport.

Summary

An understanding of the differences between physical education and sport in the United States and most foreign countries in terms of their rationale and implications is so very important. In the United States, the federal government is encouraging programs in education and physical education with international implications; it would then appear that students should have a comparative knowledge of the programs of physical education and sport in other countries. The Peace Corps and AAHPER Specialists' programs are examples of projects in dire need of teachers and coaches who have an understanding of the programs and problems of cooperating nations.

In this age of international struggle for survival, cultural and natural barriers to a world community can be broken down by world understanding through the medium of education. As an integral part of education, physical education is a very effective means of developing harmony among countries of the world. An understanding of physical education and sport in cultures other than his own should represent an important area of study for the advanced undergraduate, the graduate student specializing in physical education, and the historian of physical education and sport. A study of physical education and sports programs of other cultures may yield ideas through which our own cultures may be benefited. An investigation of physical education should not be limited to one nation and/or culture.

Selected References

Beauchamp, George A. and Beauchamp, Kathryn. *Comparative Analysis of Curriculum Systems*. Wilmette, Illinois: The KAGG Press, 1967.

Bereday, George. *Comparative Method in Education*. New York: Holt, Rinehart ;md Winston, Inc., 1964.

Boyle, Robert H. *Sport: Mirror of American Life*. Boston; Little, Brown ;md Company, 1963.

Calvert, J. S., Morgan, R. E. and Sayer, C. *Physical Education and Sport in the Soviet Union*. Leeds: The University of Leeds Institute of Education, 1961.

Cramer, J. F. and Browne, G. S. *Contemporary Education*. New York: Harcourt, Brace & World, Inc., Second Edition, 1965.

Culin, Stewart. *Games of the Orient*. (Korea, China, Japan). Rutland, Vermont: Charles E. Tuttle Company, 1958.

Draper, Mary. *Sport and Race in South Africa*. Johannesburg: South Africa. Institute of Race Relations, 1963.

Finnish Society for Research in Sports and Physical Education. *Sport and Physical Education in Finland*. Porvoo; Wernea Soderstrom Osakeyhtio, 1964.

Hackensmith, C. W. *History of Physical Education*. New York: Harper and Row Publishers, Inc., 1966.

Hunt, Sara Ethridge. *Games and Sports the World Around*. New York: The Ronald Press, 196'!.

Ickes, Marguerite. *The Book of Games and Entertainment the World Over*. New York: Dodd, Mead and Company, 1969.

King, Edmund J. *Other Schools and Ours: A Comparative Study for Today*. New York: Holt, Rinehart and Winston, 3rd Edition, 1967.

Loy, John W. and Kenyon, Gerald. *Sport, Culture and Society: A Reader on the Sociology of Sport*. New York: Macmillan Company, 1969.

Morton, Henry W. *Soviet Sport*. New York: Collier Books, 1963.

Noah, Harold J. and Eckstein, Max A. *Toward A Science of Comparative Education*. New York: Macmillan Company, 1969.

Thompson, E. M, *Other Lands Other Peoples*. Washington, D.C.: NEA, 1967.

Van Dalen, D. B., Mitchell, E. D. and Bennett, B. L. *A World History of Physical Education*. Englewood Cliffs, New Jersey: Prentice-Hall, Inc., 1953.

Vendien, Lynn and Nixon, John. *The World Today in Health, Physical Education and Recreation*. Englewood Cliffs, New Jersey: Prentice-Hall, Inc., 1968.

Miscellaneous Published Materials AAHPER, International Relations Council, 1967, 96pp. (*Proceedings of the National Conference on International Relations through Health, Physical Education and Recreation*, held May 1967 at the NEA Center, Washington, D.C.).

_____. General Division (International Relations Council's Newsletter - Three issues yearly), Washington, D. C.

_____.*JOHPER*, "International Scene." Articles on different foreign countries every 3rd or 4th issues, Washington, D. C.

American Educational Research Association. *Educational Research m Countries Other Than the United States*. The Association, Washington, D. C.. 1962.

Anthony, W. J. "Comparative Physical Education." Physical Education Association of Great Britain and Northern Ireland. Ling House, KPNottingham Place7, London, W. I. 58,175:70-73, November, 1966.

Anthony, W. J.. "Physical Education as an Aspect of Comparative Education." *Gymnasion*. II, 1966.

Australian Physical Education Association, *Report of the World Congress on Physical Education*. Melbourne, 1956.

Bereday, George F. "Reflections on Comparative Methodology in Education, 1964-1966." *Comparative Education*, 3:169-187, June, 1967.

Brinkman, William. "Comparative Education." *Review of Educational Research*. XXXIV, 1:44-61. 1964.

Butts, R. Freeman, "Civilization as Historical Process: Meeting Ground for Comparative and International Education." *Comparative Education*. June, 1967.

Clegg, A. "Visit to Canada: Impressions of a Commonwealth Visiting Fellow." *Canadian Education Research Digest*. 7:1-18, March, 1967.

Corey, R. D. "Conceptual Tools for Research in Comparative Education." *Comparative Education Review*, February, 1966, pp. 418-425.

Coserv, P. J. "At Ease, With Your International Guest." National Council for Community Services to International Visitors. Meridian House, Washington, D. C.

Downey, Lawrence W. "The Task of the Public School in the United States and Canada." *Comparative Education Review*. 4:118-120, October, 1960.

Edding, F. "Use of Economics in Comparing Educational Systems." *International Review of Education*. 1965, pp. 453-465.

Elliott, William Y. *Education and Training in the Developing Countries*. New York: F. A. Praeger Company, 1966.

Fersh, Seymour. "Studying Other Cultures: Looking Outward Is'In.'" *Yearbook - National Council for the Social Studies*. 1968.

Foshay, Arthur W. "The Use of Empirical Methods in Comparative Education." *International Review of Education*. IX, 3:257-267, 1963-1964.

Foster, Philip. "Comparative Methodology and the Study of African Education." *Comparative Education Review*. IV, 2:110-117, October, 1960.

Hans, Nicholas. "Definition and Scope of Comparative Education—A History," *Comparative Education*. London: Routledge and Kegan Paul, Ltd., 1967.

Harsky, J. E. "Development of Physical Education in Schools of Soviet Russia from 1919 to 1931." Master's Thesis, University of Pittsburgh, 1932.

Hellenic Olympic Committee. *International Olympic Academy Report of the Summer Sessions: 1962, 1963. 1964. 1965. 1966. 1967. 1968, 1969. Athens and Olympia, Greece: The Committee*. Hoffman, Verlag Karl. Gymnasion. Schorndorg/Stuttgart. (Official magazine of the International Council on Health, Physical Education and Recreation—issued 4 times yearly.)

Howell, Maxwell. Sources for Comparative Physical Education and Sport. Edmonton;, University of Alberta, Canada. Unpublished monograph listing 110 pages.

Howell, Maxwell L. and Van Vliet, M. L. *Physical Education and Recreation in Europe*. The Fitness and Amateur Sports Directorate. Canada, 1965.

Jacobs, David Hugh. "An Investigative Study of Physical Education Programs on the Primary and Secondary School Levels in England. " M. A. Thesis, Northeast Missouri State Teachers College, 1966.

Kneller, George F. "Comparative Education." *Encyclopedia of Educational Research*. Editor Chester W. Harris. 3rd Edition. New York; The Macmillan Company, 1960.

Kneller, George F. "Education in Modern and Primitive Societies; Excerpt from Educational Anthropology: An Introduction," *School and Society*, March 6, 1946.

Kobayashi, T. "Comparative Perspectives in Teacher Training Illustrated by Japan and England." *The World Yearbook of Education*. 1963.

Kazamias, A. M. "Potential Eletes in Turkey: The Social Origins of Youth." *Comparative Education Review*. 10:470-81.

Laska, J. A. L. "Use of the Education Pyramid in Comparative Education." *International Review of Education*. 1965, pp. 484-488.

Lawson, R. R. "Comparative Education at Work." *Canadian Educational Research Digest. June, 1965, pp. 114-121.*

Lloyd, John F. "British and American Education in Cultural Perspective." *Comparative Education Review*. 6,1:16-24, June, 1962.

Lupul, R. "Education in Western Canada." *Comparative Education Review*. June, 1967, pp. 144-159.

Maheu, Rene. "Sport Is Education." *UNESCO Courier*. XVII, January, 1964. pp. 4-9.

Marchiony, Joseph A. "The Rise of Soviet Athletics." *Comparative Education Review*. 7,1:17-21, June, 19G3.

Marchioni, Joseph A.. "Measures for the Further Development of Physical Culture and Sports: in the C. P. S. U. Central Committee and the USSR Council of Ministers.*" Soviet Education* 9:17-20, November, 1966.

Miyahata, T. "General Organization of Physical Education and Sports in Japan With Annotations Regarding Other Countries in Asia." Federation International d'Education Physique Bulletin. Sydevenska Gymnastik-mstitutet, Sandgat 14. Lund, Sweden, 3-4:14-23, 1962.

Moolenijzer, N. J. "Building Lasting International Relationships." *CAHPER Journal*, May, 1966, p. 64.

Nikiforov, I. I. " Physical Culture and Sports in the USSR." *New World Review*. XXVI, July, 1958, pp. 20-27.

Phi Delta Kappa. "International Education.*" Phi Delta Kappan*. January, 1970.

Phi Epsilon Kappa. "Elsewhere in the World. " *The Physical Educator*, Indianapolis, Indiana: Phi Epsilon Kappa.

Phvsical Education Yearbook. The Physical Education Association of Great Britain and Ireland. London: Ling House, 10 Nottingham Place, 1965-

Seurin, Picrre. "Comparative Study of the Organization of Physical Education and Sports in Western Countries." *Federation International d'Education Physique Bulletin.* Sydsvenska Gymnast ik-Institutet, Sandgat 14, Lund, Sweden, 1962.

Sloan, A. W. "Physical Fitness of College Students in South Africa, United States and England." *Research Quarterly*, XXIV, No, 2, May, 1947, pp. 104-108.

Sturzebecker, Russell. "Comparative Physical Education.' *Gymnasion.* IV, Nos. 3-1, Autumn-Winter, 1967, pp. 48-49.

Taylor, Fred. "Canadian Fitness and Amateur Sport Program." *Journal of CAHPER.* XXXIV, No. 3, February-March, 1968, pp. 13-14.

Washburn, J. N. "Sport as a Soviet Tool. " *Foreign Affairs.* 34:490-499, April, 1965.

Wight, R, M. "Aspects of Italian Physical Education." *Physteal Education.* Published by the Physical Education Association of Great Britain and Northern Ireland, Ling House, 10 Nottingham Place, London, July, 1966.

Zhalezniak, lu. "Physical Education; in the Subject Commission for Physical Education." *Soviet Education.* 8:40-45, June, 1906.

Comparative Physical Education and Sport

Ken Hardman
England

1. General Information

1.1. Historical Development

Comparative studies in Society and Education have their origins in intrepid explorers' and travelers' accounts of customs and practices, usually stemming from journeys based on simple curiosity in the strange and exotic and later, commercial enterprise; they preceded the nineteenth century quest for knowledge and emulation of foreign schools' practices through purposeful observation. Comparative physical education and sport is a relatively young area of study in a formal sense, although the quest for knowledge about practices and systems has been in evidence since the Prussian Count Leopold Berchtold included physical education and sport in a 400-page questionnaire for travellers in 1789. Some 20 years later, Frenchman, Auguste Basset wrote on *The Utility of Making Observations in Foreign Countries Concerning Their Different Modes of Education and Instruction*. The pioneering work of Berchtold and Basset was developed by another Frenchman, Marc Antoine Jullien, when in 1817, he published a series of questions on public education, including physical education in European countries. Jullien's work like that of others in the early nineteenth century was characterised by the pragmatism of cultural borrowing.

The pragmatism associated with detailed observation for potential 'cultural borrowing', however, was concerned more with the 'What' and less with the 'Why' and 'How'. From these seeds grew a comparative methodological movement, one which called for a more comprehensive analytical and explanatory approach. This was an approach, largely developed by Sir Michael Sadler, that was grounded in the establishment of general principles. When set in a comparative framework, it led to an analysis of similarities and differences. Historical inquiry and explanation were at the core of such comparative study, one outcome of which was that 'national character' is a major determinant in shaping a system of education.

Comparative study was progressed beyond the historical explanatory approach to a semi-scientific orientation by Moehlmann (1963), who suggested a theoretical model to ensure systematic analysis of contemporary trends and long-range cultural factors. Moehlmann argued that long-range interactive factors including population demographics, spatial (geographical) and temporal (historical) concepts, language (communication systems), art, philosophy (value choices), religion, social structure, governmental systems, economics, science and technology, health and educational process determined the profile of an education system. Systematic exploration and analysis of national practices in education were progressed through the structured approach devised by Bereday (1964) comprising four stages: **description; interpretation (or explanation); juxtaposition; and comparison.** Thus, by the mid-1960's, comparative studies in education had progressed from individual intuitive and descriptive 'raw data' and historical techniques to more sophisticated systematic methods of analysis, drawing largely from social science methods of investigation and involving interdisciplinary 'team' approaches.

In 1970, eminent American sports historian, John E. Nixon, reported an increasing interest in international aspects of physical education, testimony to which was the plethora of descriptive articles contributed to professional journals by American physical educators. In the main, these articles represented information derived from observational educational or 'touristic' visits to be shared with colleagues. They did not qualify, in Nixon's (1970) view, as comparative research reports and reflected the broader situation of comparative studies in physical education and sport trailing behind reported research in the 'parent' area, 'comparative education'. Indeed, texts concerned with comparative and international issues and dimensions were at that time a rarity. Morton (1953) and Louis and Louis (1964), had produced descriptions of sport in the Soviet Union and Nixon himself had co-edited (1968) a text with C.L. Vendien containing information on health, physical education and recreation in a number of countries around the world. As Nixon (1970) conceded, these publications were "...At best... examples of the early phases of the descriptive stage of comparative research" (p.8). However, herein lay the seeds of the growth to come, which was rather prophetically indicated by Nixon (1970) in commenting that "physical education (was) in an early stage of growth in research in comparative, international and developmental studies in the United States" (p.8). The general tone of Nixon's commentary was rather American-centric but it might well have been less so had he been aware of work of then active researchers in other countries. For elsewhere in the academic physical education and sport arena, more scholarly activity had been, and was being, carried out and reported. In the United Kingdom, for example, pioneering work had been undertaken by Molyneux (1962), Sullivan (1964) and Anthony (1966, 1969), and the latter completed a doctoral study in the genre in 1971.

After 1970, comparative and international studies in physical education and sport were subject to a relatively significant development of interest and scholarly activity, the latter being especially marked by two seminal texts in the field: Bennett, Howell and Simri (1975) and Riordan (1978). The present existence of a range of publications, an international and several national societies, seminars and conferences with a comparative focus suggest that the field of study has markedly progressed as an area of academic and professional activity. A major initiative in the international development of the comparative physical education and sport domain was the formation of the International Society for Comparative Physical Education and Sport (ISCPES) in 1978/9, which symbolically marked the coming of age of Comparative Physical Education and Sport as an area of study. Subsequent to its formation, various ISCPES publications collectively demonstrate substantial progress in nature, scope and methodological procedures and applications in the comparative genre. Significantly they also reveal enrichment through contributions from a wider academic and scholarly community beyond physical and sport educators to embrace historians, psychologists, social psychologists and sociologists and others with vested interests in socio-cultural and pedagogical domains. The maturity of ISCPES was symbolically represented in a 1995 invitation to conduct a Workshop arranged under the auspices of the Kuwait Olympic Committee, the Public Authority for Youth and Sport and the Kuwait Academy of Sciences. The Workshop aimed to bring together experts in various and different aspects of *Sport for All*. Of special interest to the partner agencies were policies and practices in other countries, which respectively impact on elite sport, women in sport and physical and sporting activity for people with disabilities.

Over the last decade or so in the Anglo-Saxon speaking world, there has been a steep decline in the number of higher education institutions offering courses or modular units under the specific nomenclature of *Comparative Physical Education and Sport*. Hence, whilst it is far from being extinct, evidence of which lies particularly in 'first order' comparisons, the body of knowledge thesis is becoming increasingly tenuous. In the United Kingdom, for example, what used to appear under the title has generally been subsumed within themes or under topics such as *International Dimensions* or features in cross-disciplinary courses variously covering "Issues", "Politics", "Economics", "Policies", "Sociological and/or "Cultural Perspectives" and so on. More usually than not, "Sport" prevails over "Physical Education" in such course units. In North America, a similar trend can be discerned particularly in re-orientation to courses in *International Studies* and *International Development* with a Sport and Physical Education focus. For all of these thematic/topic approaches, interpretation and understanding of content can be more open-ended in outcomes: comparisons can be directly and explicitly made or can be indirect, implicit or in the mind of the learner/reader.

Somewhat counter to this general trend are developments elsewhere in the world. In central and eastern Europe, where 40 years of socialism inhibited exchange of knowledge, and in some Asian and Middle Eastern countries, particularly in those countries not especially subjected to western, particularly American influences, there has been an increase in interest in international and comparative studies in the last decade or so, testimony to which are an Asian Conference on Comparative Physical Education and Sport Symposium organised by the Sport Social Science Branch of the Chinese Sports Science Society in Shanghai with published Proceedings in 1995, more recent biennial International Conferences held in the Islamic Republic of Iran since the late 1990s, journal publications, which carry international and comparative articles (continental regional e.g. *Asian Journal of Physical Education*; national and institutional e.g. *Kinesiology. International Scientific Journal of Kinesiology and Sport* of the Faculty of Physical Education, University of Zagreb, Croatia; *Acta Universitatis Carolinae, "Gymnica"*, of Charles University, Prague, Czech Republic; and *Man-Movement* of the Academy of Physical Education, Wroclaw and Polish Scientific Society of Physical Culture), and translations into Chinese, French, Japanese, Polish and Spanish languages of the Proceedings of the World Summit on Physical Education, Berlin, 1999. This more positive trend of published articles, which have a comparative, international and cross-cultural focus, can also be observed in other well established and respected international, single, multi- and cross-discipline journals, a selected list of which was included in *International Journal of Physical Education*, volume XXXVIII, Issue 3, 3rd Quarter, 2001 (see Hardman, 2001, p. 99).

A positive development in the comparative field has been the academic, professional, but most significantly, political interest generated in publication of data derived from a range of international, national and regional surveys and longitudinal literature reviews. The ICSSPE supported and International Olympic Committee (IOC) sponsored *World-wide Survey on the State and Status of Physical Education in Schools* (Hardman and Marshall, 2000) preliminary findings, disseminated at the Berlin Physical Education Summit, were used as a basis for formulation of Action Agendas and an appeal to United Nations Educational, Scientific and Cultural Organisation (UNESCO) General Conference and Ministers of Physical Education and Sport (MINEPS) III meeting in Uruguay in late November-early December, 1999. It is now a matter of historical record that the 1999 MINEPS III Declaration of Punta del Este endorsed the Berlin Agenda for Action (refer Doll-Tepper and Scoretz, 2001) and called upon member states to implement it. An international and comparative-focused study had helped to place physical education in schools on the world political agenda! A year after the publication of the world-wide survey *Final Report* (Hardman and Marshall, 2000), a Council of Europe Committee for the Development of Sport (CDDS) 'Working Group of Experts' on *Access of Children to Physical Education and Sport* picked up the baton. The Group resolved to assess the situation of school physical education and sport in the Council of Europe's member states with a view to providing recommendations for action at the Informal Meeting of Ministers responsible for Sport in Warsaw, Poland 12-13 September 2002. A follow-up survey on the situation of school physical education has been undertaken. The preliminary findings of this survey were disseminated on the occasion of the 2nd World Summit on Physical Education in Magglingen, Switzerland, 2-3 December 2005. The inclusion of school physical education on intergovernmental and non-governmental agencies' agendas demonstrates the values of engagement in comparative studies:

provision of information; increase in knowledge of one's own and others' 'worlds'; and potential facilitation of amelioration.

With the concept and contexts of globalisation has arisen renewed interest in international dimensions of physical education and sport with varying engagement of inter-governmental agencies, national and regional governments and international, national and regional non-governmental organisations as well as a range of social and educational institutions and individuals involved in either overarching or specific development initiatives. The designated 2004 European Year of Education through Sport and United Nations 2005 Year of Sport and Physical Education are symptomatic of the significance of physical education and sport to international communities. The protagonist push for harmonisation in physical education in Europe is another indicator of international interest and its process has been, and is being, aided and abetted by European Union programmes such as Erasmus and Socrates. The trend to harmonisation was clearly articulated in the 1999 Bologna Agreement to create a common model for Higher Education in Europe with institutions subsequently encouraged to develop a framework of comparable and compatible qualifications for their programmes. Hence, a three year Erasmus funded Thematic Network Project, *Aligning European Higher Education Structure in Sport Science* (AEHESIS), emerged. Drawing on the pilot project *Tuning Educational Structures in Europe* (the so-called *Tuning Project*) methodologies, the AEHESIS Project seeks to set innovative guidelines specifically for the broadly defined sport sector (Health and Fitness, Physical Education, Sport Coaching and Sport Management) for the development of curricula, and quality assurance systems for study programmes. The Project is designed to collate intelligence on the extent of implementation of the Bologna Process through identification of common or congruent elements, as well as any areas of specificity and diversity amongst higher education institutions across Europe. It is anticipated that the results of the Project might influence national policies in the sector and provide guideline models or frameworks and benchmarks for non-participating organisations. The project focuses on four main areas in the broadly defined sport's sector (refer AEHESIS Project Annual Reports for further details).

Notably for comparative genre scholars, this renewed interest in international issues marks a 'back to basics' approach within the area of physical education and sport. Whether this is indicative of 'turning back the clock' or the 'wheel coming round full circle' is debatable. What is clear is that the renewed interest in international issues is conducive to the generation of rich data, which can be compared and utilised for ameliorative development, a fundamental purpose of the comparative study domain. In essence, the situation mirrors the position on research in comparative, international and development studies some 35 years ago (refer Nixon, 1970).

1.2. Function

Comparative physical education and sport as an area of study draws from a number of disciplines and hence, is seen to be multi- and inter-disciplinary in nature and scope. Specifically as an area of scholarly activity, comparative study in physical education and sport seeks through the establishment of reliable data to: (a) provide information on the 'worlds' of others; (b) foster knowledge about one's own 'world' through confrontation with alternatives; and (c) amelioration through learning about and from others. Of crucial importance to these processes is the necessity of discovering and revealing shaping influences, which through cross-analysis, provide causal connections, and hence, explanations. It is in this way that deeper insight into, and understanding of, the processes and products of delivery are acquired.

1.3 Body of knowledge

A persistent problem is to obtain a common understanding of what constitutes comparative studies. Arguably, comparative physical education and sport might be more closely identified with method rather than with a distinct body of knowledge. The critical term is *comparative*. The International Society for Physical Education and Sport (ISCPES) defines comparative study as *investigation into and comparison of two or more units (countries, cultures, ideologies, regions, states, systems, institutions, populations)* mostly occurring in different geographical settings. Examples of phenomena to be compared include: school systems (or elements) of physical education and sport models in a macro or micro context. Usually the phenomena associated with such units are universal, but cross-culturally and cross-nationally, they may differ in focus and substance. Comparativists study how and why they differ. Comparative analyses involve those directing and initiating research, which explore the suitability of new elements from other cultures for inclusion in their programmes. Besides the comparative dimension, the domain encompasses issues related to studies of countries (so-called mono-national, first order comparative studies), education for internationalism and development assistance in its research and teaching dimensions.

1.4 Methodology

The field of comparative physical education and sport has travelled a similar route to that of comparative education, from which it has adopted the various methodological approaches to comparative study. Thus, there have been initially naive, then expert, travellers' accounts, area and national studies, followed by cultural borrowing or infusion (as in former British colonies) of ideas and systems, the international exchange of information and utilisation of cross-cultural or trans-national 'Problem' approaches, which focus on specific issues e.g. 'Excellence Systems', 'Sport for All Programmes', 'Women in Sport', 'Coach Education' etc. From the methods of analysis, which utilised historico-cultural explanatory traditions and social scientific approaches, a number of classification frameworks or schema have been developed and used to examine physical education and sports systems. They range from the simple (Vendien and Nixon, 1968; Johnson, 1981), to the detailed (Sturzebecker, 1967; Bennett, 1970) and elaborate (Morrison, 1979), but all emphasise that physical education and sport should be seen as part of the societal setting in which they exist. Vendien and Nixon and Johnson collected first hand reports, for which sections on general background as well as physical education and sports-specific information provided a framework for analysis. Sturzebecker stressed the need for delineation of 'shaping factors' controlling the nature and extent of a nation's programmes; he identified ecology, economic factors, racial-linguistic factors, beliefs/traditions/ideals, status of general education, extent of international co-operation and political factors as preliminary features to a deeper analysis of a physical education and sport delivery system. In order to produce rigour in analysis, Bennett employed seven identified influences (political, educational, scientific, economical, geographic, climatic and socio-cultural) on cultures and contributors to national differences in cross-analysis with twelve topics, covering purposes of physical education, place of physical education in society, physical activities' curriculum, facilities and equipment, organisation and administration, teacher education, teaching and coaching methods, extent of people participation, participation by females, amateurism and professionalism, research and study, and professional organisation. The framework proposed by Morrison drew heavily from other established schema in a range of related fields and disciplines. Working from the premise that physical education dynamically functions and develops in an ecological setting and interacts with social and cultural aspects within its socio-cultural setting, Morrison developed a conceptual framework for comparative study. The framework aims to show that varying circumstances combine in an interactive way to shape and form specifically a nation's delivery system in physical education and, with appropriate modifications, sport. This overview of the historical context of comparative methodologies, including frameworks or schema in physical education and sport, serves to illustrate that comparative study has moved on from early descriptive narratives of the 'what', through the formative historico-explanatory tradition, to comprehensive and systematic methods of data collection in the tradition of the social sciences to reveal the 'why' and 'how' of developed and developing systems.

At present, comparative physical education and sport studies' methodology is deemed to embrace a range of analytical tools to be applied to comparative data. Comparative study no longer attempts to define a single methodology and no one single method is developed as canon. In recent years comparative education scholars have adopted a range of methodological approaches to develop ways of dealing with complex issues. These eclectic and pluralistic approaches provide means of dealing with a broad range of issues. Empirical quantitative approaches establishing correlations have been enriched by the qualitative paradigm seeking to achieve understanding and interpretation of processes and reveal causality.

1.5. Relationship to practice

Whilst it is clear that physical education and sporting activity do have a ubiquitous global presence, they are at the same time subject to culturally specific 'local' (national) interpretations, policies and practices. Inevitably, similarities and differences are encountered at these levels. This is a feature, which demonstrates both diversity and complexity in process and product as well as in the influential factors, which have acted collectively and inter-dependently to 'shape' a delivery system. Ideological variants, for example, reinforce the argument of similarities and differences and the diversities evident at local, regional and national levels. Such diversity supports the thesis that 'localisation' within 'globalisation' can and does exist. Even in regions, where there have been common ideologies, such as the former 'socialist bloc' of central and eastern European states with their centralised systems, relevant research points to the substantial variations in aspects of the delivery services, typical of which were the variations evident in the development of young talented athletes to levels of excellence. The 'localisation/globalisation' debate is also manifest in the national settings of European Union countries, where efforts to bring about congruence and harmony in programmes have to recognise the existence of deep-seated diversities of trans-national contexts. The embedded traditions in physical education and sport in European countries are inextricably bound up with historical antecedents and are inevitably culture bound. These are features, which are fundamental to understanding, when curriculum planners strive for uniformity and standardisation.

A potential 'pitfall' within the domain of comparative and international studies lies within the sphere of the 'truth' of 'fact' often witnessed in discrepancies between principles and practices or, for example, in government policy rhetoric and its actual implementation. Illustrations of gaps between policy 'promises' and actual practice 'reality' are seen in recent international surveys of the situation of physical education in schools (refer Hardman & Marshall 2000; Hardman 2002; and Hardman & Marshall, 2005). Despite such constraints, comparative study can and does facilitate an awareness of possibilities for amelioration of existing structures and mechanisms through processes of adoption or adaptation to suit local (national), socio-cultural, economic and environmental circumstances. The international dimension within comparative research can, and does, inform policy at inter- and national governmental agency levels as testified by UNESCO, World Health Organisation, Council of Europe and European Parliament and a plethora of national governments' responses to findings from international comparative surveys.

1.6. Future Perspectives

For future developments in the comparative physical education and sport domain, mixed messages are evident. Generally, there is a shift away from the mono- and multi-national 'area' approaches of the latter years of the 20th century to thematic or topic approaches. This shift is seen in two developments: (i) the disappearance of Comparative Physical Education and Sport modules or course units from university level programmes and replacement by interdisciplinary issues-based units, which focus on **international** themes such as the situation of physical education in schools, gender or disability or topics such as politics or youth sport, with a comparative dimension or from a comparative perspective; and (ii) in titles and contents of published texts including books, journal articles and reports. However, in some regions of the world, and mainly those, which are economically emerging or developing or have recently politically and ideological re-aligned, there is interest in features and systems in national entity contexts. Central to future initiatives will be the continuing globalisation v. localisation debate, the role of ethernet communication, and increasingly sophisticated methodological procedures to enable validity and reliability of data when crossing cultural etc. divides.

2.   Information Sources

2.1. Journals

The international Society for Physical Education and Sport publishes an international journal entitled *International Sports Studies* (formerly *Journal of Comparative Physical Education and Sport*. The ISCPES Journal underwent a title change with volume 21 (1), 1999 (ISSN: 1443-0770) and change in editorship from Roland Naul to John Nauright and Dawn Penney (later replaced by Tara Magdalinski). The new editorial team, however, remained committed to the retention of the journal as a multi-disciplinary, cross-cultural and international perspectives' publication within the domain of physical education and sport. *International Sports Studies* is a refereed journal in which multi-disciplinary, cross-cultural and international perspectives are promoted as having a critical role to play in furthering understanding of complex phenomena in the arenas of physical education and sport. Recent journals have included articles on the transformations of sport in Eastern Europe; the impact of European unification on American sports; sport and national character; development of sporting excellence; physical education and sport in the East and West.

Other journals, which carry comparative, international and cross-cultural articles include:
* *International Journal of Physical Education* (ICSSPE);
* *FIEP Bulletin* (FIEP);

- *Journal of the International Council for Health, Physical Education, Recreation, Sport and Dance* (ICHPER.SD) and its autonomous regional derivatives (*African, American, Asian* and *Australian of Health, Physical Education, and Recreation*);
- *European Physical Education Review* (NWCPEA/Sage);
- *Journal of Sports History*; *International Journal of Sports Sociology*;
- *Sportwissenschaft* (Verlag Karl Hofmann);
- *International Journal of Fundamental and Applied Kinesiology* (University of Zagreb, Croatia)

A host of national journals also contain international related articles or items; the *British Journal of Teaching Physical Education*, for example, regularly features an international news corner section.

Affinity journals include: *Compare*, *Comparative Education* and *Comparative Education Review*.

2.2. Reference Books, Encyclopaedias, etc. (a selection)

Amusa, L.O., Toriola, A.L., Onyewadume, I.U. (1999). *Physical Education and Sport in Africa*. Ibadan, Nigeria, LAP Publications Ltd.

Arnaud, P., and Riordan, J. (1998). *Sport and International Politics. The Impact of Fascism and Communism on Sport*. London, Routledge.

Bartlett, R., Gratton, C., and Rolf, C. (2003). *Encyclopaedia of International Sports Studies*. London, Taylor and Francis.

Bennett, B.L., Howell, M.L., and Simri, I. (1975). *Comparative Physical Education and Sport*. Philadelphia, Lea and Febiger.

Beyer, E. (Ed.). (1987). *Tri-lingual Sport Science Dictionary*. Schorndorf, Hofmann Verlag.

De Knop, P., Engström, L-M., Skirstad, B., and Weiss, M.R. (Eds.). (1996). *Worldwide Trends in Youth Sport*. Champaign, IL, Human Kinetics Publishers Inc.

Haag, H. (Ed.). (2004). *Research Methodology for Sport and Exercise Science*. Schorndorf, Verlag Karl Hofmann.

Haag, H., and Haag, G. (Eds.). (2003). *Dictionary. Sport, Physical Education, Sport Science*. Kiel, Institut für Sportwissenschaften.

Houlihan, B. (1997). *Sport, Policy and Politics. A Comparative Analysis*. London, Routledge.

Knuttgen, H.G., Ma, C., M., and Wu, Z. (Eds.). (1990), *Sport in China*. Champaign, IL, Human Kinetics Publishers Inc.

Pühse, U., and Gerber, M. (Eds.). (2005). *International Comparison of Physical Education. Concepts, Problems, Prospects*. Oxford, Meyer and Meyer Sport (UK) Ltd.

Riordan, J., and Krüger, A. (Eds.). (2003). *European Cultures in Sport. Examining the Nations and Regions*. Bristol, Intellect Books.

Teodrescu, L., et al. (1973). *Terminologia educatiei fizice si sportului (Terminology of physical education and sport)*. Editura Stadion.

Wagner, E.A. (Ed.). (1989). *Sport in Asia and Africa: a Comparative Handbook*. Westport, Connecticut, Greenwood Press Inc.

2.3 Book Series

The ISCPES Book Series (terminated in 2004) was published by Routledge (Spon, U.K.). Structurally, the Series was divided into two types of text: volumes, which essentially have an 'area', i.e. mono-national focus, and alternately volumes which address 'problems', i.e. topics or themes in cross-cultural and/ or international settings. The vision of the template for the content of the 'area' study volumes was that each text would have a contextualising introduction, followed by chapters respectively focusing on historical developments, organisational structures, policies and programmes in physical education in educational settings, sport delivery systems, including issues of institutional development of excellence in sport, sport for all policies and practices and gender. Such a template format provides consistency within a book series and concomitantly facilitates awareness of similarities, variations and differences between countries. This template was followed by the first two titles in the Series:

Jones, R., and Riordan, J. (Eds.). (1999). *Sport and Physical Education in China*. London, E & FN Spon

Naul, R., and Hardman, K. (Eds.). (2002). *Sport and Physical Education in Germany*. London, Routledge.

The third title, in specifically addressing a gender-related topical theme, was the first volume in the Series to take a 'problem' study approach. As with its two 'area' study volume predecessors, the template for the content produces comparative awareness of situations and developments in a differentiated array of countries and cultures and provides an analytical dimension of systems and issues, which are pervasively important in global and cross-cultural contexts:

Hartmann-Tews, I., and Pfister, G. (Eds.). (2003). *Social Issues in Women and Sport – International and Comparative Perspectives*. London. Routledge.

ISCPES Monographs include:

Hardman, K. (Ed.). (1988). *Physical Education and Sport in Africa. ISCPES Monograph*. Manchester, University of Manchester. It comprises an edited collection of papers concerned with themes and issues in several African countries: Botswana, Kenya, Nigeria, South Africa and Tanzania.

Hardman, K. (Ed.). (1989). *Physical Education and Sport under Communism. ISCPES Monograph*. Manchester, University of Manchester. (This Monograph

117

is composed of papers presented at the inaugural Seminar meeting of the British Interest Network for Comparative Physical Education and Sport held at the University of Manchester in December, 1988).

A trio of Monographs published in 1996 embrace 'area' (country) and 'problem' (topic/theme/issue) approaches to comparative studies:

Hardman, K. (1996). *Foundations in Comparative Physical Education and Sport.* Manchester, Centre for Physical Education & Leisure Studies, University of Manchester.

Maeda, M., Ichimura, S., and Hardman, K. (Eds.). (1996). *Physical Education and Sport in Japan.* Manchester, University of Manchester.

Hardman, K. (Ed.). (1996). *Sport for All: Issues and Perspectives in International Context. ISCPES Monograph.* Manchester, University of Manchester.

2.4   Conference Proceedings

Between 1979 and 2000, ISCPES published the Proceedings of its eleven Biennial Conferences:
1) Wingate Institute, Israel, 1978 (published 1979).
2) University of Dalhousie, Halifax, Nova Scotia, Canada, 1980.
3) University of Minnesota, Minneapolis, USA, 1982 (published 1986).
4) Malente, Kiel, Federal Republic of Germany 1984 (published 1987).
5) University of British Columbia, Vancouver, Canada, 1986 (published 1988).
6) Chinese University of Hong Kong, 1988 (published 1990).
7) Bisham Abbey, Marlow, England, 1990 (published 1991).
8) University of Houston, Texas, USA, 1992 (published 1994).
9) Charles University, Prague, Czech Republic, 1994 (published 1996).
10) Hachi-ohji, Tokyo, Japan, 1996 (published 1998).
11) Catholic University, Leuven, Belgium 1998 (published 2000).

The Leuven Biennial Conference was the last ISCPES Conference to have published Proceedings. Thereafter ISCPES Conference papers have featured variously as a double 'special' issue of the *International Sports Studies* journal (ISCPES 12th Biennial Conference in Maroochydore, Queensland in August 2000, which had a theme of *Beyond 2000: Sport and Leisure Between Global and Local Structures*). Subsequent biennial Conference Proceedings (13th Biennial Conference, Windsor, Canada, 2001 with the theme of *The Net Effect: Intercultural Communication and Globalisation in Physical Education and Sport Science*; and 14th Biennial Conference, Melbourne 2006 with the theme of *Sport, Communities and Engagement*) have been published in CD Rom format. The Conference, scheduled for 2004 in London, Ontario was cancelled because of an outbreak of SARS.

2.5 Data Banks

Wilcox, R., (Ed.), (1986). *Comparative physical education and sport directory*. New York, Adelphi University. The *Directory* is divided into three sections:
Biographical profiles
Agencies offering information and funding potential; Journals identified as potential sources for publication; Key to Institutions of Higher Education; Key to academic, professional and research bodies
Index by nation of residence

Educational Resources Information Centre (ERIC) has over 1 million periodical articles (CIJE) and educational reports (RIE).
Heracles is a French language sport and physical education database produced by the **SPORTDOC** national network and the Institut National du Sport et de l'Education Physique in Paris.
SISA Sportlit Database has over 20,000 records (the majority is South African). It is produced by the South African Department of sport and Recreation with support from the SA national Sports Council and the SA National Olympic Committee.
SPOLIT database has may records nearly half of which are in English. It is produced by the Federal Institute of Sport Science in Cologne, Germany.
SPORTDISCUS has numerous records in a wide range of languages. It is produced by the Sport Information Centre in Gloucester, Ontario, Canada.
Sport and Leisure Research on Disc covers UK dissertations and theses at doctoral and masters levels in all areas of sport, recreation and leisure from 16 contributing universities.

2.6 Internet sources (Web sites, list serves, etc.)

AEHESIS Project: http://www.aehesis.com
EUPEA: http://www.eupea.com
ICSSPE: http://www.icsspe.org
ISCPES: http://www,iscpes.org
http://www.thenapa2.org
http://www.inclusivesports.org
http://www.erasmusmundus.be

3.0 Organisation Network

3.1 International level

A major initiative in the international development of the comparative physical education and sport domain was the formation of the International Society for Comparative Physical Education and Sport (ISCPES). ISCPES was founded, initially as the International Committee on Comparative Physical Education and Sport, in December, 1978 (the name change to ISCPES occurred at the second international seminar on Comparative Physical Education and Sport in

Halifax, Nova Scotia in 1980) on the occasion of an international seminar on comparative physical education and sport at the Wingate Institute, Israel.

Over two decades, ISCPES has become acknowledged as the lead body in comparative physical education and sport studies. This Society is a research and educational organisation, which has the expressed purpose of supporting, encouraging, and providing assistance to those seeking to initiate and strengthen research and teaching programmes in comparative physical education and sport throughout the world. ISCPES holds biennial international conferences and latterly regional conferences/workshops, has published Conference Proceedings, an international journal and monographs, sponsors (in the form of patronage), and has spawned, comparative/cross-cultural/ international research projects and has launched a Book Series.

The ISCPES Executive Board members serve for a period of four years on a 'roll off – roll on' basis to preserve an element of continuity. The Board currently comprises: Darwin Semotiuk (President, Canada), Ken Hardman (UK, Past-President), Rosa Lopez D'Amico (Venezuela), Scott Martyn (Canada), Anthony Church (Canada), Herbert Haag (Germany), Hai Ren (Peoples's Republic of China), Walter Ho (Macao), Jan Tolleneer (Belgium) and Lateef Amusa (South Africa).

In 1986, ISCPES gained membership of ICSSPE and is represented on the Associations' Board and International Committee of Sport Pedagogy (ICSP). As a constituent member organisation of ICSP, ISCPES liaises with, and has collaborated with, other international member organisations e.g. AIESEP (research and interdisciplinary Seminar in conjunction with ICSSPE Sport and Leisure Committee at the Pre-Olympic Sport Science Congress in July 1996 in Dallas, Texas); IFAPA (Sport for All Workshop in May 1995 in Kuwait); and with AIESEP, FIEP, IAPESGW and IFAPA (information exchanges, networking etc.). ISCPES also works closely with other international associations, for example: the International Society for History of Physical Education and Sport (ISHPES), a 'special' issue of the ISCPES Journal (volume XIX (2), 1997) was devoted to *Traditional Games* and edited by Gertrud Pfister, then President of the *International Society for the History of Physical Education and Sport* (ISHPES); and the International Associations for the Philosophy of Sport (IAPS) and Sociology of Sport (ISSA), both of which held regional conferences in conjunction with the ISCPES biennial Conference (international Sports Studies Conference) on the theme of *Sport, Communities and Engagement* in Melbourne, Australia, 6-8 March 2006. All of these associations contribute to comparative literature, research and study in comparative physical education and sport.

Amongst other international bodies contributing to comparative literature and with international policies in the physical education and sport domain are: the United Nations Educational, Scientific and Cultural Organisation

(UNESCO); the World Health Organisation (WHO); the International Olympic Committee (IOC); the International Federation for Physical Education (FIEP); and the International Council for Health, Physical Education, Recreation, Sport and Dance (ICHPER.SD), which has a number of Special Interest Group Commissions, of which Comparative Physical Education and Sport is one; thus, within ICHPER.SD Biennial World Congresses, Commission sessions are allocated to the comparative domain for invited presentations of relevant papers.

3.2 Regional level

Asian Society for Comparative Physical Education and Sport.

European Physical Education Associations (a forum, which comprises representatives of national Physical Education Associations).
American Alliance for Health, Physical Education, Recreation and Dance has an International Relations Council.

3.3 National level

As far as is known, the only active national 'Society' is the British Network Interest Group for Comparative Physical Education and Sport which was set up after a one-day Seminar held at the University of Manchester, Manchester, U.K. in December 1988. Subsequent Seminars have been held at St. Mary's College, Strawberry Hill, 1992 (*The Changing Face of Physical Education and Sport*), Liverpool Institute of Higher Education, 1993 (*International Sport: Past, Present and Future*), West London Institute, 1994 (*Sport in Developing Countries*) and Loughborough University, 1996 (*Sports Institutes, Sports Academies and National Sporting Identities*). For each of these Meetings, Proceedings have been published under the title of each of the respective Seminars. Other national Societies known to have existed but for a short-lived period only include the Japan Society for Comparative PE and Sport and a Comparative PE and Sport Society in the Federal Republic of Germany. Both appear to have ceased to function, though there is a more recently established German-Japanese P.E. and Sport group, which meets every two years for comparative exchanges.

3.4. Specialised Centres

Beyond Higher Education Institutions' programmes, there are no known specialised centres.

3.5 Specialised International Degree Programmes
In September 1999, an innovative European Masters in Physical Education degree programme was introduced. The programme was the culmination of two years of planning by representatives from 17 'Partner' Universities

forming the European Network of Sports Science Higher Education Institutions' (ENSSHE) PE Curriculum Development Committee, which operates within the framework of the European Union Socrates Programme. The one-year full time course involves a set of core European dimension modules, 'home' university elective modules and a comparative (European dimension) research project. To date related intensive course programmes have been held in Jarandilla, Spain, Extramadura University, Badajoz, Spain and Technical University, Lisbon, Portugal.

There is a well-established European one-year post-graduate programme co-ordinated by the Catholic University, Leuven, Belgium, that provides research and teaching methodology in Adapted Physical activity (APA), as well as the social, pedagogical, and technical aspects of physical activity adapted to the needs of disabled persons. This European Masters in Adapted Physical Activity exists alongside a recently introduced Erasmus Mundus Master in Adapted Physical Activity. Both programmes consist in total of 60 European Credits (ECTS) with English as the official language of instruction. Another disability model inspired programme is THENAPA II: "Ageing and disability - a new crossing between physical activity, social inclusion and life-long well-being". The associated thematic network is concerned to: a) define the current situation at European Higher education institutions in relation to the extent the subject of Adapted Physical Activity (APA) is included in the curricula of the future service providers; and b) create a basic profile and implement the subject of adapted physical activity for the elderly in European higher education curricula in order to compensate for the current lack of information and resources in the specific domain.

4. Appendix

4.1 Terminology

Inherent in studying phenomena from different geo-political and socio-cultural locations are inter-related challenges of interpretation of linguistic terms and conceptual variations over time and space. These are areas for concern, for language and terminology together with concepts present particular problems in studies with a comparative or international focus. In translation, some words lose their original meaning because they are culture-bound. Terms may and do differ from to country. The European region with its diversity of languages and cultures serves to illustrate the point. In France, physical education appears as *l'Éducation Physique et Sport* (*physical education and sport*) in schools; in Germany, the term *Sport/Sportunterricht* (*sport/sport instruction* or *teaching*) was generally adopted in the 1970s onwards with the *physical educator* termed the *sports teacher*; in the former divided Germany (1949-1990), the generic term for physical education in the two decades after the Second World War was *Leibeserziehung* in the then Federal Republic (West Germany) and *Körpererziehung* in the Democratic Republic (East Germany), the latter influenced by a post-world war II sovietisation process, in which *physical culture* and cultivation of the *socialist personality* had an important role throughout central and eastern Europe; since, the year 2000, several *Länder* in reunified Germany have introduced a re-conceptualised form of physical education, *Bewegungserziehung* (*movement education*). In Sweden the term in general use is *idrott i hälsa* (*sport and health*) whereas in United Kingdom, the term *physical education* features on the school curriculum time-table Taking these terminological divergences into account, it is not wholly surprising that different and various forms of the subject exist in terms of the curriculum: in strict or liberal regulatory implementation of the physical education curriculum, in general or precise prescriptions for content, in traditional and/or new aims and objectives, in central governmental and/or local school-based concepts, in teacher- or student-centred teaching concepts, in sport or movement-based skill concepts, in process and/or product approaches, in diverse and sometimes even contradicting concepts of physical education teacher training. Similar evolutionary developments can be seen elsewhere in Europe, where imported and indigenous ideas have merged in a host of 'melting pots' as the various national systems demonstrate.

These examples illustrate the difficulties not only between countries with different languages but also between countries which share a common language, but which have distinctively different ideological settings determining cultural norms and values. Thus, terminology and terminological issues are pervasive areas of debate within comparative physical education and sport studies, especially in the context of research validity when collecting and interpreting data across cultural divides. 'Back translation' of research instruments such as questionnaire and interview schedules is an imperative in cross-cultural studies. Increasingly sophisticated methodologies drawn from other disciplinary areas are being employed to assist in terminological validation of research data.

4.1. Position Statement(s)

ISCPES is a research and educational organisation. Its purpose is to support, encourage and provide assistance to those seeking to initiate and strengthen research and teaching programmes in comparative physical education and sport throughout the world. Specifically, ISCPES distributes research findings and information, supports and co-operates with local, national and international organisations with similar goals, organises and arranges meetings bringing together people from around the world working in comparative physical education and sport, and issues publications. The scope of the Society's academic mandate is affected by members' interests and research needs. Members are drawn from three major groups: social scientists, historians and pedagogists.

4.3. Varia

A set of "Presentation Guidelines" was adopted by ISCPES Executive Committee in June 1987, and subsequently published in the Society's Journal (Hardman 1987). The intention is to help comparativists in physical education and sport to formulate research proposals and standardise procedures for presentation when seeking financial etc., support from various agencies. They embrace such aspects as research project rationale, clear statement of objectives and methodology (discussion of choice of design and description of methods - including, if relevant, sampling procedures and sample units), procedures for analysis; research outputs, staffing (principal researchers and precise contribution), definition of period of research, and budget and how it is to be allocated. These guidelines conform to a structured, systematic approach to comparative research but allow for individual subject orientation.

Multi-national collaborative research projects carried out under the auspices of ISCPES include:

(i) *Education for leisure - a comparison of current physical education and recreation approaches in selected English and Canadian high schools* (B. Thompson, University of New Brunswick, Canada and Joy Standeven, Brighton Polytechnic, England). This project was extended to Ireland (P. Duffy) and the United States (R. Wilcox).

(ii) *Students' and teachers' attitudes towards interschool competition* (K. Hardman, England, M.L. Krotee, United States, A. Chrissanthopoulos, Greece, J. Piccoli, Brazil, D. Bean, Canada, N.M. Khan, Pakistan and R. Naul, Federal Republic of Germany. Subsequently a modified project on the restricted theme of *Attitudes and Participation Patterns of Youth toward Competitive Sport* was undertaken by M.L. Krotee and P.F. Blair (United States), R. Naul and W. Neuhaus (Federal Republic of Germany), K. Hardman (England), H. Komuku and K. Matsumura (Japan), P. Numminen (Finland) and C. Jwo (Taiwan).

(iii) *Sporting lifestyle, motor performance and Olympic ideals of youth in Europe* (R. Naul (Federal Republic of Germany), M. Piéron (Belgium), R. Telema (Finland), L. Almond (England) and A. Rychtecky (Czech Republic). This project was carried out as a joint study comprising scholars from ISCPES and AIESEP.

(iv) ISCPES has given its support to a research project to be conducted under the leadership of Dr. W. Ho, (University of Macao) on a global study of the teaching of physical education. This project has been endorsed by ICSP (August 2006).

For the lead comparative physical education and sport domain organisation, the recent resurgence of interest in international issues has coincided with developmental initiatives within and by ISCPES:

124

- Regional conferences held (Maracay, Maturin and Rubio, Venezuela, October 2005) and planned (Varadero, Cuba, April 2006)
- A new promotional brochure available in 6 languages
- establishment of regional and country representatives
- A graduated annual membership fee system (individual and institutional) based on national economic status
- Updating of its current web-site and review of its constitution.

References

Anthony, D.W.J. (1966). Comparative Physical Education. *Physical Education,* 58 (175), 70-73.

Anthony, D.W.J. (1969). *Comparative Physical Education.* Unpublished M.Ed. thesis, Leicester, University of Leicester.

Bennett, B.L., (1970). A Historian Looks At Comparative Physical Education. *Gymnasion,* VII, Spring, 11-12.

Bennett, B.L., Howell, M.L., & Simri, U. (1975). *Comparative Physical Education and Sport.* Philadelphia, Lea & Febiger.

Bereday, G.Z.F. (1964). *Comparative Method in Education.* New York, Holt, Reinhart & Winston.

Doll-Tepper, G. & Scoretz, D. (Eds.). 2001. *World Summit on Physical Education.* Berlin, ICSSPE.

Hardman, K. (1987). Research Proposal Presentation Guidelines. *Journal of Comparative Physical Education and Sport,* IX, (2), 27-29.

Hardman, K. (1999). Developments in Comparative Physical Education and Sport: the Contribution of ICSSPE. *International Journal of Physical Education,* Volume XXXVI, (3), 3rd Quarter, 88-113.

Hardman, K. (2001). *International Journal of Physical Education,* volume XXXVIII, Issue 3, 3rd Quarter, 96-103.

Hardman, K. (2002). *Council of Europe: Committee for the Development of Sport (CDDS) European Physical Education/Sport Survey.* MSL-IM 16 (2002) 9. Strasbourg, Council of Europe.

Hardman, K. & Marshall, J.J. (2000). *World-wide Survey of the State and Status of School Physical Education. Final Report.* Manchester, University of Manchester.

Hardman, K. & Marshall, J.J. (2006). Update on Current Situation of Physical Education in Schools. *ICSSPE Bulletin,* 47, May 2006.

Johnson, W. (1980). *Sport and Physical Education Around the World.* Champaign, IL, Stipes Publishing Co.

Louis, V., & Louis, L. (1964). *Sport in the Soviet Union.* London, Pergamon Press.

Moehlmann, A.H. (1963). *Comparative Educational Systems.* New York, Center for Applied Research in Education, Inc.

Molyneux, D.D. (1962). *Central Government Aid to Sport and Physical Recreation in Countries of Western Europe.* Department of Physical Education, University of Birmingham.

Morrison, D.H. (1979). Towards a Conceptual Framework for Comparative Physical Education. In M.L.

Morton, H.W. (1953). *Soviet Sport.* New York, Collier Books.

Nixon, J.E. (1970). Comparative, International and Developmental Studies in Physical Education. *ICHPER Journal,* VIII (1), Spring, 4-9.

Petry, K., Froberg, K., and Madella, A. (Eds.). (2004). *Report of the First Year.* AEHESIS Thematic Network Project. Cologne, the Department of Leisure Studies, German Sport University.

Petry, K., Froberg, K., and Madella, A. (Eds.). (2005). *Report of the Second Year*. AEHESIS Thematic Network Project. Cologne, the Department of Leisure Studies, German Sport University.

Petry, K., Froberg, K., and Madella, A. (Eds.). (2006). *Report of the Third Year*. AEHESIS Thematic Network Project. Cologne, the Department of Leisure Studies, German Sport University.

Riordan, J. (1978). *Sport in Soviet Society*. Cambridge, Cambridge University Press.

Sturzebecker, R.L. (1967). Comparative Physical Education. *Gymnasion*, IV, Spring-Autumn, 48-49.

Sullivan, D.T. (1964). *A Comparative Study of Physical Education in the USSR and in England*. Unpublished M.A. Thesis, University of London.

Vendien, C.L. & Nixon, J.E. (1968*)*. *The World Today in Health, Physical Education and Recreation*. Englewood Cliffs, New Jersey, Prentice-Hall Inc.

Selection #6
W(h)ither Comparative Physical Education and Sport?

Ken Hardman
England

Introduction

The title of this article has been chosen in the light of developments and trends in the domain of Comparative Study since 1999 when my article on *Developments in Comparative Physical Education and Sport: the contribution of the "International Society for Comparative physical Education and Sport"* (ISCPES) featured in the *International Journal of Physical Education*, Issue 3, 3rd Quarter, pp.88-113. In that article, it was suggested that there is a closer affinity of comparative physical education and sport with methodological procedure than with its identification as a distinct body of knowledge. It was also intimated that despite increased scholarly activity in the domain over the last thirty years of the 20th century, the comparative dimension still had "not received the attention that it deserves" (Hardman, 1999, p.104). This point of view was reinforced two years later when Birte Kaulitz (2001), also in the *International Journal of Physical Education*, commented: "the comparative dimension is often neglected" in Germany, where "few scholars contribute studies and research projects to this field of sports sciences" (p.104). This present review will further address the situation and again will draw from developments specifically associated with the International Society for Comparative Physical Education and Sport (ISCPES); it will also refer to comparative study-related endeavours elsewhere.

1. ISCPES Journal – new direction

A new editorial team (John Nauright and Dawn Penney) succeeded Roland Naul in January 1999 and the ISCPES journal entered a new stage in its development, first in a switch to an Australian based publisher but then secondly, and more significantly, with a change in the name of the Journal to *International Sports Studies* following a contentious decision by the ISCPES Executive Board at its May 1999 inter-biennial meeting. The new editorial team, however, remained committed to the retention of the journal as a multi-disciplinary, cross-cultural and international perspectives' publication within the domain of physical education and sport. The renamed journal included a restyled book reviews section, typified by reviews of pairs of books, under the guidance of Douglas Booth.

The content of the 'inaugural' edition included two comparative dimension articles (Rees, Brandel-Bredenbeck and Brettschneider on sports stereotyping among American and German adolescents; Wright on students' practice teaching experiences in Singapore, the United Kingdom and the United

States). Two other articles took a mono-national approach: Phillips and Nauright employed a global capital and local audiences analysis in focusing on suburban-based clubs' supporters' responses to threatened merger changes in Australia and alluded to some comparisons with other countries, whilst Light, drawing from his rugby coaching experience in Japan, addressed the construction of embodied masculinity in Japanese University Rugby. The results of collaborative research feature alongside individual research contributions in the second issue of *International Sports Studies*: Chow and Fry contribute to the debate on practice teaching experiences and extend it to new training settings in different cultural contexts, Australia and Hong Kong; Lake and Patriksson address physical and health education curricula issues in an examination of links between physical activity and alcohol consumption in England and Sweden; the notion of 'first order comparison', where there is a single entity approach and the comparative perspective is with the reader, lies with the articles respectively by Oku who demonstrates that Nigerian women suffer from similar inadequate sporting opportunities as women do in other countries and by Booth who examines antinomies of multi-cultural sporting nationalism in Australia and South Africa. The first issue in 2000, guest edited by Tara Magdalinksi, was intended to raise awareness of sport in religious communities, particularly those generally designated as 'minority'. The contributions here provide an historical perspective in a variety of religious and national and cultural contexts: Jewish American Women (Borish); Catholics in Northern Ireland (Cronin); the Jewish Community in Shanghai (Anthony Hughes); and Islam (Smith). In the second year 2000 issue, there is an emphasis on the comparative dimension in all articles included: Booth examines comparative method in sports history through analysis of methodological issues and is followed by Light's study of masculinity among Australian and Japanese rugby players (thus, expanding on his earlier contribution on masculinity among Japanese University rugby players in volume 21 (2)) from a comparative perspective; Trangbæk explores how Swedish Gymnastics was introduced in different ways for women in middle and working classes and rural situations in England and Denmark; Toriola et al provide a comparative analysis of youth sport programmes in Botswana and Nigeria; and Thompson and Soós the review comparative impacts of globalisation and localisation on youth sport in New Zealand and Hungary. With Dawn Penney's resignation, reluctantly accepted by the ISCPES Executive Board with due full recognition of her major contribution to raising the scholarly image of the Journal, this second issue of the year marked the end of the co-editorial arrangement. The immediate future of the Journal, however, remained secure in the hands of Editor, John Nauright, ably supported by Tara Magdalinski and Douglas Booth. Notice was given in the editorial preface that a double issue was being planned for 2001 with two main thematic strands: women and sport and the Olympics. In the event, a double 'special' issue was indeed published, but it consisted of papers delivered at the ISCPES 12th Biennial Conference in Maroochydore, Queensland in August 2000. I shall return to this issue later in this review.

The 'Special' issue in effect replaced the established ISCPES practice of publishing Biennial Conference Proceedings. Essentially, the fourteen papers making up volume 23 (1/2) can be divided into two groups; the first group examines issues of sport and space (Vertinsky), sport writing (Markula) and biography (Denison) and elite sport issues (Schweinbenz; and de D'Amico and O'Brien); the second group covers topics related to the state of school physical education in continental regional (Hardman) and developing countries (Chappell; and Kloppers) contexts, elderly people's engagement in cultural and physical activities (Mertens), sports marketing in Bahrain (Al-Khaja) and sports developments in China (Yan Ho; and Whitby). Collectively, these papers reveal diversity of interest among researchers from various discipline and area backgrounds and with a vested interest in comparative and international studies in physical education and sport. This diversity of interest is also evident in volume 24 (1), in which the editor alludes to the significance of historical awareness to contemporary studies and the necessity of taking account of historical processes at a number of levels when considering local or regional issues. The latter is particularly apposite in Ha and Xu's article on physical education teachers' values in Shanghai and Hong Kong, two cities with very different politico-ideological and economic historical situations; the former is relevant to Gems' piece on American influences on sport specifically in the areas of colonialism and reconstruction in the Philippines as well as to the history of doping in sport provided by Yesalis and Bahrke. The lead contribution in this issue, by Bradshaw, comprises an analysis of theoretical stances within international literature on women and sport. An innovation in issue two of 2002 was a 'State of the Field' article, initiated in order to examine significant issues within comparative physical education and sport. The first 'State of the Field' issue included was by Bang-Chool Kim, who examined the differences between teaching and writing of sport history in Korea and the United States. The comparative dimension persists in articles by Wrynn, who focuses on links between American and European sports scientists in the period 1926-1966, and by Nash with her study of soccer coaching in Scotland and the United States. The content of this edition is completed with Miah's discussion on the reaction of men's tennis to the impact of recent technology on the game.

In this fourth stage of its development, the ISCPES Journal significant name change has been accompanied by an orientation more towards historical and sociological processes and issues than in previous stages. In part, this orientation tendency may well reflect the genre of the Journal as perceived by the 'market' of potential contributors; it may also in part reflect the scholarly interests of the editor and editorial support team, who in their endeavours to raise the academic profile of the Journal, have been proactive, and rightly so, in seeking contributions, which meet with strict review criteria, from relevant academic contacts. Hitherto as asserted previously, the ISCPES Journal has persistently suffered from limited numbers of submissions received from aspiring contributors. Reminders of this not insignificant constraint are seen in the ISCPES Executive Board Meeting Summary of Minutes, 21 May, 2001, in which it was recorded that difficulties were still being experienced in obtaining copy and in the frequent Journal editorial requests for support for, and submissions to, the Journal, though the editorial preface in volume 22 (2) reported a "slow but steady stream of submissions" (p.4). The concern about both quantity and quality of submissions is evident in other minuted ISCPES Executive Board deliberations and was instrumental in an Editor's recommendation for an award for a 'best article' published in the Journal. The ISCPES General Assembly of August 2000 in Maroochydore, Queensland, Australia, adopted a proposal to establish the Earle F. Zeigler[1] Journal Article ("Best Article") Award, the first of which covering the period 1999-2002 was scheduled for announcement in July 2003 at the ISCPES Biennial Conference in London, Ontario, Canada. Because of the cancellation (due to the SARS outbreak in the province) the London Conference was cancelled and the announcement withheld. Interestingly in relation to the number of articles being submitted as well as the quality, and in the light of perceptions on the situation of the comparative dimension indicated in the introductory statement, further evidence of the concern is seen in editorial preface policy-related commentaries throughout the current developmental stage. The first issue of the renamed journal (volume 21 (1), 1999), referred to barriers in extending discussion beyond discipline boundaries because of deterrent contexts to multi-disciplinary and cross-institution research and writing and the perceived hierarchical lower status of work "'outside' or at the peripheries of those disciplines" (Penney and Nauright, 1999, p.4). This 'lower status' is reminiscent of Birte Kaulitz's (2001) reference to "second class treatment" (p.104) and the neglect of comparative study in Germany. The ICSSPE Journal editors sought to counter the adverse perceptions on status through enhanced content of future issues. Later (volume 22 (2)), the policy shifted to one of consolidation of "a strong academic journal" (Nauright, 2000, p.4). The 'State of the Field' initiative referred to earlier is an example of innovation intended to push international and comparative sports studies forward and attract readers to the Journal. Despite continuing concerns, the editorial policy initiatives have, without doubt during this present stage, served to further develop *International Sports Studies* as a more highly respected academic publication.

2. ISCPES Biennial Proceedings – end of the road!

The 11th ISCPES Biennial Conference held in Leuven in July 1998 proved to be the last ISCPES Conference to have published Proceedings. The title of the Conference "Old borders, new borders, no borders", as the Proceedings' editors (Jan Tolleneer and Roland Renson) remind us in their prefatory statement, was intended to be understood not only in its geographical meaning but also in its broader senses applying to the relationship between different disciplines, embracing movement culture. It is this broader sense that is the pervasive feature of Part A, *Disciplines crossing borders*, the first of five, which make up the Proceedings. Collectively, three Conference key-note presentations by John Bale, Garry Chick and Richard Holt, which form Part

A, address methodological issues, which transcend comparative and cross-cultural studies, and which represent mutual dependence and interdependence of perspectives grounded in geography and evolutionary anthropological and historical roots. In essence, Part B, *Countries getting closer*, embraces a common theme of globalisation and localisation: American hegemony and international sport (Clumpner); convergence and diversification of national sport experiences in the global village (Yan Ho); fitness as a cultural phenomenon (Volkwein); western and eastern fitness exercise integration trends (Ren); sport in China (Jones); football and nationalism (Verwimp); and globalisation and localisation, which the authors (De Knop and Harthoorn) conclude are a manifestation of increasing differentiation in sport. Part C, *The past explaining the present* provides a number of case studies with a historico-comparative flavour: bi-cultural influences on physical education in Quebec (Lèbe); sport in French colonies (Combeau-Mari and Dumont); naturism in France and Germany (Villaret and Delaplace); physical education teacher training in Spain and Italy (Aja and Teja) and United States and Japan (Takeshita and Watanabe); American sporting influences in England (baseball - Bloyce; horse-racing - Vamplew); Olympics-related issues (Universiades - Renson and Verbeke; nationalism in Atlanta - O'Brien; and differentiated concepts of amateurism - Wassong). Part D, *Sports challenging the world*, is composed of papers, which variously depict sport-related policies in different countries and collectively show that sport as a cultural phenomenon has its own dynamics: Germany, France and Great Britain - inclusion (Hartmann-Tews); Flanders - sports participation (Van Heddegem, De Martelaer and De Knop); Canada - government policy (Semotiuk); Europe - football league structures (Duke); Germany and Japan - rugby players' attitudes to fouls (Teipel and Kondo); New Zealand - youth sporting culture (Thomson); Germany and England - women's sport and leisure careers; Olympic Movement barriers for women (Odenkirchen); and comparative research design (Haag). The final Part, *The world confronting physical education*, contains papers, which variously address conceptual, contextual and political issues in and out of the classroom and beyond the school: Penney (conceptual and structural borders in an English context with added experiences in Australia) and Kloppers (restructuring of physical education in South Africa) focus on developments in physical education; Fouqué (health education components within physical education curricula in Sweden and Northrhine-Westphalia) and Morales-Figueroa, Krotee and Myeres (physical education programmes in Puerto Rico, the United States and Europe) provide comparative analyses; Schimmel and Chandler (curriculum influences) and Magdalinski and Nauright (corporate invasion of the classroom) raise the spectre of influences of Olympism and olympologies on physical education programmes; Mette, Trangbæk and Laursen physical education teachers' views on delivery and environmental circumstances and conditions (ageing and working); Burnik, Doupona and Bon discuss provision for, participation in and evaluation of, sport education in the University of Ljubijana, Slovenia; and Willy Laporte poses a challenge for comparative studies in the process of harmonisation of physical education teacher education programmes in Europe.

It is perhaps rather ironic that the ISCPES Executive Board post-Leuven decision not to publish future Biennial Conference Proceedings (the decision was taken in due awareness of financial expedience but more importantly on the grounds of alleged realities of the academic credibility and currency of published conference papers) followed what to all intents and purposes was a set of highly regarded, peer reviewed papers, which addressed a range of pertinent international, trans-national and cross-cultural issues and set out new perspectives for further research. The Leuven Conference Proceedings with papers drawing from disciplines and areas associated with social sciences and humanities and with methodologies variously embedded in comparative, cross-cultural, international and 'first order' (single entity) approaches typically represent the eclectic nature of the domain of comparative physical education and sport. This eclecticism is both a strength and weakness: the strength lies in its broad constituency and capability of addressing a wide range of issues in different and varying historical, socio-cultural, psycho-social and pedagogical contexts; the weakness, somewhat paradoxically, lies with this broad constituency, which appears not to have specific, clearly defined boundaries and has no obvious academic peg to hang its scholarly hat on. In other words, its eclectic nature does not overtly lend itself to being a scholarly and academic comfort zone.

3. ISCPES Book Series – rise and fall

As indicated in the review in the *International Journal of Physical Education*, (XXXVI (3)) ISCPES, with the support of publishing House E & FN Spon (later Routledge), launched a Book Series. The expressed concept of the Book Series was alignment of each volume with the overall purposes of comparative and cross-cultural study and progression of comparative and international studies beyond description in order to facilitate deeper analytical awareness and understanding in a variety of geographical political area and thematic issues settings. Individually and collectively, the primary purpose of the titles was to extend knowledge of national systems and 'problem' themes and topics in the areas of physical education and sporting activity with the volumes, when taken together, providing an integrated basis for informed comparisons, thereby serving the overall purpose of contributing to critical awareness and analysis amongst confirmed and potential comparativists and young scholars at under- and post-graduate levels. Physical education and sporting activity have a ubiquitous global presence; at the same time, they are subject to culturally specific 'local' (national and/or community) interpretations, policies and practices. Inevitably, therefore, similarities and differences are encountered at these 'local' levels.

Structurally, the Series was divided into two types of text: volumes, which essentially have an 'area', i.e. mono-national focus, and alternately volumes which address 'problems', i.e. topics or themes in cross-cultural and/ or international settings. The vision of the template for the content of the 'area' study volumes was that each text would have a contextualising introduction, followed by chapters respectively focusing on historical developments, organisational structures, policies and programmes in physical education in educational settings, sport delivery systems, including issues of institutional development of excellence in sport, sport for all policies and practices and gender. This template was set by the first title in the Series, *Sport and Physical Education in China* (edited by Robin Jones and Jim Riordan) and was followed by *Sport and Physical Education in Germany* (edited by Roland Naul and Ken Hardman). Such a template format provides consistency within a book series and concomitantly facilitates awareness of similarities, variations and differences between countries. The third title, *Sport and Women: Social Issues in International Perspective*, (edited by Ilse Hartmann-Tews and Gertrud Pfister) in specifically addressing a gender-related topical theme, was the first volume in the Series to take a 'problem' study approach. As with its two 'area' study volume predecessors, the template for the content produces comparative awareness of situations and developments in a differentiated array of countries and cultures and provides an analytical dimension of systems and issues, which are pervasively important in global and cross-cultural contexts. The introductory chapter to this volume sets *Women and Sport* in comparative and international perspective in a framework of issues, aims and theoretical approaches and is followed by contributions on Norway, the United Kingdom, Germany, France, Spain, the Czech Republic, Tanzania, South Africa, the United States, Canada, Brazil, Colombia, Iran, People's Republic of China, Japan and New Zealand with a concluding chapter on comparative and international findings on women's inclusion in sport.

Regrettably, I have to report that in spite of positively favourable peer reviews representative of a number of international and national journals with either a discipline or an area focus on each of the three volumes in the Series, the publisher has terminated the ISCPES Book Series contract on "commercial grounds"; the Series has proven to be a rather short-lived 'flagship' specifically for studies in Comparative Physical Education and Sport.

4. ISCPES Conferences and Symposia – competition and selectivity

ISCPES Conferences have been held on a regular biennial basis since the inaugural Seminar, held at the Wingate Institute in 1978, up to and including the successful 12th Conference, held in Maroochydore on the Sunshine Coast, Queensland, Australia in 2000. The theme of the 12th Biennial Conference on *Beyond 2000: Sport and Leisure Between Global and Local Structures* proving to be particularly attractive to sport sociologists. Because of the conference competition linked with major international events, such as the ICSSPE Pre-

Olympic Scientific Congress and Commonwealth Games Sports Science Conferences held in 'even' years on a four-yearly basis, the ISCPES Executive Board agreed and was supported by the General Assembly to switch its biennial conference programme to 'odd years', commencing with a hastily (just over 6 months from concept to event) organised 13th Biennial Conference in May, 2001 in Windsor, Ontario, Canada. Whilst this Conference with its theme *The Net Effect: Intercultural Communication and Globalisation in Physical Education and Sport Science* was very well organised, the consequences of insufficient lead-in time were mirrored in the small contingent (less than 30) of delegates. At the Windsor Conference, it was decided to hold an ISCPES Seminar within the Commonwealth Games Conference in Manchester, UK in July 2002 as an interim phasing out even years/phasing in odd years measure; furthermore London, Ontario, Canada was selected as the venue for the 14th Biennial Conference albeit with some concerns about hosting two ISCPES Conferences in Canada within a space of two years. The Manchester ISCPES Symposium took place over two days with a range of themes embracing comparative/international perspectives on physical education, sport in developing countries, health and physical activity, excellence in sport and sport as business as well as a skills teaching workshop inspiringly led by Roy Clumpner. As mentioned above, the 14th Biennial Conference on *Global Issues in Sport and Physical Activity* planned for 4-7 July 2003 in London, Ontario was cancelled or, more accurately, postponed (until 2-5 July 2004) for medical security reasons. However, at the time of notice of cancellation less than 50 delegates had registered to attend. Further problems for the rescheduled conference may arise from competition with the European College of Sport Science (ECSS) Annual Congress in July 2004 in Clermont Ferrand, France and the International Council of Sport Science (ICSSPE) Pre-Olympic Congress in early August, 2004 in Thessalonika, Greece. In times of funding limitations experienced by institutions, individuals are becoming increasingly constrained with regard to conference etc. attendance because of the high costs involved: greater selectivity prevails and contribution and exposure to perceived hierarchically higher status of scholarly work is at the core of selective decision-making and taking.

5. Other spheres of Comparative Studies Endeavours (re-orientation and diversity)

In the Anglo-Saxon speaking world, there has been a steep decline in the number of higher education institutions offering course programmes or modular units under the specific nomenclature of "Comparative Physical Education and Sport" hence, whilst it is far from being extinct, evidence of which lies particularly in 'first order' comparisons, the body of knowledge thesis is becoming increasingly tenuous. In the United Kingdom, for example, what used to appear under the title has generally been subsumed within themes or under topics such as "International Dimensions" in

Physical Education and/or Sport or features in cross-disciplinary courses variously covering "Issues", "Politics", "Economics", "Policies", "Sociological and/or Cultural Perspectives and so on. More usually than not, "Sport" prevails over "Physical Education") in such course units. In North America, a similar trend can be discerned particularly in re-orientation to courses in "International Studies" and "International Development" with a Sport and Physical Education focus. For all of these thematic/topic approaches, interpretation and understanding of content can be more open-ended in outcomes: comparisons can be directly and explicitly made or can be indirect, implicit or in the mind of the learner/reader. Typical of the genre trend are the selected texts, in date order, listed immediately below:

Houlihan, B., (1997). *Sport, policy and politics. A comparative analysis*. London, Routledge.

Arnaud, P., and Riordan, J., (1998). *Sport and international politics. The impact of fascism and communism on sport*. London, E & FN Spon.

Coakley, J.J. (1998). *Sport in society. Issues and controversies*. Boston, Massachusetts, WCB, McGraw-Hill.

Riordan, J., and Krüger, A., (1999). *The international politics of sport in the 20th century*. London, E. & FN Spon.

Horne, J., Tomlinson, A., and Whannel, G., (1999). *Understanding sport. An introduction to the sociological and cultural analysis of sport*. London, E & FN Spon.

Bednarik, J., (Ed.), (2001). *Some economic aspects of sport in Slovenia*. Ljubljana, University of Ljubljana, Faculty of Sport.

Riordan J., and Krüger, A., (Eds.), (2003). *European cultures in sport. Examining the nations and regions*. Intellect Books, Bristol, UK

Somewhat counter to this general trend are developments elsewhere in the world. In central and eastern Europe, where 40 years of socialism inhibited exchange of knowledge, and in some Asian and Middle Eastern countries, particularly in those countries not especially subjected to western, particularly American influences, there has been an increase in interest in international and comparative studies in the last decade or so, testimony to which are an Asian Conference on Comparative Physical Education and Sport Symposium organised by the Sport Social Science Branch of the Chinese Sports Science Society in Shanghai with published Proceedings in 1995, more recent biennial International Conferences held in the Islamic Republic of Iran since the late 1990s, journal publications, which carry international and comparative articles (continental regional e.g. *Asian Journal of Physical Education*; national and institutional e.g. *Kinesiology. International Scientific Journal of Kinesiology and Sport* of the Faculty of Physical Education, University of Zagreb, Croatia; *Acta Universitatis Carolinae, "Gymnica"*, of Charles University, Prague, Czech Republic; and *Man-Movement* of the Academy of Physical Education, Wroclaw and Polish Scientific Society of Physical Culture), and translations into Chinese, French, Japanese, Polish and Spanish languages of the Proceedings of the World

Summit on Physical Education, Berlin, 1999. This more positive trend of published articles, which have a comparative, international and cross-cultural focus, can also be observed in other well established and respected international, single, multi- and cross-discipline journals, a selected list of which was included in *International Journal of Physical Education*, volume XXXVIII, Issue 3, 3rd Quarter, 2001 (see Hardman, 2001, p. 99).

A positive development in the comparative field has been the academic, professional, but most significantly, political interest generated in publication of data derived from a range of international, national and regional surveys and longitudinal literature reviews. The ICSSPE supported and International Olympic Committee (IOC) sponsored *World-wide Survey on the State and Status of Physical Education in Schools* (Hardman and Marshall, 2000) preliminary findings, disseminated at the Berlin Physical Education Summit, were used as a basis for formulation of Action Agendas and an appeal to United Nations Educational, Scientific and Cultural Organisation (UNESCO) General Conference and Ministers of Physical Education and Sport (MINEPS) III meeting in Uruguay in late November early December, 1999. It is now a matter of historical record that the 1999 MINEPS III Declaration of Punta del Este endorsed the Berlin Agenda for Action (refer Doll-Tepper and Scoretz, 2001) and called upon member states to implement it. An international and comparative-focused study had helped to place physical education in schools on the world political agenda! A year after the publication of the world-wide survey *Final Report* (Hardman and Marshall, 2000), a Council of Europe Committee for the Development of Sport (CDDS) 'Working Group of Experts' on *Access of Children to Physical Education and Sport* picked up the baton. The Working Group resolved to assess the situation of school physical education and sport in the 48 member states of the Council of Europe with a view to providing informed recommendations for discussion and action at the Informal Meeting of Ministers responsible for Sport in Warsaw, Poland 12-13 September 2002. In the event, the survey data collected for the assessment (Hardman, 2002) prompted a Council of Europe Deputy Secretary General's (Maude De Boer-Buquicchio) comment that "the crux of the issue is that there is too much of a gap between the promise and reality" and drew ministerial *Conclusions* acknowledging a serious decline in the quality and the time allocated for teaching physical education and sport for children and young people in schools as well as inadequate opportunities to participate in recreational sport out of school; additionally, they indicated a need to study ways in which the provision of physical education and sport can be improved in Council of Europe member countries for all children and young people, including those with disabilities.

The international interest in physical education in schools extends beyond UNESCO and the Council of Europe as witnessed in the attention being paid to the situation by the World Health Organisation (WHO) as well as by some national governments and non-governmental agencies. As I prepare this manuscript, a communication from central government's (England)

Department for Culture, Media and Sport (DCMS) Information Centre intimates that it is interested in how many hours on average per week children spend on school sports in other EU countries and whether extra curricular sporting activities are promoted; it also expresses an interest in information on the existence of infrastructures in each country for sports colleges and specialist training for physical education teachers. The interest stems from the Department's aim

> to enhance the take up of sporting opportunities by 5-16 year olds and to increase the percentage of school children in England who spend a minimum of two hours each week on high quality PE and school sport within and beyond the curriculum. What we would like to do is compare UK targets with that of targets in other EU member states" (DCMS, 2003).

In addition to the essentially significant contribution made by ICSSPE, amongst non-governmental agencies, which have either shown, or continue to show, interest in the issues surrounding school physical education are the International Olympic Committee (IOC)[2], Trim and Fitness Sport for All Association (TAFISA)[3], European Non-governmental Sports Organisations (ENGSO)[4], European Physical Education Associations (EUPEA)[5] and European Network of Sport Science, Education and Employment (ENSSEE)[6] at international level. The inclusion of school physical education on intergovernmental and non-governmental agencies' agendas demonstrates the values of engagement in comparative studies: provision of information; increase in knowledge of one's own and others' 'worlds'; and potential facilitation of amelioration.

Concluding Comments

There are mixed messages in regard to the situation of Comparative Physical Education and Sport. Arguably, the situation of comparative physical education at institutional level (i.e. ISCPES) is somewhat fragile at the present time. When seen together, the figures for attendance at the ISCPES 2001 Windsor (actual) and 2003 London (intended) Biennial Conferences and the low membership number levels are indicative of either problems for, and perhaps within, ISCPES or of a generally low status and esteem perception of the genre of comparative study, which continues to challenge the re-oriented ISCPES Journal editorial team. Moreover, the attraction (or not so in this case) of the genre is not dissimilar to that within the International Council of Health, Physical Education, Recreation, Sport and Dance (ICHPER.SD), in which the 'Special Interest Group' for Comparative Studies also suffers from low levels of interest and support. Additionally, the cessation of publication of ISCPES Conference Proceedings and termination of the ISCPES Book Series are suggestive of disinterest in the product, if not the process. For protagonists of the genre, there is sufficient evidence to generate considerable disquiet about the situation. However, as observed earlier, other more academically respected journals do include articles with a comparative/cross-cultural/international perspective or dimension, which have drawn from comparative research methodologies. Moreover, as also observed, an increased interest in thematic topics, which portray either 'first order' or 'true' comparative dimensions, is evident in recent text-book publications and developments in programmes in higher education institutions. There is a sense of *déjà vu* about the 'mixed messages' situation as identified in the introduction to this article with the references to increased interest in scholarly activity on the one hand and neglect on the other.

"Whither Comparative Physical Education and Sport in ISCPES" can play a crucial role here in helping to determine or shape the future of the genre directionally or it can stand by and watch it wither. A fundamental question is what should be done to secure a higher status for comparative studies in physical education and sport? One answer is to accept the situation for what it is and suffer the consequences. The other is to confront the situation and address available options to help resolve some of the problems. The example pertaining to the situation of physical education in schools clearly suggests that comparative data are one imperative in bringing about national, continental regional and international advocacy and action involving significant players and institutions at governmental, inter-governmental and non-governmental levels separately and collectively in striving for amelioration, a key purpose of comparative study! The Berlin Physical Education Summit *Agenda for Action for Government Ministers*, the Punta del Este *Declaration*, the Council of Europe's Warsaw Meeting *Conclusions* and UNESCO's *'Round Table' Communiqué* together with various WHO, IOC, ICSSPE and EUPEA initiatives amongst others demonstrate that there is now an international consensus that issues surrounding physical education in schools deserve serious consideration in order to solve existing and future problems. It is imperative that watching briefs on what is happening (or not as the case may be) in physical education and sport across Europe (beyond the Forum of European Physical Education Association's efforts to monitor the situation) are maintained. Both the Council of Europe's ministerial *Conclusions* and the UNESCO 'Round Table' *Communiqué* called for monitoring systems to be put into place to regularly review the situation of physical education in each country. Indeed, the Council of Europe referred to the introduction of provision for a pan-European survey on physical education policies and practices every five years as a priority! (Bureau of the Committee for the Development of Sport, 2002a; 2002b). Such provision, if realised, will mean the collection of comparative data, which in essence will allow both vertical and horizontal comparisons: the former facilitating a time-period comparison, the latter a contemporary comparison; together they facilitate identification of trends and tendencies.

Notes

1. Earle F. Zeigler, internationally renowned scholar, one of the founders of ISCPES and former co-editor of the Journal.
2. ICSSPE World-wide Survey sponsorship and Berlin PE Summit patron.
3. TAFISA Conference Cape town, South Africa, 2002, Declaration on Sport for All, which includes references to physical education in schools.
4. ENGSO Malta Forum, October 2002, pledged its support for physical education in schools through appropriate partnership advocacy initiatives and demonstrated interest in the EUPEA's recently published *Code of Ethics and Good Practice Guide for Physical Education* to inform its own planned code of ethics and practice for personnel involved in sport.
5. EUPEA 1st Symposium, 9th November 2002 in Brussels on the topical theme of *Quality Physical Education* resulted in the emergence of a number of perceived challenges. In summarising the deliberations of the Symposium, EUPEA Vice-President Chris Laws (2002) concluded that in striving for a relevant physical education curriculum there is a role for all European Physical Education Associations to act to provide *"quality experiences for all children"*. Clearly there is concurrence here with the UNESCO *Communiqué* and the Council of Europe's ministerial *Conclusions*.
6. ENSSEE 7th Forum, 26-29 September 2003 in Lausanne on the theme of *Sport World and Academic World – What Relationship?"* had a main strand, which addressed physical education-related issues in Europe: employment and qualifications; harmonisation of physical education teacher education from a comparative perspective; and the development of an action plan on policies and content for physical education.

References

Bureau of the Committee for the Development of Sport. (2002a).

Draft conclusions on improving physical education and sport for children and young people in all European countries. MSL-IM16 (2002) 5 Rev.3. 16th Informal Meeting of European Sports Ministers, Warsaw, Poland, 12-13 September. Strasbourg, Council of Europe.

Bureau of the Committee for the Development of Sport. (2002b).

Draft conclusions on improving physical education and sport for children and young people in all European countries. Revised by the Drafting Group. MSL-IM16 (2002) 5 Rev.4. 16th Informal Meeting of European Sports Ministers, Warsaw, Poland, 12-13 September. Strasbourg, Council of Europe.

DCMS, (2003). *Personal Communication.*

De Boer-Buqicchio, M. (2002). Opening Address. 16th Informal Meeting of the European Ministers responsible for Sport. Warsaw, 12 September.

Doll-Tepper, G., and Scoretz, D. (2001). Proceedings, "World Summit on Physical Education". Schorndorf, Verlag Karl Hofmann.

Hardman, K., (1999). Developments in Comparative Physical Education and Sport; the contribution of the "International Society for Comparative Physical Education and Sport". *International Journal of Physical Education*, XXXVI (3), 3rd Quarter. pp.88-116.

Hardman, K. (2001). Comparative Physical Education and Sport. *International Journal of Physical Education*, XXXVIII (3), 3rd Quarter. pp.96-103.

Hardman, K. (2002). Council of Europe Survey. Committee for the Development of Sport (CDDS) European Physical Education/Sport Survey. Report on Summary of Findings. Strasbourg, Council of Europe.

Hardman, K., and Marshall, J. (2000). World-wide survey of the state and status of school physical education, Final Report. Manchester, University of Manchester.

Kaulitz, B., (2001). Comparative Physical Education in German publications from mid 1999 until mid 2001. *International Journal of Physical Education*, XXXVIII (3), 3rd Quarter. pp.104-113.

Laws, C. (2002). Report on 1st EUPEA Symposium, Brussels, 9th November 2002. *Personal Communication.*

Part Three
Developing a Body of Knowledge
About Comparative Physical Education and Sport

Selection #7
What Can We Do
About What We Don't Know?

or
Why the Area of International & Comparative Physical Education and Sport Should Employ a Systems Approach to Gather, Assess, and Relate Its Scholarly Development to a Specialized Inventory of Scientific and Scholarly Findings About the Entire Field of Physical Activity Education and Sport

Earle F. Zeigler
Canada

Introduction

The basic premise of this analysis of the present situation is that the large majority of our dedicated practitioners simply *"don't know what they don't know"* about the best ways to carry out their professional practice!

> Note: *This assertion actually applies to the entire field, and here it is being addressed to those who have expressed an ongoing interest in international and comparative physical education and sport.*

Granted that this assertion may sound simplistic and impossible to prove, but it is simply an axiomatic statement to make in today's increasingly complex society. Our well-intentioned professionals have been gradually and steadily overwhelmed by available periodical literature, monographs, and books. This is true whether one is talking about (1) our own field, (2) our allied professions, and (3) our related disciplines. Also, quite probably, most of our practitioners don't fully appreciate this fact either.

"How can this be?", you may ask. It is so—to repeat myself—because the average practitioner simply *"doesn't know what he/she doesn't know!"* Yet, despite this suggested lack, much of this available information could be highly valuable, interesting, and useful to the professional practitioner in physical activity education and educational sport.

It can be argued in rebuttal that such material is often not geared to the interests of professionals who are fulfilling many duties and responsibilities in the various positions they hold. However, this problem is also occurring in the field's allied professions (e.g., recreation management,

142

health education). Whatever the case may be there, there is undoubtedly much overlapping material emanating from these fields that could be helpful to physical education and sport, as well as that emanating from the scholarly production of our related disciplines (e.g., physiology, psychology, history, sociology). Further, much of the available material—when a person by intent or chance happens to discover it—is unintelligible to us, partially understandable, or not available in a condensed, understandable form to the professional in physical education and sport. Thus, one can only conjecture in what form such information will be (or unfortunately *won't be*) conveyed to the public on whose behalf the allied professions presumably carry out their work.

To make matters worse, because of provinciality and communication barriers, our field is usually missing out on important findings originally published in some of the leading tongues in which scholarly work relating to our profession is being reported regularly (e.g., German, Russian, Japanese, and Finnish). Further, because of a plethora of rules, regulations, and stipulations, people may not be receiving information about substantive reports of various government agencies at all levels. The essence of much of this information should become part of personal retrieval systems of those carrying out scholarly work in our subdisciplinary and subprofessional areas of investigation (see Definition of Terms below). It is true, of course, that since 1970 Cambridge Scientific Abstracts (CSA) has offered libraries a service for their users called Physical Education Index that includes abstracts of scholarly articles and research added to monthly. Also, bibliographies of scholarly publications are occasionally made available. However, busy professionals rarely would know how--or take the time--to dig out exactly what they need at the moment.

Still further—and this is really *the* most important point to be made—the profession simply does not know where it stands *cumulatively* in regard to the steadily developing body of knowledge in the many subdisciplinary and subprofessional aspects of physical education and sport. This is why the play on words in the title of this publication is deemed to be correct: We do not know what we do not know! Nowhere does the field have an inventory of scholarly, scientific findings arranged as ordered principles or generalizations to help professionals in their work—be that as teacher, coach, performer, scholar, researcher, supervisor, or administrator. Thus, I believe it is reasonable to state that we now urgently need something like the law profession's *Lexus-Nexus*, or a variation of that service geared to our needs. (See <www.lexus-nexus.com>.)

This deficiency can—and indeed must—be rectified in the near future. Then the professions (?)—AAHPERD, *established as physical education only in 1885*!—should carry such an inventory forward on a yearly or semiannual basis of renewal for all *registered* practitioners to have available on demand. Comprehension of this knowledge in readily available form would be vitally important to the professional practitioner, of course, but the essence of it would ultimately be most important to all people as part of their general education. Initially, however, the profession needs such information to form the basis—the theory, intellectual "underpinning," evidence, body of knowledge—for an evolving professional (practitioner's) loose-leaf handbook that would immediately become an essential component of every person's professional practice in the field of physical education and educational sport. Finally, to implement the proposed development, it would be necessary to gradually implement a systems approach that should result in the rapid development and use of theory and research related to our unique profession.

Along with many other fields, the field of physical education and sport has simply not yet appreciated the need to implement a "total system" concept. However, there are many urgent reasons why a holistic view should be taken if the profession hopes to merit increased public support in the future. Such an approach would soon concern those involved with implementation of the necessary components of a viable system—input, thru put, output, and subsequent user reaction for corrective purposes.

In this analysis of the present situation, after the introductory statement the following topics will be considered in the ordered listed below:

1. Definition of Professional and Disciplinary Terms
2. Past Development and Status of the Field
3. Common Denominators in Program Development
4. A Diagrammatic Representation of the 20th-Century Development of Physical Education/Kinesiology
5. Formulation of a Plan for an inventory
6. An Urgent Need Right Now
7. How an Inventory Could be Constructed
8. The Need for a Systems Approach
9. What Appears to be Needed
10. Summary (to this Point)
11. Professional Essentials: From Bits to Wisdom
12. Definition of Computer Terms
13. How Knowledge Has Been Communicated Historically
14. The Form in Which Knowledge Is Available
15. Where Our Knowledge Is Located
16. A Broad Assessment of the Field's Body of Knowledge)
17. How the Proposed Taxonomy Might Fit into a Model for Optimum Development of a Field Called "Physical (Activity) Education and (Educational) Sport"
18. A Multidiscipline Moving to Cross discipline Status Prior to Inter discipline Status
19. Other Techniques and Services That Are Needed
20. What Ordered Principles or Generalizations Are
21. A Plan Leading Toward an Ever-Expanding Body of

Knowledge Through the Implementation of a
Systems Approach

Definition of Professional and Disciplinary Terms

The basic terms employed here are defined here so that they will be clear to all. Also, since they are often used ambiguously at present, certain terms have been given a specific meaning that needs further clarification. The following, then, are brief definitions of terms used in what is believed to be a logical order for their presentation.

Sport and Physical Education. The term adopted to describe the field by the National Association for Sport and Physical Education (NASPE within AAHPERD).

Physical Activity and Recreation. The term adopted to describe the field by the American Association for Physical Activity and Recreation (AAPAR within AAHPERD)

Research Consortium. The term used to describe a unit composed of scholars and scientists within AAHPERD that serves to encourage and promote scholarly endeavor related the purposes of the Alliance.

Developmental Physical Activity in Sport, Exercise, and Related Expressive Movement. A term recommended for what might be called the *disciplinary* aspect of the field of physical education and sport.

Note: If the term "developmental physical activity" were ever accepted by the field for its disciplinary aspect, logical accompanying terms for the prospective profession and its practitioners might be "physical activity education" and "physical activity educators."

Sub disciplinary Aspects. Those aspects of developmental physical activity (as defined above) that make up a substantive segment of the essential components of the body of knowledge upon which professional practice in physical education and sport is based (e.g., the functional effects of physical activity, which some call exercise physiology).

Subprofessional Aspects. Those aspects of developmental physical activity (as defined above) that make up the remaining segment of the essential components of the body of knowledge upon which professional practice in

145

physical education and sport is based (e.g., program development, measurement and evaluation).

Allied Profession. One of the professions within the American Alliance for Health, Physical Education, Recreation, and Dance that is closely related to the profession of sport and physical education.

Related Discipline. A field of scholarly endeavor or branch of learning, the findings from which should be employed by professionals in physical education and sport as they perform their professional duties and responsibilities (e.g., psychology, history).

Taxonomy. A classification into categories based on natural relationships.

Inventory. A listing, accounting, or catalogue of ideas, facts, things (and as used here of ordered principles and generalizations).

Ordered Principles or Generalizations. A series of verified statements or findings in a 1-2-3-4 arrangement.

Systems Approach. A plan designed for the management of an operation or organization that involves the determination of exactly what is to be accomplished and how such an achievement of objectives may be executed successfully.

Past Development and Status of the Field

Before proceeding with the case being made that teachers and coaches in physical education and educational sport "don't know what they don't know" about the best way to carry out their professional practice, we need to review how the field got itself to this point. In a report to The American Academy of Physical Education (Zeigler, 1979), I traced the history of the development of three categories or subdivisions of the field: (1) the potential body of knowledge as characterized by its subdisciplinary areas, (2) the concurrent professional components of the developing field (found in all subject-matter fields to some extent), and (3) the potential allied professions (such as may also exist for other emerging fields of study of a quasi-disciplinary and quasi-professional nature).

A reasonably balanced disciplinary development was envisioned in the 1960s in the field of physical education, but whether this movement will result ultimately in a more significant professional development for the field remains to be seen. Because there have been so many different interpretations with varying and at times conflicting emphases, the aims and objectives of physical education and its allied professions in the 20th century in North America should be reviewed. The goals of the allied professions (AAHPERD) stated here as "common denominators" are to provide (1)

146

movement fundamentals, (2) regular exercise, (3) health and safety education, (4) physical recreation, (5) physical fitness, (6) competitive sport, and (7) therapeutic exercise (when needed). They are probably accepted by the majority in the several allied professions. If this listing of common denominators is reasonably acceptable, then this presumed agreement—having coming about gradually over a period of decades—has offered certain approaches, emphases, and courses of action for our scholars and researchers to pursue in their work over the past 50 years or so (See Figure 1 below).

During the first half of this century our leaders have espoused a plethora of objectives for the field as they sought to make a case for our greater or lesser "intrusion" into the school, college, and university curricula. Because of our typical defensive posture—a stance almost automatically assumed still today by the large majority—our leaders have felt it necessary to proclaim that an excellent health and physical education program can produce truly remarkable results in children and young people. However, the evidence to support the arguments for these possible accomplishments has not been readily available in sufficient quantity or quality. Quite often we have used missionary zeal to make up for the lack of supportive scientific data. Be that as it may, these educators were dedicated leaders with a certain amount of vision regarding their chosen profession—and they did actually point the way for the coming generation. Notable among these leaders who have defined a variety of objectives, starting in the early 1920s, were Hetherington (1922), Bowen and Mitchell (1923), Wood and Cassidy (1927), Williams (1927), Hughes (with Williams) (1930), Nash, 1931, Sharman (1937), Wayman (1938), Esslinger (1938), Staley (1939), McCloy (1940), Clark (1943), Cobb (1943), Lynn (1944), Brownell & Hagman, Scott, Bucher, Oberteuffer (all in 1951. There have been many fine, earlier statements and some later ones as well (e.g., the names of Metheny, Shepard, Brightbill, and Sapora are also shown in Figure 6.1 below). One could categorize and then enumerate the objectives proposed for the field by category. The resultant list would be impressive as to our subject matter's potential educational contribution. Our professional task today is to ascertain in a scholarly and scientific manner what the effects of planned, developmental physical activity are under a myriad of conditions. Additionally, we need to become more alert in our interpretation of the various social forces impacting on our work as to its effect on acceptable program development for the normal, accelerated, and special populations at all levels for all ages (Zeigler, 2003).

In the late 1950s, Hess (1959) completed a study in which he investigated the objectives of physical education in the United States from 1900 to 1957 in the light of certain historical events. While we must grant a certain subjectivity to this type of historical analysis, this investigation does nevertheless offer us a point of departure when we seek to compare (1) the results of Hess' study, (2) the stated objectives expressed by the various

Figure 6.1

Common Denominators in Physical Education
Program Development in the 20th Century

Statement of Objectives by Leaders (1922-1950s)

Hetherington, Wood & Cassidy, Williams, Hughes.
Bowen & Mitchell, Nash, Sharman, Wayman, Essinger,
Staley, McCloy, Clark, Cobb, Lynn, Bownell, Scott,
Bucher, Oberteuffer, Metheny, N. Shepard, Brightbill,
Sapora

Developing Allied Professions

1. Health Education
2. Safety Education
3. Recreation & Park Administration
4. Dance (Education)
5. Athletics
6. Exercise Therapy

Common Denominators in Program Development

1. Movement Fundamentals
2. Regular Exercise
3. Health & Safety Education
4. Physical Recreation
5. Physical Fitness
6. Competitive Sport
7. Therapeutic Exercise
8. Others? (Zeigler, 1977)

Hess's Objectives of the 20th Century in the Field of Physical Education

Hygiene or Health Objective (1900-1919)
Socio-Educational Objective (1920-1928)
Socio-Recreational Objective (1929-1938)
Physical Fitness & Health Objective (1939-1945)
"Total Fitness & International Understanding (1946-1957)
Disciplinary Development; Sport Experience 1960-???

148

leaders listed, (3) the influence of the several (now) allied professions that were growing rapidly during this 50-year period (keeping in mind that many physical educators favored "being all things to all people"), and (4) the ever-present pivotal social forces operative in the society. The major objectives of the various periods, as identified by Hess, are the following:

1. The hygiene or health objective (1900-1919)
2. The socio-educational objectives (1920-1928)
3. The socio-recreational objectives (1929-1938)
4. The physical fitness and health objectives (1939-1945)
5. The "total fitness" and international understanding objectives (1946-1957) (See Figure 1 at bottom left.)

(**Note:** It was next to impossible for Hess to achieve historical perspective for the 1950s, of course, but he could certainly list several "leading" objectives [which he did]. Also, we should not forget the overlapping nature of these objectives from one period to another—or even to the next period beyond that.)

The influence of physical education's allied professions on the objectives of physical education is an interesting question in itself. Each of these professions had dedicated adherents who were working to have their embryonic profession both well and fairly represented within the health and physical education curriculum of the first half century. At the same time they were looking forward to the day when separate, fully independent status might be granted to their particular field (or subject-matter) with resultant increased curricular time allotment. These allied professions have been identified as the following:

1. Health education
2. Safety education (including driver education)
3. Recreation and parks administration
4. Dance (education)
5. Competitive athletics (interscholastic & intercollegiate *and* intramurals and recreational sports, with the latter now striving for its own professional identity and with a significant number wanting to call it "campus recreation")
6. Adapted or special physical education (See left middle of Figure 1.)

Common Denominators in Program Development.

Interestingly, even as each of these allied professions (listed immediately above) was developing to a point where it saw clearly its own program objectives (and therefore felt it necessary to break free from a direct relationship with physical education), each nevertheless has had a greater or lesser influence on the stated objectives of physical education in the 20th century. These presumably consensual objectives offer an indication of this influence on what toward the middle of the century was designated as physical education at all educational levels. Further, it is highly interesting to note that—even today with only slight modification—these "common denominators" of human motor performance within what is here being called "physical activity education" in sport, exercise, and expressive movement are still intact and we find considerable agreement on them all over the civilized world:

1. That regular physical education and sport periods be required for all children and young people up to and including 16 years of age.

2. That human movement fundamentals through various expressive activities are basic in the elementary, middle, and high school curricula.

3. That physical vigor and endurance are important for people of all ages. Progressive standards should be developed from prevailing norms.

4. That remediable defects should be corrected through exercise therapy at all school levels. Where required, adapted sport and physical recreation experiences should be stressed.

5. That a young person should develop certain positive attitudes toward his or her own health in particular and toward community hygiene in general. Basic health knowledge should be an integral part of the school curriculum.

(Note: This "common denominator" should be a specific objective of the profession of sport and physical education only as it relates to developmental physical activity.)

150

6. That sport, exercise, and expressive movement can make a most important contribution throughout life toward the worthy use of leisure.

7. That boys and girls (and young men and women) should have an experience in competitive sport at some stage of their development.

8. That character and/or personality development is vitally important to the development of the young person, and therefore it is especially important that all human movement experience in sport, exercise, and expressive movement at the various educational levels be guided by men and women   with high professional standards and ethics.

(See right side of Figure 1 above.)

Note: See, also, Zeigler, 1989, pp. 185-186, for an elaboration of these proposed common denominators.)

A Diagrammatic Representation of the 20th-Century Development of Physical Education/Kinesiology

In an effort to make this initial historical analysis even more clear, I combined the narrative with appropriate diagrams dating back to 1900 and concluded with diagrammatic figures and tables indicating what should now begin to happen. My hope is that physical education-kinesiology will now sharpen its focus and delimit its aims and objectives as it seeks to serve humankind more efficiently and effectively in the 21st century.

Stage I–Physical Education–circa 1900-1930. In this analysis of the emerging physical education field dating back at the beginning of the 20th century within the public education system primarily, three subdivisions (or categories) of the field will be traced as follows:

1. The *potential body-of-knowledge* as characterized by its sub-disciplinary areas (e.g., anatomical and physio-logical aspects)
2. The *concurrent professional components* of the developing field such as exist in all subject-matter fields (e.g., curriculum, methods of instruction
3. The *potential allied professions* (e.g., health education, competitive athletics)

(See Figure 2 below; note that the sub-disciplinary names in the diagrams use the names of other disciplines (e.g., physiology, psychology), but that toward the end of the study a recommendation is made to only employ those names that do *not* "give our field away" to another established discipline.)

Figure 2 describes the situation for the period extending from app. 1900 to app. 1930 (or Stage 1). It indicates that the sub-disciplinary areas are "blurred" and almost indistinguishable within the center of the circle depicting physical education. It is true that professional students of that time received instruction in anatomy and physiology, as well as in chemistry and physics, prior to the required professional physical education courses identified, for example, as physiology of exercise, kinesiology, anthropometry, physical examination and diagnosis, massage, history of physical training, emergencies, and medical gymnastics (*Oberlin College Catalogue* for 1894). However, the strong point to be made here is that there were (1) basic science courses and (2) professional physical education courses. Instruction in the so-called "academic courses" was almost completely lacking. It was true, very importantly, that certain professors (instructors) had areas of specialization (e.g., Fred Leonard in physical education history; Delphine Hanna in medical gymnastics), but the very large majority of these people *saw themselves as physical educators*—not as specialists in some other disciplinary subject-matter within the college or university.

> (Note: We should mention the "M.D. phenomenon" in our early history. For example, a person such as James H. McCurdy, M.D., recognized that our embryonic profession needed people with "scientific ability who will increase our knowledge with reference especially to bodily growth, to personal hygiene, to physiology of exercise, etc." [McCurdy, 1901, pp. 311-312].)

The "potential allied professions" were also "blurred" and almost indistinguishable within the center of the circle depicting physical education in Figure 2. For example, in the *Wellesley College Catalogue* for 1910, athletics (no.1 under potential allied professions) is included in the requirements for the Bachelor of Arts degree in Physical Education under the heading of "Professional Courses" by virtue of a two-hour course in "organized sports," a three-hour course in "athletics" (presumably track and field), and a three and one-half hour course in "outdoor games and athletics."

Health education (no. 2) is included as "Reg. A.B. Hygiene" for one hour, and dance (education) (no. 3) is listed as "dancing" for one or two hours. Recreation (no.4) could conceivably be regarded as <u>physical</u> recreation insofar as sports activities were offered within the physical education curriculum. Adapted exercise (therapy) (no. 5) appeared as "corrective gymnastics and massage" for one hour. Finally, the only reference to safety education (no. 6) was a course experience called "emergencies" for one hour. Thus, if you will check Figure 2 above again, you will note (1) that the sub-disciplinary areas (A, B, C, D, E, and F) are very close together in the center of the core depicting physical education as a field; (2) the potential allied professions (shown as 1, 2, 3, 4, 5, and 6) are firmly attached, or closely spaced

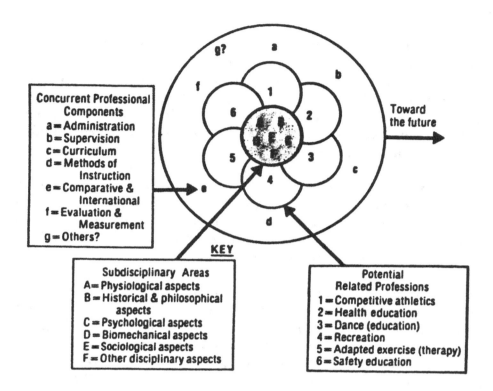

Figure 6.2

Stage One--1900-1930

next to, the core of the diagram; and (3) the concurrent professional components (a, b, c, d, e, f, and g) are simply indicated as belonging in the larger circle (similar to the way that they will be shown in subsequent diagrams).

Stage 2—Physical Education—circa 1930-1960. In Figure 3 below, which represents roughly the period from 1930 to 1960, we find that there has actually been considerable change within the field still known as "physical education." However, the sub-disciplinary areas are beginning to emerge from the core depicted in Figure 2 above. The typical tests and measurements course, for example, was gradually characterized by an improved laboratory experience, often largely physical fitness/exercise physiology in nature. These were soon supplemented by motor learning and kinesiology laboratory experiences as well. There was kinematic analysis of human movement in sport and exercise, but the first doctoral study involving kinetic analysis had not yet been carried out. Sport and physical education sociology had not yet appeared on the scene, nor had the social psychological analysis of sport and physical activity surfaced to any recognizable extent.

There were a great many historical theses, including many biographies, but by and large the historical studies were not characterized by the use of an *interpretive criterion* to evaluate the evidence that had been gathered. The biographical studies were interesting and usually substantive, but the subject of such an investigation typically emerged with such a large halo around his/her head that one wondered whether the author was somehow a relative of the subject of the thesis! Early philosophical studies were not impressive theoretically, although in the mid-1940s and the fifties they improved and were similar to studies being carried out in educational philosophy. Occasionally the question was being asked by scholars like C.H. McCloy, and others who decried "nonscientific" studies, as to how long a field could expect to prosper as a profession when the bulk of its research was carried on through the medium of doctoral dissertations.

Shifting attention to the designated "concurrent professional components," there were a large number of doctoral studies that could be characterized as *administrative* in nature. Many of these were helpful and provided useful information, but as Spaeth reported, "there is an almost total lack of theoretical orientation in the design of research and interpretation of the findings in the sample of administrative research studied." She stated further, "the administrative research lacked the methodological rigor necessary for contributions to the development of scientific knowledge about administrative performance" (Spaeth in Zeigler and Spaeth, 1975, p. 44). With exceptions, of course, much the same can probably be said for the studies carried out in the components identified as "supervision," "curriculum," and "instruction."

154

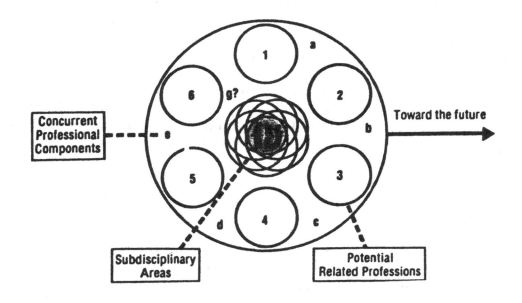

Figure 6.3

Stage Two--1930-1960

It is important to keep in mind, however, that these are usually types of investigation employing a variety of techniques under descriptive research methodology. In such cases it is often not possible nor desirable to emerge from these studies with a coefficient of correlation or a multiple correlation—not to mention results available from employment of a factor-analysis technique. International and comparative research in sport and physical education was practically nonexistent from the standpoint of the use of even relatively complex social science methodology and accompanying techniques. The final category listed here ("measurement and evaluation") was viewed more as part of the sub-disciplinary efforts of our experimentally oriented scientists. It was therefore tied in with those interested in the physiological, kinesiology, and psychological aspects (i.e., motor learning) of physical education. Today it is being used more as a tool subject that may be used by almost any researcher in the field carrying out an investigation based on the natural sciences, the social sciences, or even the humanities.

Finally, then, in this period from 1930 to 1960, the "potential allied professions" will be considered briefly. Further examination of Figure 3, which is called Stage 2 of this 20th-century analysis, indicates that the "allied professions," which were firmly attached to (and literally part of) physical education, had by then moved out of its inner core. By 1960, these potential allied professions—i.e., competitive athletics, school health education, dance (education), (community) recreation, adapted exercise (therapy), and safety education—have clearly established their own identities. Indeed, in some cases they had even established a separate identity within the field of education, not to mention the recognition that had been accorded to them in the society at large.

Stage 3—Physical Education (and Sport)—circa 1960-1970. Some people can recall vividly the events of the 1960s both within society in general and within physical education specifically. Our graduate study programs were attacked by President Conant of Harvard University; responded to by Dean Arthur Esslinger, University of Oregon on our behalf. The field soon developed an incomplete understanding of the need for a substantive body-of-knowledge to under gird our professional efforts. A notable undertaking, still operative in an altered format, was the Big Ten Body-of-Knowledge Project as conceived by Arthur Daniels, Indiana University) and followed through to fruition by King McCristal (UnIversity of Illinois) and some of us who were present at the time. The sub-disciplinary areas included in this undertaking were (1) sociology of sport and physical education; (2) administrative theory; (3) history, philosophy, and comparative physical education and sport; (4) exercise physiology; (5) biomechanics; and (6) motor learning & sport psychology (Zeigler, ed., 1975, p. 292).

The sub-disciplinary areas shown in Figure 4 below are similar, the only difference being that certain sub-disciplinary areas are indicated as concurrent professional components (e.g., administrative theory). The

156

significant point to be made, however, is that the sub-disciplinary areas themselves have moved from the central core of physical education in the earlier diagrams to a position not unlike the positions held earlier by the potential allied professions. These sub-disciplinary areas (e.g., so-called sociology of sport) were indeed moving strongly away from physical education toward the end of the 1960-1970 decade. The position of sport sociology, soon followed by other sub-disciplinary societies being established. reminded one of the "floating apex" of Peter Principle notoriety. They had gone off to function by themselves without any under girding organizational support of the mother discipline of sociology—much less the field of physical education. Thus, it was essentially unrecognized by the societal entities that they purported to describe—i.e., sport or sociology.

Further examination of Figure 4 in regard to the movement of the potential allied professions shows that all six of the field have moved further in the direction of establishing their own identity even within educational circles. It is impossible to describe *precisely* where each of these professions concerned was located, but it was clear that further movement away from the field of physical education had been taken.

Examination of the concurrent professional components for the period from 1960-1970–components which by their very nature are inextricably linked to the professional development of physical educators—brings to light some interesting developments as well. For example, we saw the introduction of a more theoretical orientation in these topics on the part of a relatively few graduate programs. Typically, the concept of supervision had merged more completely with the larger realm of overall administration. The subject of curriculum (i.e., program development) received somewhat more attention generally, and several scholars led the way in giving this topic a more theoretical orientation than previously. The same can be said for the topic "methods of instruction," but this professional component did not receive noticeably more attention during this decade. (A few professors reacted to what they considered to be the overemphasis of the sub-disciplinary orientation by a very small segment of the total population of physical educators in the United States. As a result, they cast their lots with what they called a "professional preparation" approach to both undergraduate and graduate education in the field. It could be argued that this "move" was simply an improved, more precise approach to what the large majority of college and universities had been emphasizing for decades.

Stage 4—Physical Education (and Sport—circa 1970-2000. Stage 4, as explained in Figure 5 below, treats the period from 1970 to 2000 and, as we can readily appreciate, it is extremely difficult to gain a true perspective on the happenings of this recent 20-year period. Nevertheless, some of the developments that began in previous decades did indeed continue along apace, and so several reasonably accurate observations may be possible.

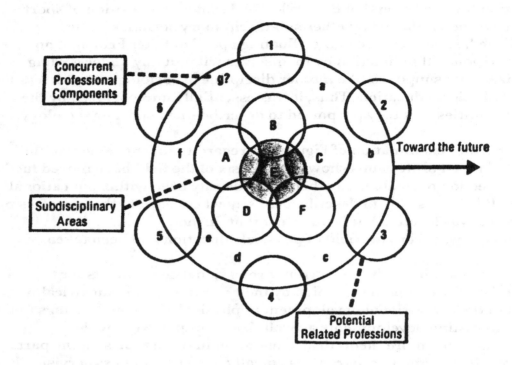

Figure 6.4

Stage Three--1960-1970

For example, the sub-disciplinary areas that were moving strongly away from involvement with physical education at the professional-conference level have continued with their movement in the direction of the respective mother disciplines (e.g., sport history and sport philosophy). However the movement of those who called themselves sport philosophers was "sharper" in nature, whereas the North American Society for Sport History still provides a "comfortable atmosphere" for those with an historical interest in physical education to convene. This trend has continued despite the fact that the very large majority of these people received their graduate training in what were called physical education units and—where some money was still available—received their travel funds from the same units as well.

Also, although many within the larger professional associations in both the United States and Canada have been aware of this departure of many scholars, it has been difficult to know whether to ignore this development or to attempt to reverse it. We did witness the creation of a number of sub-disciplinary *and* sub-professional "academies" within our professional association. In the United States the AAHPERD, recognizing the growing impact of the term "sport," established the entity now known as the National Association for Sport and Physical Education. (It should be noted that, still in the 1990s, the large majority of conferences held on other continents, including those with a worldwide orientation, typically employ the word "sport" in their terminology in one way or another along with the term "physical education."

Viewed overall, it can be argued that the six potential allied professions have almost completely consolidated their positions either within or outside of educational circles. The American *Association* for Health, Physical Education, and Recreation recognized this independent growth of the allied professions by changing its name to the American *Alliance* for Health, Physical Education, and Recreation. Then, just before the turn of the 1980s decade, the Alliance Board of Governors officially added the word "dance" to the official title and it became AAHPERD. This action culminated a period in which a number of dance units within colleges and universities moved, or sought permission to move, out of the physical education unit per se to some other educational entity on campus (e.g., music). Thus, whether the topic is about competitive athletics, health education, dance (education), recreation (education), safety education, or even adapted exercise (therapy), it became obvious that most of those people who came to relate primarily to one or the other of these allied professions want to be free from what they identify as the "PE" or "fizz-ed" stigma.

During this recent period, there doesn't appear to have been a considerable amount of change in the concurrent professional components shown in Figure 5 as Stage 4 of this 20th century "plus" analysis. The term "management" began to gain acceptance in the latter half of the 1970s in the

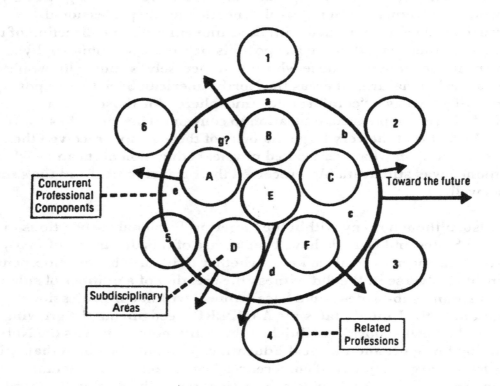

Figure 6.5

Stage Four--1970-1990

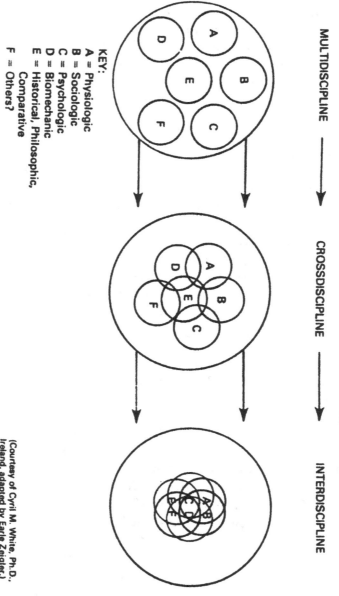

MULTIDISCIPLINE → CROSSDISCIPLINE → INTERDISCIPLINE

KEY:
A = Physiologic
B = Sociologic
C = Psychologic
D = Biomechanic
E = Historical, Philosophic, Comparative
F = Others?

(Courtesy of Cyril M. White, Ph.D., Ireland, adapted by Earle Zeigler.)

Figure 6.6

Physical Education: A Multi-Discipline on the Way toward Becoming a Cross-Discipline

business world with the term "administration" in decline. Sport management curricula in universities began to spring up in the 1980s. However, it was only after the establishment of the North American Society for Sport Management (and its official journal) in the latter half of the decade that there was evidence of the need for improving both the theoretical and practical components of professional preparation in this aspect of the field.

Also, a small, stalwart band of curriculum theorists continued to strive for careful investigation into the intricacies of this aspect of physical education's professional program. Further, and fortunately for those interested in professional preparation, the inclusion of curriculum (or program) development and instructional methodology, coincided with higher education institutions' continuance of their drive for an improved level of instructional competency by all professors. This movement had been sparked originally by the clamor of students in the 1960s. Then it was perpetuated by the continuing "aim to please" trend within universities occasioned by ongoing financial constraints that began in the 1970s as they strove to preserve the student head-count. Such constraints had become even more constricting by the beginning of the 1990s.

The remaining two professional components to be considered within Stage 4 are "international and comparative" and "measurement and evaluation." First, there was a relatively small, ever-loyal, insightful group of professionals keeping the former area alive within the "physical education and sport" component of the Alliance, as well as the ongoing International Council for Health, Physical Education, and Recreation (ICHPER.) Also a relatively small, but dedicated international group of professionals functioned as the International Society for Comparative Physical Education and Sport. However, the amount of scholarly investigation carried out overall in this aspect of our professional endeavor must be categorized as minimal throughout the 1970-2000 period. Physical education's professional growth internationally was undoubtedly limited, this at a time when it appears vital that there be more not less involvement with our colleagues abroad. However, there is no doubt but that a good deal of cross-fertilization does occur with the international meetings and symposia, as well as in the sub-disciplinary societies at their international meetings. The knowledge engendered at these international conferences is often available through journals to practicing professionals everywhere, but the extent to which they are read is debatable. It was obvious at that time that much more needed to be done in this regard.

Measurement and evaluation, typically packaged earlier in the required tests and measurement course, was still an important part of undergraduate professional preparation in physical education at the end of the 1970s. However, during that decade it became diffused in many programs at the graduate level into the various sub-disciplinary or subprofessional streams available. Thereafter a similar development occurred at the undergraduate level at well. There are some universities that offer it as an area of specialization at the graduate level, and there are universities who maintain a "measurement and evaluation professor" (i.e., allot a percentage of this person's workload) to service students and/or colleagues needing advice insofar as research design and statistical techniques are concerned. The feeling seems to be that it is a physical impossibility to do a good job of packaging the several, broad research methodologies and the multitude of accompanying research techniques under one specific course. There is some merit in this argument, but I believe that the student is being shortchanged with this approach and resultantly does not understand the "big picture" in regard to overall scholarly research.

Stage 5—Physical Education/Kinesiology—2000-????. We have finally arrived at the point where we are in a position to conjecture *about*, and possibly prescribe *for*, the future of the field of physical education-kinesiology as we move along in the 21st century. By combining these two terms in this way, the current position seems to be that "physical (activity) education" is what the professional practitioner does, and kinesiology, or the study of movement, is where the under girding knowledge resides.

Before continuing, it will be necessary to retrogress for a moment to Figure 4 (Stage 3—1960-1970) above where it was explained that the various sub-disciplinary groups began to move significantly away from what might be called the "central core" of the physical education profession during that decade. It was at that point that Cyril White, an Irish sport sociologist studying at Illinois, offered the idea that our field might be moving from status as a *multidiscipline* to that of a *cross discipline* on the way toward becoming an *inter discipline* (Zeigler, 1975, pp. 350-51). He postulated that the profession's "future development to interdisciplinary level will require a far greater degree of sophisticated research abilities and orientations than the field at present possesses." The idea was intriguing, but it simply was not happening that way at that time, and thus seemed completely out of phase with the development taking place. Somewhat later, Philip Sparling (then of Georgia Tech) opined that the field was moving in the opposite direction. Time has shown that Sparling may indeed have been right in his judgment! (See Figure 6 below.)

To compound further what is already a complex situation, we as a field are not moving rapidly enough to what may be called true professional status. By that is meant a profession that is recognized both within education and in society at large as one that "professes" physical (activity) education to people of all ages and conditions based on the study of developmental physical activity. Those teachers functioning in the public schools can, of course, comfort themselves with an understanding that they will be sheltered indefinitely by the protective arm of the teaching profession. Others in the

163

field professing some aspect of physical (activity) education (i.e., strength fitness coaching) have taken these other more specific professional titles believing that society at large will not recognize physical activity education as that profession which it could or should be—i.e., the leading force physical activity education in exercise, sport, and related expressive movement. Whatever the facts in the matter may be, there is no escaping one discouraging fact that—despite our *unique* mission—we are, along with art and music typically at the bottom of the totem pole in educational circles. Additionally, we are missing the opportunity to become the profession of which we are capable and, along with this omission, are thereby deprived of any accompanying social recognition and support that would otherwise be our lot.

It is for these reasons, therefore, that a Stage 5 is postulated here for the profession's consideration. Vigorous steps need to be taken by the leading professional associations (i.e., NASPE) and the newly created American Association for Physical Activity and Recreation (AAPAR) both within the Alliance (the latter a combination of several former groups), along with university and college personnel active in the independent National Association for Kinesiology and Physical Education in Higher Education (NAKPEHE) in higher education circles. It is conceivable and possible that a strong, coordinated thrust would lead to a trend that would be soon recognized and could lead to a much stronger profession under girded by a body-of-knowledge generated by the scholars and researchers of our present *cross discipline*. The field might then relatively soon be on the way to becoming an *inter discipline* as postulated by White.

This recommended development is explained in Figure 7 below. The reader will notice immediately as the diagram is examined that the *sub-disciplinary areas*, instead of continuing along with their movement for greater identification with the *related* disciplines, have been persuaded to function more strongly *within* the field of physical education/kinesiology and are firmly attached to the profession's core—explained as a developing body-of-knowledge about the theory and practice of movement or physical activity in exercise, sport, and related expressive movement. Obviously, persuading these groupings (NASPE, AAPAR, NAKPEHE [outside of AAHPERD!]) to move solidly and soundly to a position of direct alliance or affiliation will be a tall order, but it could be done by means of persuasion, encouragement, influence, and even "bribery" if necessary.

The present situation cries out for the following to occur:

(1) the scholars and researchers of our field identifying and
     working strongly with the professional associations and

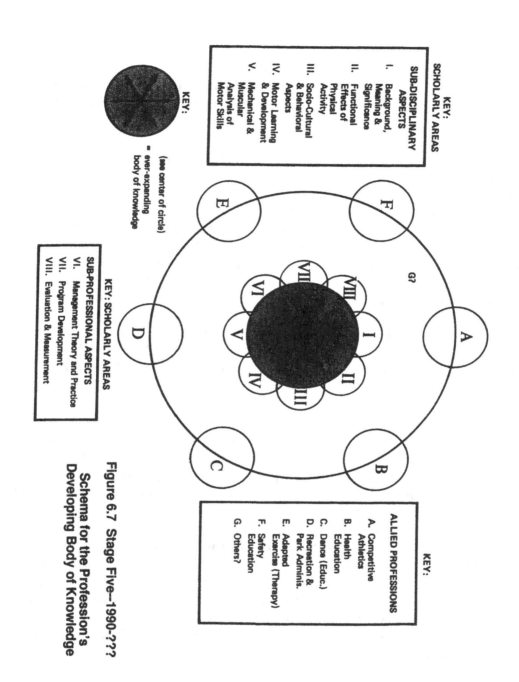

KEY:
SUB-DISCIPLINARY ASPECTS
SCHOLARLY AREAS

I. Background, Meaning & Significance
II. Functional Effects of Physical Activity
III. Socio-Cultural & Behavioral Aspects
IV. Motor Learning & Development
V. Mechanical & Muscular Analysis of Motor Skills

KEY:

■ (see center of circle)
= ever-expanding body of knowledge

KEY: SUB-PROFESSIONAL ASPECTS
SCHOLARLY AREAS

VI. Management Theory and Practice
VII. Program Development
VIII. Evaluation & Measurement

KEY:
ALLIED PROFESSIONS

A. Competitive Athletics
B. Health Education
C. Dance (Educ.)
D. Recreation & Park Adminis.
E. Adapted Exercise (Therapy)
F. Safety Education
G. Others?

Figure 6.7 Stage Five—1990-???
Schema for the Profession's
Developing Body of Knowledge

165

(2) the leaders of the professional associations recognizing that the future of the profession *requires* the under-girding sound knowledge that only scholars and researchers can provide.

As matters stand, neither set of groupings (guided by their own leaders) sees the need for such a development. We has been hand-wringing over the dispersion that is occurring, but the leaders haven't made it clear that the profession needs a concerted effort to assure a future that embodies professional status of a higher order. Frankly, keeping all of the characteristics typically ascribed to a full-fledged profession in mind, the field of physical (activity) education and (educational) sport—in addition to being a subject-matter within the teaching profession—is presently a "glorified trade" with potential to become a true profession!-If or **when** it organizes itself sufficiently to provide its practitioners with tenable theory about lifelong developmental physical activity based on ongoing high-level scholarly endeavor, that could make all the difference Further, any such resultant body-of-knowledge needs to be made available as *ordered generalizations* that can be readily understood and applied by our professional practitioners.

If the *sub-disciplinary areas* of our to-be-hoped-for cross-discipline/inter discipline can be brought to conform with the proposal made in Figure 7, what about the *concurrent professional components*? In this instance we are fortunately not in a position where we will have to retrieve these elements from other professional organizations far removed from our midst. Our task here is to simply follow the lead to a greater extent of those scholarly people who have played leadership roles in (1) curriculum and program development, (2) instructional methodology, (3) measurement and evaluation, (4) (international and comparative physical education and sport, and (5) management theory. If their investigations are well executed, such scholarly efforts need to be recognized equally along with the work of those in the sub-disciplinary areas. Thus, these components have been left importantly within the circle that describes the total field of physical education/kinesiology.

Within AAHPERD we are, of course, faced with the continuing problem of our relationship with what have been described as the (potential) *allied professions*. The Alliance has made steady progress in this regard; on October 1, 1992 a three-year transition to full implementation of a new organizational model was undertaken. It was "intended to maximize autonomy of functioning for the national associations (the Alliance program arm), maintain autonomy for the district associations, and at the same time preserve the Alliance umbrella and the potential for synergistic mission accomplishment inherent in such an organization" (*Update*, April, 1993, 1).

This plan was executed to insure that these related professions stay firmly allied to the Alliance. We can do this best, of course, (1) by making the members of these associations (e.g., the National Dance Association) feel completely at home within the Alliance and by demonstrating through our actions that we are proud of the early role that physical education played in assisting them to develop to the point where separate professional status was the next feasible step for them to take; (2) by improving the quantity and quality of our own scholarly endeavor so that they will feel proud to be allied with us; and (3) by relating in cross-disciplinary fashion to those scholars in each of these related professions at those points where joint research effort can be rewarding to all involved.

The sub disciplinary areas identified at that time included the physiological, historical and philosophical, psychological, biomechanical, and sociological aspects. (There may be other disciplinary aspects that should be considered today.) The concurrent or sub professional components were determined to be administration and supervision; curriculum and methods of instruction; comparative and international relations; measurement and evaluation, etc. (The potential allied professions that had begun to emerge early in the 20th century were competitive athletics, (school) health education, dance (education), recreation, special physical education (adapted or corrective exercise), and safety education.

Summarizing Statement. The evidence indicated the following for the four time periods examined (i.e., from 1900-1930, 1930-1960, 1960-1970, and 1970-2000):

> (1) that there had been a strong disciplinary thrust in the 1960s that tended to swing the field's research efforts away from a scholarly consideration of problems faced by the practicing professional in the field (e.g., evaluation, program development, management);

> (2) that during the 1970s the sub disciplines that were moving from physical education continued to move toward their "mother" disciplines (*not* their counterparts within schools of professional education);

> (3) that the six potential allied professions continued the consolidation of their positions outside physical education departments and similar units at college and university levels; and

> (4) that there was little change in the so-called concurrent, sub professional components as delineated above (e.g., instructional methodology).

By this latter point (#4), it is meant that people specifically interested in these aspects of the field maintained a relationship with the field of physical (activity) education and (educational) sport represented by the National Association for Sport and Physical Education within the larger Alliance (now the AAHPERD).

Tracing the history of the field throughout the 20th century permitted me to develop insight into what might be recommended as the best curricular taxonomy to be adopted for the future—or at least until changing conditions warrant a further reappraisal. In developing such a proposal, the recommendations of earlier national conferences on professional preparation in physical education held in North America were reviewed. Specifically, a careful analysis was carried out of the recommendations for physical education emanating from the 1967 Graduate Study Conference sponsored by the AAHPER (the acronym used before Dance was added in the masthead. I correlated this developing analysis with the thought of the late Laura J. Huelster, Professor-Emerita, University of Illinois, Urbana-Champaign (the chair of the 1967 national graduate study conference).

An examination of the proposed taxonomy's outline, upon which the recommended inventory was to be based, reveals that there is a balanced approach in regard to the emphasis placed on the sub disciplinary and sub professional aspects. By this is meant that full status is accorded to the latter aspects on the assumption that appropriate research methodology and accompanying techniques will be developed and fully employed to provide the field with its body of knowledge in these sub professional aspects (e.g., program development, measurement and evaluation). The position taken was that the then-growing rift in the field, as identified by the 1979 study, should be narrowed considerably and even eliminated if possible. The recommendation was that a reasonable, workable taxonomy should be integrated with an evolving inventory through the implementation of a systems approach in an effort to close the gap between the profession and what was emerging from the field's contributing sub-disciplines (e.g., exercise physiology, sport sociology.

Building on the 1979 historical analysis, in Table 1 above (see left-hand column) there is a classification of the areas of scholarly study

With this recommendation of taxonomy for the profession in Table 1 above, therefore, a strong recommendation is being made that *the field of physical (activity) education and (educational) sport—developmental physical activity as explained 'disciplinarily' in Table 1—should promote and develop its own unique disciplinary effort.* At the same time, the field should work cooperatively with what are here being called its allied professions (e.g.,

Table 1
DEVELOPMENTAL PHYSICAL ACTIVITY IN SPORT, EXERCISE, AND RELATED EXPRESSIVE MOVEMENT

Areas of Scholarly Study & Research	Subdisciplinary Aspects	Subprofessional Aspects
I. BACKGROUND, MEANING, & SIGNFICANCE	-History -Philosophy -International & Comparative Study	-International Relations -Professional Ethics
II. FUNCTIONAL EFFECTS OF PHYSICAL ACTIVITY	-Exercise Physiology -Anthropometry & Body Composition	-Fitness & Health Appraisal -Exercise Therapy
III. SOCIO-CULTURAL & BEHAVIORAL ASPECTS	-Sociology -Economics -Psychology (individ. & social) -Anthropology -Political Science -Geography	-Application of Theory to Practice
IV. MOTOR LEARNING & CONTROL	-Psycho-motor Learning -Physical Growth & Development	-Application of Theory to Practice
V. MECHANICAL & MUSCULAR ANALYSIS OF MOTOR SKILLS	-Biomechanics -Neuro-skeletal Musculature	-Application of Theory to Practice
VI. MANAGEMENT THEORY & PRACTICE	-Management Science -Business Administration	-Application of Theory to Practice
VII. PROGRAM DEVELOPMENT	-Curriculum Studies	-Application of Theory to Practice

(General education; professional preparation; intramural sports and physical recreation; intercollegiate athletics; programs for special populations--e.g., handicapped--including both curriculum and instructional methodology)

VIII. EVALUATION & MEASUREMENT	-Measurement Theory	-Application of Theory to Practice

recreation) and its related disciplines (e.g., exercise physiology). The rationale for our profession's strong promotion of its own unique disciplinary effort is simple and straightforward: if people in our field always speak of exercise physiology, sociology of sport, psychology of sport, etc., it will just be a matter of time before certain trained scholars in these related disciplines wake up to the research opportunities available in developmental physical activity in exercise, sport, and related expressive activities. One reason for the hastening of this transformation is undoubtedly the increasing attention the media pay to sport and exercise because of their overall cultural importance.

Such realization has its good side, of course, but at the same time it is deleterious to physical (activity) education's and (educational) sport's own desire for professional status and recognition. In the past 40 years or so, we have witnessed the organization of a multitude of what I am calling sub disciplinary societies. The membership of these sub disciplinary societies (e.g., the North American Society for Sport History, the North American Society for Sport Psychology) came initially to a great degree from the field of physical education, people holding degrees in physical education with a few courses in their background from a related discipline (e.g., physiology, psychology, philosophy, history). For a variety of reasons, a smaller percentage of the membership of any of these societies came from the related discipline itself.

Of course this trend did (and still does!) seem to represent a conscious position taken by many working at the college and university level who on occasion seemed ashamed to be receiving their paychecks from what an entity called the department of a physical education. Some of this contingent quite obviously wanted to call themselves exercise physiologists or sport philosophers (or whatever, respectively). The important point was that the name of the related discipline was mentioned and the name of physical education was omitted—especially when research grants were being applied for. The term "kinesiology" subsequently "came to the rescue." It had often been used before, or in place of, the term "physical education." In discussion with a number of these men and women, some argued that our field is really not a discipline in itself, that it is actually a subdivision of the education profession. These people have a right to their beliefs, of course, but this development has caused a "debilitating fractionation" that resulted in our emerging field's status being downgraded. (In the Province of Newfoundland in Canada recently, for example, the new premier of the province was characterized by the press as a "gym teacher and fiddler" because he was teaching physical education and played the violin as a hobby.

I am taking the position here, however, that the ultimate goal of the field should be full-fledged status as a profession. I argue that educating people of all ages—"womb to tomb" either within the educational system or in the public domain—can be carried out best by us—*with the help of the allied professions and the related sub-disciplines*. Further, if our field's members must wait for other in the related disciplines to do this for them on a piecemeal basis, such development and possible accompanying recognition of the importance of purposeful physical activity within the lifestyle of the "evolving human animal" will come belatedly. Still further, it would be less effective because of poor interdisciplinary and inter-professional articulation. In fact, one of our allied professions with AAHPERD has already moved in the direction of physical education and educational sport's duties and responsibility outside of the formal educational system AAPAR (as explained under Definitions above). This development can be beneficial so long as these two associations work cooperatively—one within education and one in society at large—to provide physical activity experiences for all people of all ages and conditions under the rubric of *developmental physical activity*.

Formulation of a Plan for an inventory

What Can We Do About What We Don't Know?, the title of this monograph, brings us directly to the idea of developing some sort of an inventory of scientific findings about a subject-matter, in this case developmental physical activity in exercise, sport, and related expressive movement. This idea is not unique to our field. Bernard Berelson and Gary Steiner implemented such an inventory more than 40 years ago for what they called "the behavioral sciences." In their publication, *Human Behavior: An Inventory of Scientific Findings* (1964), the editors and various associates reported, integrated, assessed, and classified "the results of several decades of the scientific study of human behavior (p. 3). The basic plan of this formidable undertaking was fundamentally sound. Thus, many of their ideas concerning format could be employed in the development of a scientific inventory of findings about developmental physical activity. Actually, it could well be carried out in all of the world's existing disciplines and then updated at regular intervals on a worldwide basis in one or more agreed-upon languages. Of course, varying emphases and certain significant differences might be introduced, but the basic approach is still valid. Berelson and Steiner summarized their task as the development of *"important statements of proper generality for which there is some good amount of scientific evidence"* (p. 5).

The allied professions of health, physical education, and recreation (dance education was not indicated separately at the time) can take some pride in the fact that certain early steps had indeed been taken about this same time of an "inventory nature." It was titled "The Contributions of Physical Activity to Human Well-Being" (*Research Quarterly*, 1960). This fine contribution of the Research Council, chaired by Dr. Raymond Weiss, of the (then) American Association for Health, Physical Education, and Recreation described the status of the profession's research knowledge at that point. The Council's intent was "to inquire into the validity of objectives which have been endorsed in our allied professions. The supplement will serve to consolidate the evidence for these objectives and to point the way for further research" (Foreword). The allied fields referred to were health education, physical education, and recreation. Each section's title began with the words "The Contributions of Physical Activity to . . ." The specific topical headings included were physical health, social development, psychological development, skill learning, growth, and rehabilitation. Despite the seeming importance and helpfulness of this document to practicing professionals, only a paucity of evidence existed then in comparison to the availability of supportive evidence now, some 45 years later. Thus, it is understandable that this synthetic presentation was characterized by excessive generality at various points.

The idea to develop an inventory of scientific findings about developmental physical activity had its origins in the period now referred to as the "knowledge explosion of the 60s," with the accompanying sub disciplinary and sub professional specialization that occurred then. The *Research Quarterly* supplement should have been very helpful to the conscientious professional, but perhaps it wasn't enthusiastically received either because it did not include the "ordered principles or generalizations approach" found in the Berelson and Steiner volume, or because people were not fully aware of the potential value of such an inventory as it might evolve. Whatever the situation, such a supplement—even without the ordered principles and generalizations—was not updated every ten years (as was the original intention) to reflect later developments.

Becoming increasingly aware of the potential for our field's advancement that this approach offered any profession, I consulted with Dr. Laura J. Huelster of Illinois (U-C) some 35 years ago about developing a proposal to carry out such an undertaking using the Berelson and Steiner format as it might be applied to developmental physical activity. Textbook publishers were wary of such an undertaking because of relatively unfortunate sales experiences with what they called "typical subject-matter encyclopedias." However, the editors and publishers of Lea and Febiger, Philadelphia, did consent to follow the format outlined in Table 1 above *if and only if* the volume was turned out as an introductory text for the field. Thus in 1982, *Physical Education and Sport: An Introduction* appeared as an introductory text *but unfortunately the publisher would **not** agree with the idea of including ordered principles or generalizations as recommended by Berelson and Steiner.*

However, in a 1994 publication (Stipes), working a group of scholars from each of the sub disciplinary and sub disciplinary areas included in Table 1, we were able to describe more succinctly what we believed the foundations of the field of physical education/kinesiology consisted of at that time in North America. Also, we used "our own" designated sub professional and sub disciplinary titles, respectively. In providing a synoptic overview of the field, this volume at least was prepared in such a way that it could possibly meet the needs of at least four different groups of people:

   (1) those who are using it as an introduction to a field in which they are being prepared professionally,
   (2) those who are mature professional students and scholars and who are preparing for written and oral examinations at the master's and doctoral levels,
   (3) those who are already professional practitioners and/or scholars who wish to review a recent summary of the body of knowledge of the profession and the discipline, and
   (4) those who are using it from the standpoint of general education, as part of a broad liberal arts and science background.

Oddly enough—and it has become very distressing—it is still today very difficult to know just what name to give the field. It is called "sport and physical education" within the National Association for Sport and Physical Education, one of the allied professions of the American Alliance for Health, Physical Education, Recreation, and Dance. Recently established, however, there is now the American Association for Physical Activity and Recreation (AAPAR) with the AAHPERD, with the former being oriented more to the educational environment. In Canada the professional association is still called the Canadian Association for Health, Physical Education, Recreation, and Dance, but the term "physical and health education" prevails at the public- and secondary-school levels. "Physical education and sport" is still well recognized around the world, but the term "sport" is making strong headway as a singular (or perhaps composite) title in the European Union.

In this analysis we are offering "physical (activity) education and (educational) sport" as a "holding-pattern" term, to borrow from airline nomenclature. However. it is true that the entire list of names that one will find applied to the field in North America is overly long, numbering more than one hundred! Without listing them all, we still see the terms physical education (by itself), sport and physical education (NASPE), kinesiology (at the university level by itself), human kinetics and physical education, sport and exercise sciences, physical activity studies, physical and health education (in Canada), etc.

Analysis of the present situation indicates that the field needs redirection and rejuvenation. The American Alliance for Health, Physical Education, Recreation, and Dance has had excellent leadership and has over the course of time has fully recognized that each of these terms deserves a separate identity and represents a separate profession—all of which are also almost inextricably allied. (Whether they are truly separate professions depends, of course, on the definition of the term employed.) In Canada there is a separate parks and recreation profession, but physical and health education remain closely intertwined as an instructional unit in the public schools. Dance educators are active within the Canadian Association for HPERD. There is also a variety of separate sub disciplinary societies, and many scholars affiliate with more broadly based North American societies as well.

In Table 1 above—the proposed taxonomy for the field—the reader was urged to recognize that a balanced approach between the *sub disciplinary* areas of our field and what might be identified as the *sub professional* elements was being recommended. By this Dr. Huelster and I meant that what many have called professional writing (e.g., curriculum theory investigation) should be regarded as scholarly endeavor—*if it is well done*—just as what many have considered to be scholarly, scientific endeavor (e.g., functional effects of physical activity) is regarded as professional writing too (writing that should ultimately serve the profession). Some may feel that this tends to redress the present imbalance too much, but we believed that our field, involved with lifelong developmental physical activity as it is, is indeed unique in this regard. Accordingly, we believe that the widening (psychological?) gap or rift in the field between the so-called scholars and researchers and the so-called practicing professionals should be significantly narrowed at the very least—if we wish to move toward a relatively ideal state early at some point in the 21st century. The hope is that this proposal, if well received, may help to close the presently widening gap.

Our position was that we must promote our own discipline of physical education/kinesiology (the term presently in vogue in higher education in the U.S.A. in the AAKPE and the NAKPEHE) as described below, while at the same time working cooperatively with the related disciplines (e.g., physiology, psychology, history, sociology) to the extent that these scholars shown interest is shown in our problems. However, as pointed out above, if we continue to speak of sociology of sport, physiology of exercise, etc., it will just be a matter of time before these other disciplines and professions awake to the importance of what we believe to be our professional task—the discovery, gathering, and dissemination of knowledge about, and the promotion of it to the extent that such promulgation is socially desirable, developmental physical activity through the media of exercise, sport, physical recreation, and expressive movement. It is our contention that the present trend, truly a debilitating fractionation, will in time if unchecked result in our developing field being regarded as simply one more trade within the field of education, and not a very important one at that.

The position being taken here is that our field (emerging profession?) has the inherent potential to serve the high goal of enriched living and well-being for all people. It can provide an opportunity for the improvement of the quality of life and, additionally, there is now evidence that regular exercise throughout one's life will lengthen one's life span as well. Few other professions can make such a claim, but we can do this best with the help of our allied professions and related disciplines. Moreover, no other profession will do this for us, but—because of our inactivity or misdirected activity—other professions and trades are now fulfilling some of our duties and responsibilities in a piecemeal fashion. This can only result in knowledge, competencies, and skills serving belatedly and ineffectively to help people improve the quality of their lifestyles. The posing of this dilemma for our field points up what is an urgent need right now.

An Urgent Need Right Now

What is needed right now, and is not presently available, is a steadily growing inventory of scholarly and scientific findings about developmental physical activity in exercise, sport, physical recreation, and expressive movement arranged as ordered generalizations to help our various professional practitioners in their daily work (be they teachers, coaches, scholars, laboratory researchers, managers, supervisors, performers, or others engaged in positions of a public, semipublic, or private nature (e.g., YMCAs, commercial fitness establishments).

Working with a selected group of scientists and scholars, I sought to make some headway in this direction with the publication foundations text in 1994 (Stipes). What was included was decided in the following ways:

> (1) by review of the historical development of the field in the twentieth century;
> (2) by consideration of the material that has been included in earlier, similar texts;
> (3) by careful observation of the strong trend that developed in the 1960s in certain quarters—a trend that swung the pendulum too far in many instances in the direction of the related disciplines (and away from the consideration of our field's professional problems);
> (4) by review of the recommendations emanating from a variety of conferences devoted to undergraduate and graduate curricular analysis; and
> (5) by conjoint effort of the Editor and the late Laura J. Huelster (who played a key roles in many of these conferences and who along with the Editor had observed the occurrences of the past five decades with increasing concern).

Further, in any analysis of this emerging field that traces the developments of the twentieth century, three categories or subdivisions of the field should be investigated:

> (1) the growing and potential body of knowledge being

created by researchers and scholars drawing upon
research methods and techniques of the subdisciplinary
areas;

(2) the similar development of knowledge emanating from
the concurrent professional components of the developing
field (as exist in all subject-matter fields to a greater or
lesser extent); and

(3) the knowledge becoming available from what may be
called the allied professions (as may exist also in other
emerging fields).

In the 1994 offering to the field, therefore, the reader first found a
prologue in which the urgent need for retention of a social-science
perspective for physical education and kinesiology is explained. Then the
editor presented an introductory chapter explaining the background, present
status, and intercultural significance of the field in North America for which
this volume had been specifically designed. Next seven additional chapters
were presented, all eight of which (together) offer succinct delineation of the
fundamental sub disciplinary areas of the field as explained in Table 1 above.
James S. Skinner discussed the Functional Effects of Physical Activity; A. V.
Carron, the Social Psychological Aspects; Susan L. Greendorfer, the
Sociocultural Aspects; Michael G. Wade, Motor skill Acquisition; Glynn A.
Leyshon, The Human Locomotor System; and Marion J. L. Alexander,
Biomechanics: The Mechanics of Human Movement.

The last three chapters explained the various concurrent subsumed
professional components: Daniel G. Soucie discusses Management Theory
and Practice; Ann E. Jewett, Curriculum Theory & Program Development;
and B. Don Franks, Measurement and Evaluation. (The editor offered a final
prologue that summarized, drew some obvious conclusions, and looked to
the future.

It is unfortunate, nevertheless, that we still have a situation today in
which—even though facts and figures have become increasingly available—
the professional practitioner is quite probably still at a loss when asked a
specific question about (1) the latest development or (2) some new
information about an aspect of daily work performance. A reasonable answer
to any question of this nature could be obtained by tracking down the needed
information in the journal where this information was made available, or
from a sub disciplinary specialist or a sub professional specialist (e.g., in
motor learning or in program development, respectively), but very few
people have such a journal or the availability of expert opinion close at hand.
To be sure, we have witnessed the development of such on-line services as
MEDLINE, QL, ERIC, AND *PSYCH. ABSTRACTS* to which requests can be
made electronically for an abstract or even an entire article, and also the
practitioner can make a request for a particular article in a library (if such a
service is reasonably close by and available). But where, specifically, can the

answer to a specific question or material about a specific topic be obtained right now when (or if) it is needed? This lack points up the need for some type of knowledge inventory.

How an Inventory Could Be Constructed

The type of inventory being recommended could be developed through the combined effort of people in physical activity education and educational sport, the allied professions, and the related disciplines. In the latter two instances, help would have to come from those who might have any interest in the provision of such developmental physical activity knowledge for practicing professionals and the public. The goal would be to present an evolving inventory of knowledge on the subject of developmental physical activity in sport, exercise, and related expressive activities. That is to say, the present state of knowledge and scholarly thought would be assessed. Those who prepare this information would be writing as reporters and integrators, presenting *what they know* and *what they think they know* based on the available evidence. Every effort would have to be made to avoid presenting *what they hope will be known* (unless it's under a completely separate category). Down through the years there appear to have been frequent occasions in many professions where this latter approach has been followed, where people make declarative statements presuming honestly—and occasionally dishonestly—that such thoughts are indeed based on documented evidence.

A second type of service that might also be provided is one similar to Lexus-Nexus in law where a practitioner facing a situation where specific theoretical or practical knowledge is needed in regard to a specific problem or issue that has arisen in the ongoing work of the practitioner with a client or student. Such a situation could be handled in several ways, but basically the practitioner as a member of AAHPERD would have such a service available (perhaps having paid an additional fee along with his/her regular membership fee).

In the first instance, the provision of an inventory, the member could call up series of verified findings, principles and/or generalizations in an ordered 1-2-3-4 arrangement, typically with the citation of sources which generated the information. For example, several general theoretical propositions relative to human behavior are offered below according to several categories as adapted from Berelson and Steiner. From the area of small-group research (face-to-face relations), the following theory (assumptions or testable hypotheses) might be included in an inventory:

      1. That the manner in which the administrator leads his
         or her department is determined more by existing

regulations of the educational institution itself, and the expectations of faculty and staff, than the manager's own personality and character traits.

2. That a department head will find it most difficult to shift the department away from established norms.

3. That the department head will receive gradually increasing support from staff members to the extent that he or she makes it possible for them to realize their personal goals.

4. That an administrator who attempts to employ democratic leadership will experience difficulty in reaching his or her own personal goals for the department if there are a significant number of authoritarian personalities in it (adapted from Berelson & Steiner, pp. 341-346, the original being much more detailed with direct sources based on specific research).

In reporting the available material, the language used should be as free as possible from scientific jargon. It should be understandable to the intelligent lay person and, of course, to people in the allied professions and academic colleagues in the related disciplines. This would be no mean task, because the findings would range from sport history to exercise science to curriculum investigation in a field that presently includes many areas (and sub areas!) of specialization. In any case, what would be presented is currently not available elsewhere in this form. This type of inventory would therefore represent a truly significant contribution to the field of physical activity education and educational sport and to the allied professions. It would even be helpful to scientists and scholars in the related disciplines to a degree—and, of course, to the public at large to a great extent.

To explain this process a bit further, the reader should keep in mind that it may be necessary to select a particular study for inclusion in the inventory from among many similar report available in the literature of developmental physical activity—and also from studies carried out in closely related fields that have a direct bearing on the topic at hand. The synthesizer would be looking primarily for theory, findings, principles, generalizations, and propositions that apply to this field (i.e., what we might call "the art and science of developmental physical activity in exercise, sport, and related expressive movement").

After accepting a finding for inclusion, it would be necessary to condense it and other similar findings to one distinct principle or generalization. Next, the investigator would organize the material into subheadings that could subsequently be arranged in a logical, coherent, descending manner (e.g., Proposition A1, then A1.1, A1,1a, A1.1b, A1,1c, etc., depending upon the complexity of the proposition at hand). Finally, the resultant material would be reviewed and analyzed in order to eliminate certain technical language that might only confuse the majority of people for whom the inventory is primarily intended.

The goal of this project would be an inventory representing a distillation of the literature of developmental physical activity exercise, sport, and related expressive movement that would communicate what scholars believe is known about the field to those professionals who are not research scholars in the specific sub disciplinary or sub professional area described. This is not to say that such an inventory could not be helpful to the scholar in his or her own specialty, *but that this is not the basic objective of the inventory*. Further, to some extent there would at first be reliance on secondary summaries of the empirical literature but these should be kept to a minimum. However, such reliance would be necessary because of the great bulk and variety of material. However, the investigators could also obtain the benefit of the evaluative judgment of the specialist who may have originally developed a summary or evaluation. Such material would be temporarily helpful in those instances where gaps in the field's own literature still exist— and there are undoubtedly many of these.

Then, too, as more evidence is forthcoming, it would provide a base for improved professional operation as the fundamental theory grows broader and deeper. Even then, the scholar, as well as the professional user of the generalized theory, would appreciate the necessity of using some qualifying statements in the development of ordered principles or generalizations (e.g., "under certain circumstances"). This inventory could be made available as *an evolving professional handbook* on the assumption that the steadily growing body of scientific findings about developmental physical activity as applied to this field is truly needed now—whether they appreciate this fact or not!—by the many professionals in the field—be they teachers, coaches, administrators, researchers, supervisors, performers, or those serving at YM-YWCAs, commercial fitness centers, racquet clubs, etc.

The Need for a Systems Approach

To this point an effort has been made to present the "background," the "why" and the "how" of a proposed inventory of scientific findings covering developmental physical activity as defined by this profession. It has been recommended further that such an inventory be based on a newly conceived taxonomy including both the sub disciplinary and sub professional aspects of the field.

The first such inventory would obviously have certain gaps or deficiencies. There would be no need for apology, however, because such an effort would represent a meager beginning compared to what may be possible in 10, 20, or 50 years. However, this great development will not come about unless substantive change occurs in present practice. To this end, I am recommending the gradual implementation of what has been termed a "systems approach." Whether the reader of these words is a professional practitioner, a scholar and researcher in a related disciplines, or a member of the general public, he or she may already be able to visualize to a greater or lesser degree the development needed to make available a sound, complete body of knowledge about developmental physical activity. The argument here is that using a systems approach would undoubtedly result in a more rapid development through the use of theory and research related to this unique profession.

Along with many other fields, physical activity education and educational sport does not yet appreciate the need to promote and subsequently implement a "total system" concept. However, there are many reasons why this field urgently needs to take a holistic view as the profession seeks to merit increased support in the future. The promotion of this "evolving entity" of developmental physical activity—characterized as it is with so many dynamic, interacting, highly complex components in exercise, sport, and related expressive movement—would require the cooperation of innumerable local, state (provincial), national, and international professional associations so that full support for the total professional effort could be provided.

The model presented here to help achieve a common purpose for developing and using theory and research (see Figure 8 below) explains a system with interrelated components that should be functioning as a unit—admittedly with constraints—much more effectively than they are at present. Although in practice the execution of such an approach would be very complex, the several components of the model are basically simple. As can be observed from Figure 8 below, the cycle progresses from input to thru put to output and then, after sound consumer reaction is obtained and possible corrective action is taken, goes back to input again (possibly with altered demands or resources).

What Appears to be Needed

To this point I have expressed serious concern about the need for physical (activity) education and (educational) sport to move more rapidly to true professional status. The profession—if we seek to develop it so that we may call it a "true" profession—will not be sheltered indefinitely by the protective arm of the teaching profession. Tenured contracts are being broken, and we all recognize the instability of art, music, *and* physical education (not athletics) when financial constraints are imposed. Also, those "professing" physical activity education and educational sport outside of the educational system have not yet joined with those inside to demand state-by-state (or province-by-province) certification as practicing professionals.

Figure 8

A Systems Approach to the Development and Use of Theory and Research in Sport and Physical Education

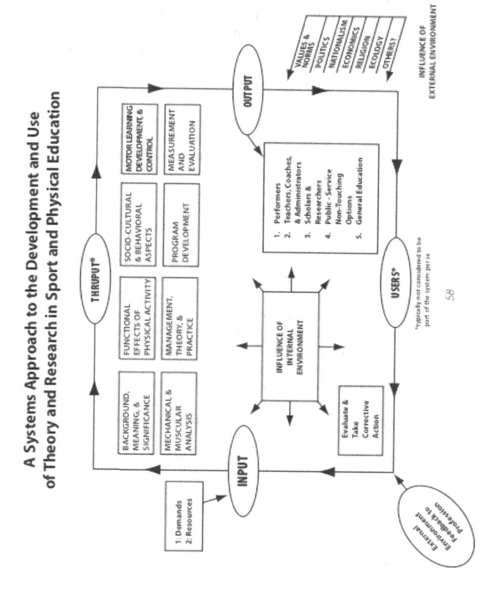

Further, more positive, substantive, and enlightened effort within the field should be directed toward what has above been called sub disciplinary and sub professional scholarly endeavor. Moreover, the professional practitioner should learn to trust and employ the results of such research. Until this happens, society will simply not recognize the field as that profession in our culture which is the leading force in disseminating sound knowledge about, and teaching sound practice in, developmental physical activity in exercise, sport, and related expressive movement.

It is for these reasons, as well as for additional reasons that will be introduced below, that I am making a strong recommendation for the consideration of the combined forces of the profession through North America. This recommendation is simply that an all-out effort be mounted to reverse the present trend toward the "outward dispersion" of the allied professions and the sub disciplinary areas of scholarly study and research— or at least to bring these elements to where the "centrifugal and centripetal" forces maintain a desirable position insofar as the evolving profession is concerned. Figure 7 above had explained diagrammatically the specific recommendations to be achieved in the field (profession?) of physical activity education and educational sport by the mythical year 2025. Instead of a continuation of the present trend toward ever-greater identification with related disciplines (e.g., sociology, physiology, psychology), the designated areas of scholarly study and research (e.g., the socio-cultural and behavioral aspects, the functional effects of physical activity) have been brought back with this recommendation to a point where they are firmly attached to the profession's core, characterized in Figure 7 as a "developing body of knowledge about the theory and practice of developmental physical activity."

It must be emphasized that achieving such a state does not imply little or no involvement with colleagues who identify primarily with the departments housing these related disciplines. It simply means that those who consider themselves full-fledged members of this field or profession should:

> (1) have the greatest knowledge and wisdom about its problems,
> (2) develop the greatest expertise in solving these applied problems, and
> (3) have the greatest interest in—and loyalty to—this profession and its attendant problems.

Summary (Interim)

To this point I have argued:

> (1) that the evolving profession should develop a revised

taxonomy of developmental physical activity in exercise, sport, and related expressive movement as soon as possible,

(2) that the profession should plan to develop an inventory of scientific findings arranged as verified, ordered principles or generalizations because developments of the past 40 years in our allied professions and related sub disciplines have exceeded this profession's capability to assimilate the scientific findings that have accumulated,

3) that the field should implement a systems approach—on the North American continent at least—to effect the development of an inventory before others carry out the profession's task for it, and

(4) that the evolving profession of physical education and sport mount an all-out effort to reverse the present trend toward dispersion of the allied professions and the sub disciplinary areas of scholarly study and research.

At present the field is hampered immeasurably by a lack of focus on its unique mission. This continues the prevailing confusion and vitiates the profession's overall effect. (It also causes confusion for those in the allied professions, the related disciplines, and the general public, because they see gaps to be filled and almost necessarily are moving steadily to somehow fill those "cracks and crevices" for the benefit of all.

To fulfill its role best, our profession must *primarily* focus on developmental physical activity for the accelerated, the normal, and the exceptional or special populations of all ages. Working in this direction will help the profession's focus to become sharpened. Concurrently we will be able to continue efforts to coordinate the efforts of the many splinter groups now often working at cross-purposes with poor or nonexistent inter-group communication.

The profession's system of providing service to people of all ages and abilities can only be realized if the sub disciplinary and sub professional inputs are sufficient and timely. Further, the entire profession can only prosper if a satisfied public rewards it with a continuing demand for services. Only then will the public purse strings open to provide the necessary funding for the delivery of such quality service.

Professional Essentials: From Bits to Wisdom

In the remainder of this historical and descriptive analysis, I will explain how an inventory of scientific findings as explained here could fit into a broader scheme whereby the entire profession's ability to serve effectively and efficiently could be raised to a new, hitherto undreamed of level. To review briefly what was described above, present developments in the field of physical education and educational sport have convinced me that the leaders of professional associations in the United States such as the National Association for Sport and Physical Education with Alliance (AAHPERD)—and the recently organized American Association for Physical Activity and Recreation (AAPAR, also within AAHPERD should forthrightly ask themselves what the future holds for our profession (i.e., physical [activity] education). This statement applies to the Canadian Association for Health, Physical Education, Recreation, and Dance (CAHPERD/l'ACSEPLD as well.

If we able to begin achieving the specific objectives, and are moving toward the long range aims outlined in this analysis (i.e., about how we can best upgrade our profession and the service it is prepared to offer its members), then we will have begun to live up to the potential that is fundamentally inherent in developmental physical activity in exercise, sport, dance, and play to become a "socially useful servant" designed to improve the quality of people's lives.

The answer seems obvious as to what will happen to the profession if it doesn't meet this objective. Thus I believe that the choice is before us right now. Either we move ahead steadily and consistently to become a full-fledged, recognized profession, or we will most certainly struggle along in our present uneasy role as a teaching-coaching occupation with some of the characteristics of a trade. Ongoing lesser status within the teaching ranks will continue unless we move forward strongly! In my opinion there can be no middle ground on this subject.

If we choose the "professional route"—the move to insure a "from bits to wisdom" approach outlined here that merges scientific findings with computer technology—as opposed to what I call our present "trade route," we will most definitely have to resolve collectively that there is a need for a metamorphosis along the lines recommended here. We all recognize what a full-fledged profession can accomplish in a society (e.g., law, medicine). Further, we must recognize fine professional practice can *only* be built on *a sound body of knowledge that is readily available to practitioners.*

Emerging professions such as we still are, should be aware of the extent to which they have achieved what society demands of a respected profession. The now legendary—to the medical profession at least—Abraham Flexner (1915) recommended six criteria as being characteristic of a profession. However, in 198, Bayles maintained that there was still no definition of the term that was generally accepted. However, Bayles did suggest an approach whereby necessary features were indicated along with a number of other common features that would tend to elevate an occupation to professional status. The three necessary aspects or components of a profession that are generally recognized are:

1. the need for an extensive period of training,

2. a field with a significant intellectual component that must be mastered before the profession is practiced, and,
3. a recognition by society that the trained person can provide a basic, important service to its citizens.

Specifically, then, I am concerned about the body of knowledge that the profession of physical activity education and educational sport does (or does not) have available at the present. I am further concerned about:

1. *Who* is developing it;
2. *How* it is being developed;
3. *In what form* it is being made available; and
4. *How* we should be going about providing such knowledge to our professional practitioners.

Proceeding from the general to the specific, therefore, I will seek to answer the following questions:

1. What are the definitions of the terms used with this topic?
2. How has knowledge been communicated historically?
3. How individual humans actually gain knowledge?
4. In what form is knowledge available?
5. Where our knowledge is located (i.e., what we think we know about "developmental physical activity in exercise, sport, and related expressive movement")?
6. What do we know? (A Broad Assessment of Our Field's "Body of Knowledge" Expressed as Principal Principles)
7. How can the proposed disciplinary taxonomy fit into a Model for Optimum Development of a Field Called "Physical (Activity) Education and (Educational) Sport"?
8. What other techniques and services do we need to achieve this objective that is demanding attention?
9. How might we as a type of profession obtain what appears to be needed to make this plan a reality?
10. Keeping present status in mind, how should we proceed initially as we move toward our eventual goal?, and
11. What might the future hold for us if we carry out this task successfully?

Definition of Computer Terms

There are a number of definitions of computer terms that should be reviewed for a full understanding of the ideas to be included in the following discussion (some were originally taken from the *Dictionary of Computing*, 1983):

Bits = acronym (plural) for binary digit (i.e., the binary digit used in the number system most commonly employed in computers; a bit is either 0 or 1).

Data = facts, that which is given (e.g., a, 4, abc) (T. Haggerty).

Information = information is data (raw facts) placed in context so that it (the information) changes the receiver's perceptions, beliefs, or knowledge base (T. Haggerty).

Note: Information may be created, transmitted, stored, retrieved, received, copied, processed, or destroyed.

Knowledge = facts, truths, or principles resulting from study or scientific investigation.

Inventory = a listing, accounting, or catalogue of ideas, facts, things, principles, or generalizations.

Taxonomy = a classification into categories based on natural relationships (e.g., chemical elements).

Hypothesis = a theoretical assumption used as a basis for investigation.

Theory = a systematic arrangement of facts with respect to some real or hypothetical laws (e.g., Einstein's Theory).

Principles or Generalizations (Ordered) = a series of ordered statements or findings in a 1-2-3-4 arrangement (Berelson and Steiner, 1964).

Expert Systems = computer programs built for commercial application using the programming techniques of AI (i.e., the product-directed approach to Artificial Intelligence) for problem-solving (e.g., a hypothetical medical expert system for diagnosing liver cancer) (Schank, 1984).

Note: Knowledge engineering is the sub discipline of AI concerned with the building of expert systems.

Systems Approach = an analysis that stresses the necessity for maintaining the basic elements of input-process-output and for adapting it to the larger environment that sustains the organization (Rosenberg, 1978, p. 430).

Finally, however, regardless of the above, the finest professional people are those to whom we turn for wisdom (i.e., the quality of being wise; the faculty to discern right or truth and to judge or act accordingly).

How Knowledge Has Been Communicated Historically

In 1970 Asimov warned that a "fourth revolution" in the realm of communications was rapidly occurring within the social development of people on earth. These revolutions in chronological order have been as follows:

1. The invention of speech,
2. The invention of writing,
3. The mechanical reproduction of the printed word, and
4. The development of relay stations in space.

To most of us the idea of relay stations in space seems most beneficent. The eventual result of this advancement means that all people will be confronted with a blanketing communications network that is steadily and increasingly making possible interpersonal relationships hitherto undreamed of by humans. However, Asimov (1970) at this time was predicting that this fourth revolution means that a great danger lies before us as well. His point is that we are being well informed about the world's tragic happenings before we have created a "fully cooperative world situation," or at least a situation where truly responsible world government has been developed. Obviously, this is a factor that must be reckoned with in our quest for the greater dissemination of knowledge.

How Individual Humans Actually Gain Knowledge

More specifically, how do people gain knowledge of any type? For example, how do we "know what we know" about society in general, about the process of education, or specifically about developmental physical activity in sport, exercise, or dance?

Royce (1964) offers considerable insight into this question when he offered a model explaining that throughout history knowledge has been gained in four different ways as follows: (1) thinking (known more formally as rationalism); (2) feeling (or intuitionism), perhaps "intuiting" would be a better term here; (3) sensing (or empiricism); and (4) believing (or authoritarianism). This is described more graphically in Figure 9 below.

The Form in Which Knowledge Is Available

Keeping the above four ways in which humans gain knowledge in mind, we should review briefly the actual form in which knowledge is available to us. Keep in mind that knowledge has been defined above as "facts, truths, or principles resulting from study or scientific investigations." Also, a hypothesis is a "theoretical assumption used as a basis for investigation. Further, "a theory is "a systematic arrangement of facts with respect to some real or hypothetical laws."

On this basis, one category might be the "depth," "quality," "intensity," or "power" of the facts or truths provided. Moving from the elementary to the most complex, then, this categorization of the form in which knowledge is available could reasonably progress in the following progression:

1. common sense,
2. informational articles,
3. descriptive studies based on specific concepts,
4. ad hoc theories or hypotheses with a fairly low level of abstraction,
5. "middle range" (Merton) incomplete "segmental" theories, and
6. explicit, complex, grand theories based on a model and a perspective (e.g., Parsonsian theory in sociology, Marxian theory).

A second category, on a more practical basis for the seeker of knowledge in the form of specific facts or truths (possibly through the use of the computer and an on-line service), would be that made of the actual informational material. Here the searcher for available knowledge might turn (through the use of a specific on-line service) to the following:

1. a bibliographic listing,
2. an abstract of the item in question,
3. a specific page from the article, or
4. the entire article or publication.

Of course, if the listing is not available through an on-line service, the professional person or investigator will have to go to a library to track down the actual article in a magazine or journal, or possibly in the book or monograph in which it appears.

Where *Our* Knowledge Is Located

People joke that Julius Caesar is purported to have said, "A funny thing happened as I entered the Forum!" Our field that was known as physical education in—say 1960—might say today, "A funny thing happened since we started down the path toward becoming a discipline— and also striving to be recognized as a profession!" That "funny thing" is that still today we simply do not know where we stand in regard to the steadily increasing body of knowledge about "developmental physical activity in exercise, sport, and expressive movement." Like "Julius," we too could be "eliminated!"

,

Figure 9

How Humans Gain Knowledge

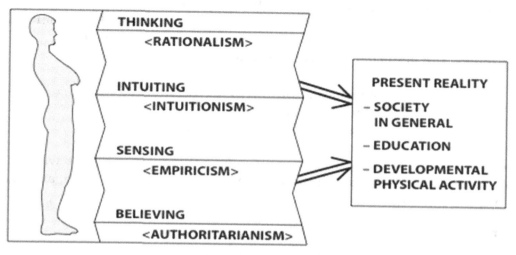

(Adapted from Royce, 1964)

69

189

Although other established or embryonic professions, may be facing an identical or similar problem, that's their particular worry at this stage of society's development. Our own problem is that our professional practitioners are gradually and increasingly being overwhelmed by information, opinions, and facts available in newspapers, periodicals, monographs, proceedings, and books. Resultantly they see their workload responsibilities in a blurred manner.

However, although much of this vast quantity of material is often interesting, valuable, and occasionally vitally important, it is typically not presented in such a way as to be readily useful to the physical educator/coach as a practitioner. Interestingly, this information and knowledge is also available to us under a great variety of headings through such on-line services as SIRC, SIRLS, ERIC, The Physical Education Index, Sport Dokumentation (FRG), and now Sport Search through Human Kinetics Publishers. Nevertheless, the generic questions to be answered are roughly:

1. "What information is it I am looking for?",
2. "Where is it located?", and
3. "What does it say and in what form?"

Obviously, also, if very few people are availing themselves of this widely dispersed, documented material, we must discover why this is so, and then try to improve the situation.

What Do We Know? (A Broad Assessment of Our Field's Present Body of Knowledge)

Despite what has been said to this point, we can affirm with considerable assurance that the steadily growing body of knowledge has now provided our field with a more substantive knowledge base than existed at the middle of the 20th century. In addition to the "principal principles" listed by Professor Arthur Steinhaus, with reasonable assurance resulting from consistent data analysis over the years, I am now suggesting that physical education's "principal principles" have increased in number from four to thirteen! Building on the work of Steinhaus and others since that time, I have assembled some 13 recommended principles as aspects of our field's body of knowledge. Ordered generalizations can be developed under each of these headings as a guide to future research.

It is perhaps pointless to attempt to determine precisely to what extent this increase (i.e., from four to thirteen) can be attributed more to the efforts of the profession's natural science scholars than to those of the more recently added social science and humanities scholars. Also, we must not forget the contributions emanating steadily from our allied professions and related disciplines. That there is some overlap in "what we believe we now know" seems obvious, but this increase in the number of "principal principles"—as the idea was originated by Dr. Steinhaus—points to the wisdom of searching for evidence wherever it is to be found from whatever discipline.

In concluding his now "historical proclamation" in 1951, Steinhaus summarized as follows:

1. The principle of overload charters physical education as a unique force in the growth and development of man;
2. The principle of reversibility discloses the fleeting effect and dictates its practice at every age;
3. The principle of integration and integrity raises physical education to the human level and governs its contribution to mental strength and morality; and
4. The principle of the priority of man makes physical education a socially useful servant, possessed of capacity to produce a better generation (p. 10).

In the 13 "principal principles" postulated below, I have included Steinhaus's principles. Note, however, that his "principle of integration and integrity" has been divided in two, thereby creating two separate principles. As I recommend this list for consideration and possible adoption as areas for which "ordered generalizations" could be provided initially if the field moves to develop the inventory recommended, I believe we should all express sincere appreciation to the many scientists and scholars—within our field, the allied professions, and the related disciplines—whose efforts have made the following statement of these 13 principal principles possible at this time.)

Principle 1: The "Reversibility Principle". The first principle affirms that circulo-respiratory (often called cardiovascular) conditioning is inherently reversible in the human body; a male, for example, typically reaches his peak at age 19 and goes downhill gradually thereafter until eventual death. This means that you must achieve and maintain at least an "irreducible level" of such conditioning to live normally.

Principle 2: The "Overload Principle". The principle here is that a muscle or muscle group must be taxed beyond that to which it is accustomed, or it won't develop; in fact, it will probably retrogress. Thus, a human must maintain reasonable muscular strength in his/her body to carry out life's normal duties and responsibilities and to protect the body from deterioration.

Principle 3: The "Flexibility Principle". This principle states that a human must put the body's various joints through the range of motion for which they are intended. Inactive joints become increasingly inflexible until immobility sets in. If inflexibility is a sign of old age, the evidence shows that

191

most people are becoming old about age 27! Maintenance of flexibility in body's joint must not be neglected.

Principle 4: The "Bone Density Principle". This principles asserts that developmental physical activity throughout life preserves the density of a human's bones. The density of human bones after maturity is not fixed or permanent, and the decline after age 35 could be more rapid than is the case with fat and muscle. After prolonged inactivity, adequate calcium in your diet and weight-bearing physical activity is absolutely essential for the preservation of your bones. Remember that prevention of bone loss is much more effective than later efforts to repair any bone damage that might have been incurred.

Principle 5: The "Gravity Principle". This principle explains that maintaining muscle-group strength throughout life, while standing or sitting, helps the human fight against the force of gravity that is working continually to break down the body's structure. Maintaining muscle group strength and tonus and the best possible structural alignment of one's bones through the development of a proper "body consciousness" will help a person to fight off gravity's potentially devastating effects as long as possible.

Principle 6: The "Relaxation Principle". Principle 6 states that the skill of relaxation is one that people must acquire in today's increasingly complex world. Oddly enough, people often need to be taught how to relax in today's typically stressful environment. Part of any "total fitness" package should, therefore, be the development of an understanding as to how an individual can avoid chronic or abnormal fatigue in a social and physical environment that is often overly taxing.

Principle 7: The "Aesthetic Principle". This principle explains that a person has either an innate or culturally determined need to "look good" to himself/herself and to others. Socrates is purported to have decried "growing old without appreciating the beauty of which the body is capable." This is evidently a "need" to make a good appearance to one's family, friends, and those who one meets daily at work or during leisure. Billions of dollars are spent annually by people striving to "make themselves look like something they are not" naturally. Why do people do this? Quite probably, they go through these "body rituals" to please themselves and because of various social pressures. Thus, if one is physically active, while following the above six principles, one's appearance can be improved normally, naturally, and inexpensively.

Principle 8: The "Integration Principle". Principle 8 asserts that developmental physical activity provides an opportunity for the individual to get "fully involved" as a living organism. So many of life's activities only challenge a person fractionally in that only part of the individual's sensory equipment and even less of the motor mechanism are involved. By their very nature, physical activities in exercise, sport, play, and expressive movement demand full attention from the organism—often in the face of opposition—and therefore involve complete psycho-physical integration.

Principle 9: The "Integrity Principle". The "integrity principle" goes hand in hand with desirable integration of the human's various aspects [so-called unity of body and mind in the organism explained in Principle 8 immediately above]. The idea of integrity implies that a completely integrated psycho-physical activity should correspond *ethically* with the avowed ideals and standards of society. Fair play, honesty, and concern for others should be uppermost in one's individual pattern of developmental physical activity.

Principle 10: The "Priority of the Person Principle". Principle 10 affirms that any physical activity in sport, play, and exercise sponsored through public or private agencies should be conducted in such a way that the welfare of the individual comes first. Situations arise daily in all aspects of social living where this principle—stressing the sanctity of the individual—is often forgotten. In a democratic society, a man or woman, or boy or girl, should never be forced or encouraged to take part in some type of developmental physical activity where this principle is negated because of the desire of others to win. The wholeness of one's personal life is more important than any sport in which an individual may take part. Sport must serve as a "social servant."

Principle 11: The "Live Life to Its Fullest Principle". This principle explains that, viewed in one sense, human movement is what distinguishes the individual from the rock on the ground. Unless the body is moved with reasonable vigor according to principles 1-6 above, it will not serve a person best throughout his/her life by helping a person to meet the normal daily tasks and the unexpected sudden demands that may be required to take advantage of life's many opportunities or to protect a person from harm.

Principle 12: The "Fun and Pleasure Principle". Principle 12 states that the human is normally a "seeker of fun and pleasure," and that a great deal of the opportunity for such enjoyment can be derived from full, active bodily movement. The physical education profession stresses that the opportunity for such fun and pleasure will be missing from life if a person does not maintain at least an "irreducible minimum" level of physical fitness.

Principle 13: The "Longevity Principle". This final principle affirms that regular developmental physical activity throughout life can help a person live longer. The statistical evidence is mounting that demonstrates the wisdom of maintaining an active lifestyle throughout one's years.

Succinctly put, all things being equal, if a human is physically active, he or she will live longer (Zeigler, 1994).

How the Proposed Disciplinary Taxonomy Might Fit into a Model for Optimum Development of a Field Called "Physical (Activity) Education and (Educational) Sport"

Carrying the above recommendation one step further, we now need to show how the proposed taxonomy of our profession's body of knowledge (Table 1 above) might relate to a model that might be employed for the optimum development of the profession. (See Figure 10 above.) Actually this model could well be employed for development of any profession, but in this case it is applied specifically to our field that is currently known in the United States, for example, as "sport and physical education" within the National Association for Sport and Physical Education within the American Alliance for Health, Physical Education, Recreation, and Dance. In Canada in the schools it is typically still called "physical and health education," whereas in the universities the designation ranges from physical education to human kinetics or kinesiology.

Note that this model includes the following subdivisions:

1. societal values and norms,
2. an operational philosophy for the profession,
3. a developing theory embodying assumptions and testable hypotheses,
4. professional, semiprofessional, and amateur involvement as practitioners,
5. professional preparation and general education, and
6. scholarly endeavor and disciplinary research.

Societal values and norms are placed at the top of the model. This is based on the theory that:

1. a society's values and norms have a watershed quality,
2. in the final analysis progress will be made toward their achievement, and
3. they exert control and conditioning over the lower levels in the social system as the culture moves gradually and unevenly toward what might be considered progress.

Directly below in the model was the overriding philosophy of sport and physical education in a society, or the values according to which the

Figure 10

A Model for Optimum Development of a Field Called "X"

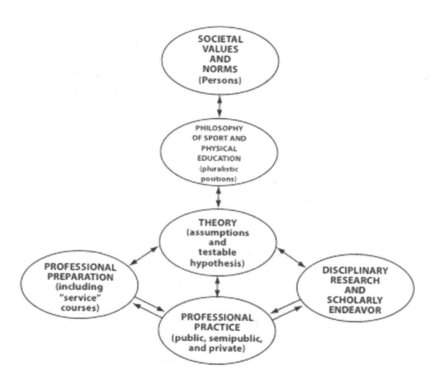

77

195

profession conducts its practice. At this level we appreciate that especially in a democracy pluralistic philosophies are allowed to exist (Zeigler, 1977, pp. 7-9).

The third level involves the assumptions and testable hypotheses of a steadily evolving theory—a knowledge base upon which professional practice is predicated and executed. This theory should comprise a coherent group of general and specific propositions that can be used as principles to explain the phenomena observed in developmental physical activity in exercise, sport, and related expressive movement.

The fourth level in the model is depicted as professional, semiprofessional, and amateur involvement in the practice of the profession. This is subsumed under the categories of public, semipublic (or semiprivate), and private involvement or practice. To the left of this is the area of professional preparation and general education. Professional preparation should include

1. the performer,
2. teachers/coaches,
3. administrators/supervisors,
4. teachers of teachers/coaches,
5. scholars and researchers, and
6. people in alternative professional careers.

So-called general education in physical (activity) education and (educational) sport should be elevated so that it is regarded as part of a broad liberal arts and science background rather than merely as a "service" course. To achieve this it will be necessary to provide a sound educational experience in the theory and practice of human motor performance in exercise, sport, and related expressive movement.

To the right at the fourth level is the area of disciplinary research and scholarly endeavor as explained detail in Table 1 above. *Once again* the reader should note carefully that by the year 2025 I am recommending a complete changeover from the use of the terms belonging to the related fields (e.g., physiology, sociology) to those terms that are solely ours and that will in time help us earn the status that can and should be rightfully ours (Zeigler, 1982, pp. 39-41).

If these ideas, or a reasonable facsimile thereof, are acceptable to the profession, the taxonomy (taxonomical model?) recommended in Figure 9 above explain what the field would look like diagrammatically in the future? In Figure 10 below the specific recommendations to be achieved are explained.

It will be noticed immediately that, instead of a continuation of the present trend toward ever-greater identification with related disciplines, the designated areas of scholarly study and research (e.g., the socio-cultural and behavioral aspects, the functional effects of physical activity) have been brought back within the field of sport and physical education. The recommendation is that they should be firmly attached to the profession's core, characterized in Figure 10 as a "developing body of knowledge about the theory and practice of sport and developmental physical activity."

I must emphasize at once that achieving such a state does not imply little or no involvement with colleagues who identify with and are paid primarily by the departments housing these related disciplines. It simply means that those who consider themselves full-fledged members of the physical (activity) education and (educational) sport profession should:

> (1) have the greatest knowledge and wisdom about its
>   problems
> (2) should develop the greatest expertise in solving
>   these applied problems, and
> (3) have the greatest interest in—and loyalty to—this
>   profession and its attendant problems (Zeigler,
>   1983, 63-64).

Other Techniques and Services That Are Needed

"What else is needed other than the development of a sound body of knowledge?" you may ask. Basically, what we need most urgently as well are better ways to actualize our potential first during the period of our professional preparation and thereafter for the rest of our lives. We need improved competency development training in what I have called:

> (1) personal skills,
> (2) conceptual skills,
> (3) technical skills,
> (4) human skills, and
> (5) conjoined skills
>   (some combination of
>   nos. 2-4 above).

This thought is stressed, because I have been concerned that those responsible for the management-development aspects within professional education add laboratory experiences to that phase of their professional programs to prepare university students in the field (Zeigler and Bowie, 1995).

Additionally, and most importantly, we need greatly improved and more readily accessible information services. These can be categorized in a fourfold manner, although they are not always discrete or completely distinguishable one from the other as follows:

1. On-Line Services (via a modem and personal computer) for bibliographic data, abstracts, complete articles, etc. (i.e., electronic libraries). Obviously these are already available to us through (for example) SIRC and SIRLS in Canada and ERIC in the United States through Knowledge Index of DIALOG. However, professionals are often not yet geared up to use such services because of lack of money, equipment, etc.

2. Electronic Bulletin Boards (via a modem and personal computer, also at all levels—i.e., local, regional, national and—possibly—international). If these were to be developed and become fully operative, professionals could quite easily get the benefit of ongoing dialogue with colleagues at all levels and of varying abilities. Additionally, there should be an opportunity for our professional associations (AAHPERD in the U.S.A. and CAHPERD in Canada to work cooperatively with designated universities insofar as the concept of an 'electronic university' is concerned. Such an arrangement would mean that students could elect credit courses leading to various degrees. Further, in-service courses and clinics could be made available regularly to mature professionals who need assistance and possible upgrading in a variety of degree programs. (At present there is an organization called Electronic University operating out of San Francisco that offers college credit courses through a linkage with some 25 colleges and universities in the United States.)

3. Comprehensive Professional Handbook available to all. Such a handbook would be open-ended and loose-leaf for updating and expansion at 6-month intervals. This handbook would be developed on the basis of ordered principles or generalizations at a nominal cost to members of the leading professional association (e.g., AAHPERD in the USA and PHE Canada, but would also be made available on a sales-for-profit basis to any other interested person.

4. Interactive, Electronic Data Base (from which the Professional Handbook in #3 above is developed). With this service a professional seeking an answer to a problem (urgent or otherwise) could "carry on a conversation with Hal" (remember 2001 and 2010!), and at the present time would be given the best available answer to his/her problem in return at the so-called "making-sense" level.

> Note: Here, of course, we are getting into the realm of
> Artificial Intelligence, or AI, the so-called 5th generation
> computers. As Schank (1984) told us, there are three fairly
> distinct levels of understanding that can be differentiated
> (i.e., making sense, cognitive understanding, and complete
> empathy). At the "making sense" level, computers can

198

make sense because they are given "rules for how to produce certain outputs on the basis of having processed corresponding inputs" (p. 57). The "cognitive understanding" level is harder because it requires a computer to understand how it comes to a new conclusion about a problem with certain information it has processed. Some second-level AI programs have been developed, but whether that level can be surpassed (and how we will be certain that progress has been made toward the achievement of "complete empathy") are problems or questions to which there are no answers currently available. Thus, we need to appreciate that we are probably still years away from AI in the field of physical education and sport at this second or "cognitive understanding" level. *Nevertheless, the time is past when we should have at least made more significant progress at the first (making-sense) level.*)

5. Finally, keeping in mind the potential services available if and when Electronic Bulletin Boards and on-line services become available at all levels, a topflight practitioner wants and needs wisdom as he or she confronts truly difficult problems in carrying out professional responsibilities and duties. Here we need the opportunity to discuss difficult and intricate problems with specialists in each of the many sub disciplinary and sub professional aspects of our field. Such specialists would help us to reach the "complete empathy" level that may never be possible with reactive computers functioning at the cognitive understanding level. Of course, each of us must work to develop the required maturity that will afford a modicum of wisdom—the faculty to discern right or truth and to judge or act accordingly based on the advice obtained from specialists.

How to Obtain What Appears to Be Needed

Moving to obtain what appears to be needed for our profession is "much easier said than done!" However, I would recommend that AAHPERD in the USA or CAHPERD in Canada (hopefully working cooperatively) should take the lead in promoting this development that could be coordinated on a North American scale.

A first step that may be difficult, of course, will be the mos careful definition of exactly what it is that we do—or have responsibility for—as professional persons. Can we agree, for example, that our task is to practice professionally the application of developmental physical activity in exercise, sport, and related expressive movement with normal, accelerated, and special populations of all ages so as to enhance their quality of life?

Next I believe that we will need advice and financial assistance from governmental or private funding agencies—and, of course, also from the appropriate offices offering these services in the various provinces and territories in Canada and educational departments at the various levels in the USA.

It seems self evident further that we will need to work cooperatively with the Education Resources Information Center (ERIC) in the United States in the development of a complete, on-line data base, and in Canada with the Sport Information Resource Centre (SIRC of Fitness and Amateur Sport) and the Sport Information of Recreation and Leisure Studies (SIRLS of the University of Waterloo) in Canada. Also, we will need to request cooperation and assistance from both allied and related disciplines and their respective professional associations (e.g., in Canada the Canadian Society for Exercise Physiology, the Canadian Education Association, the Canadian Medical Association, the disciplines of physiology, psychology, history, sociology, and/or their counterparts in the USA).

Finally, and this is not all inclusive listing, of course, we could well need cooperation and assistance from selected people in our profession and others in allied and related professions and disciplines in regard to the development of an electronic bulletin-board consulting service.

How to Proceed From This Point

How shall we begin right now to implement this plan to help our developing profession obtain sound theory and knowledge to achieve its lofty goals? Some wise person is purported once to have said, "If you want to accomplish something big in this life, do not expect people to roll stones out of your path; in fact, do not be surprised if they heap boulders in your way."

Frankly, at this point I am not looking for stones of any size to be heaped on our path in the years immediately ahead. However, based on past experience, I just know that they are going to be there. The powers that be are simply not going to say "Eureka, that's the answer! Here's two million dollars to organize, develop and begin the administration of a plan to bring together the body of knowledge about developmental physical activity that will make physical education and sport a full-fledged, respected field." I don't propose to repeat here and now what might be their arguments and rebuttals to any proposals. Further, I would not be the least surprised if we as professionals were somehow to prove to be our own worst enemies as we traverse this rocky path.

Nevertheless, without attempting to enumerate specifically where any stumbling blocks might confront us, I would like to propose four major processes that were first spelled out almost 50 years ago (March and Simon,

1958, pp. 129-131). These processes could be employed chronologically, as we seek to realize the desired objective as follows:

1. Problem-solving: Basically, what is being proposed here is a problem for our profession to solve or resolve. We must move as soon as possible to convince others of the worthwhileness of this proposal. Part of our approach includes assurance that the objectives are indeed operational (i.e., that their presence or absence can be tested empirically as we progress). In this way, even if sufficient funding were not available—and it well might not be—the various parties who are vital or necessary to the success of the venture would at least have agreed-upon objectives. However, with a professional task of this magnitude, it is quite possible, even probable that such consensus will not be achieved initially.

2. Persuasion: For the sake of argument, then, let us assume that our objectives on the way toward the achievement of long range aims are not shared by the others whom we need to convince, people who are either inside our own profession or are in allied professions or related disciplines. On the assumption that the stance of the others is not absolutely fixed or intractable, a second step of persuasion can (should) be employed on the assumption that at some level our objectives will be shared. We can also hope that any disagreement over sub goals can be mediated by reference to common goals. (Here we should keep in mind that influencing specific leaders in each of the various "other" associations with which we are seeking to cooperate can be a most effective technique for bringing about attitude change within the larger membership group of each larger association [as recommended by J. J. Jackson].)

> Note: If persuasion works, then the parties concerned
> can obviously return to the problem-solving level (#1).

3. Bargaining: Moving along to the third stage of a theoretical plan, let us assume that the second step (persuasion) didn't fully work. This means obviously that there is still disagreement over the operational goals proposed at the problem-solving level (the first stage). Now the profession has a difficult decision to make: do we attempt to strike a bargain or do we decide that we simply must "go it alone?" The problem with the first alternative is that *bargaining implies compromise*, and compromise means that each group involved will have to surrender a portion of its claim, request, or argument. The second alternative may seem more desirable, but following it may also mean eventual failure in achieving the final, most important objective.

> Note: We can appreciate, of course, that the
> necessity of proceeding to this stage, and then
> selecting either of the two alternatives, is

obviously much less desirable than settling the
matter at either the first or second stages.

4. Politicking: The implementation of the fourth stage (or plan of
attack) is based on the fact that the proposed action of the first three stages
has failed. The participants in the discussion cannot agree in any way about
the main issue. It is at this point that the organization (or professional
association) involved has to somehow expand the number of parties or
groups involved in consideration of the proposed project. The goal, of course,
is to attempt to include potential allies so as to improve the chance of
achieving the desired final objective. Employing so-called "power politics" is
usually tricky, however, and it may indeed backfire upon the group bringing
such a maneuver into play. However, this is the way the world (or society)
works, and the goal may be well worth the risk or danger involved.

> Note: Obviously, we hope that it will not be necessary
> to operate at this fourth stage continually in
> connection with the development of our profession. It
> would be most divisive in many instances and time
> consuming as well. Therefore, we would be faced with
> the decision as to whether this type of operation would
> do more harm than good (in the immediate future at
> least).

What the Future Might Hold for Physical (Activity) Education and (Educational) Sport If It Achieves Its Desired Objective

In this historical and descriptive analysis I have discussed the means
whereby the physical (activity) education and (educational) sport field could
move to obtain an ever-expanding body of knowledge based on ordered
generalizations. In this way the United States and Canadian professional
associations (AAHPERD & CAHPERD) could soon take the lead nationally
and internationally by moving steadily ahead toward the achievement of this
objective. Our field could thereby become a leader according to all
recognized standards of excellence.

Penultimately, may I suggest that you think ahead to the year 2050—a
year when many of us may be memories only. When we pass on, our
historians may well record the answers to the following questions:

1. In the early 20th century were the professional organizations known
as the American Alliance for Health, Physical Education, Recreation, and
Dance and the Canadian Association for Health, Physical Education, and
Recreation (l'ACSEPLD en français) able to jointly achieve a focus about their
unique mission?

2. If the answer to Question #1 is "yes," were professionals in the field
able to coordinate the efforts of the many splinter groups in both countries—

now often working at seemingly cross purposes—to achieve the field's avowed goals?

3. If the answers to Question #1 and #2 are "yes," did the profession, the federal governments, and the various states, provinces,territories, and commonwealths work cooperatively in this endeavor?

4. If the above questions can be answered affirmatively, did the field of physical (activity) education and (educational) sport and others concerned employ a systems approach to develop an inventory of ordered scientific findings about the possible role of developmental physical activity in improving the quality of people's lives?

5. If the answers are still affirmative, did this body of knowledge arranged as ordered principles or generalizations continue to grow? Further, was it gradually made readily available on an "interactive data" basis to practitioners seeking to serve Americans and Canadians of all ages and conditions through the medium of developmental physical activity?

6. Assuming affirmative answers above, did a satisfied public truly recognize the importance of the profession and reward it with a continuing demand for high-level services?

Concluding Statement

The large majority of professionals in the field of physical (activity) education and (educational) sport—or whatever we eventually decide to call ourselves—will need to agree that it is time for this vital development described here. The opportunity to achieve such a fine, purposeful goal of solid professional status lies before us right now as we are confronted by the urgent need for professionals in the field of physical (activity) education and (educational) sport to undertake such information processing to keep them up to date. Borgmann (1992) calls the provision of this service one hypermodern tendency of a postmodern world (p. 82). If we lay the proper foundation in the years immediately ahead, the answers to the six questions delineated above about our future can all be loudly and clearly "Yes"— strongly in the affirmative!

References

Asimov, I. (1970). The fourth revolution. *Saturday Review*, Oct. 24, 17-20.

Berelson, B., & Steiner, G. A. (1964). *Human behavior; An inventory of scientific findings.* New York: Harcourt, Brace & World.

Bayles, M. B. (1981). *Professional ethics.* Belmont, CA: Wadsworth.

Berelson, B. & Steiner, G. (1964). *Human behavior: An inventory of scientific findings.* NY: Harcourt, Brace and World, pp. 365-373.

Borgmann, A. (1992). *Crossing the postmodern divide.* Chicago: The University of Chicago Press,

Dictionary of computing. (1983). NY: Oxford.

Flexner, A. (1915). Is social work a profession? In *Proceedings of the National Conference on Charities and Correction.* Chicago, IL: Hildmann, pp. 578-581.

Haggerty, T. His interpretations and definitions for the terms "data" and "information" were added on July 24, 1985.

March, J. G. & H. A. Simon. (1958). *Organizations.* New York: Wiley.

Research Council of the American Association for Health, Physical Education, and Recreation. (1960). The contributions of physical activity to human well-being. *Research Quarterly*, 31, 2, 261-375.

Rosenberg, J. M. (1978). *Dictionary of business and management.* New York: Wiley.

Royce, J. R. (1964). Paths to knowledge. In *The Encapsulated Man.* Princeton, NJ: Van Nostrand.

Schank, R. C. (1984). *The cognitive computer.* Reading, MA: Addison-Wesley, p. 33.

Zeigler, E. F. (1977). *Physical education and sport philosophy.* Englewood Cliffs, NJ: Prentice-Hall.

Zeigler, E. F. (1979). The past, present, and recommended future development in physical education and sport in North America. In *Proceedings of The American Academy of Physical Education* (G. M. Scott (Ed.), Washington, DC: The American Alliance for Health, Physical Education, Recreation, and Dance.

Zeigler, E. F. (1980). A systems approach to the development and use of theory and research in sport and physical education. *Sportwissenschaft*, 10, 4, 404-416.

Zeigler, E. F. (Ed.) (1982). *Physical education and sport: An introduction.* Philadelphia: Lea & Febiger.

Zeigler, E. F. (1983a). Relating a proposed taxonomy of sport and developmental physical activity to a planned inventory of scientific findings. *Quest*, 35, 54-65.

Zeigler, E. F. & Bowie, G. W. (1983b). *Developing management competency in sport and physical education.* Philadelphia: Lea & Febiger.

Zeigler, E. F. (1994) (ed. & au.). *Physical Education and Kinesiology in North America: Professional & Scholarly*

Foundations. Champaign, IL: Stipes.

Zeigler, E. F. & Bowie, G. W. (1995). *Management competency development in sport and physical education*. Champaign, IL: Stipes.

Zeigler, E. F. (2003). *Socio-Cultural Foundations of Physical Education and Educational Sport*, Aachen, Germany: Meyer and Meyer Sport.

Zeigler, E. F. (2005) *History and Status of American Physical Education and Educational Sport*. Victoria, Canada: Trafford.

Part Four: A Descriptive Research Format, Recommended Research, and Exploratory Studies

Selection #8
An Approach to Comparative Research
In Physical Education and Sport

Eric F. Broom
Canada

In the essentially sedentary, repetitive, and impersonal life of modern industrial societies, it is desirable that everyone–adults and children alike–participate in some form of sport or physical recreation. Since the end of World War II, ever-increasing numbers of adults in these societies have available the necessary discretionary income and time to engage in such activities. However, cultural differences between Western Europe and North America have resulted in inequalities in the provision of opportunities for adults to learn and engage in sports and physical recreation.

The provision of opportunities for adult participation appear to be directly related to the interpretation of the role of the central administration of sport and physical recreation. A wide divergence in the interpretation of this role exists between Western European and North American countries. In a number of Western European countries, of which Great Britain and West Germany are good examples, the central administration of amateur sport and physical recreation embraces a wide range of services. The governing bodies of amateur sport and physical recreation, and the coordinating associations, have particularly in the last 25 years increasingly concerned themselves with more than the control and organization of competition.

They have developed coaching schemes, national coaches, training and accreditation of coaches, and instructional and other promotional activities. These services nurture the provision of opportunities for participation by post-school populations. Inevitably, the administrative demands of such a wide range of services rapidly outgrew the capacity of spare-time officers. To coordinate and service the provision of amateur sport and physical recreation many Western European countries have established Sports Federations.

In North America, particularly in the United States, the corresponding agencies which administer and coordinate amateur sport and physical recreation confine their activities primarily to the control and organization of competition. Beyond the high school, coaching is predominantly associated with universities.

However, in Canada the central administration of amateur sport and physical recreation is a combination of the British and American systems, and in the last decade the governing bodies have attempted to increase the range of their activities. Recent Federal Government proposals indicate a desire for a further expansion of services, similar to those offered in Great Britain and West Germany.

Statement of the Problem

The central problem of this study is to identify, categorize, analyze, and compare the major characteristics of the central administration of amateur sport and physical recreation in Great Britain, West Germany and Canada.

Sub -Problems

1.   What are the key features in the organizational structure of the central administration of amateur sport and physical recreation in Great Britain, West Germany and Canada?
2.   What are the key features in the functional role of the central administration of amateur sport and physical recreation in Great Britain, West Germany and Canada?
3.   How may the efficacy of the central administration of amateur sport and physical recreation in Great Britain, West Germany and Canada be assessed in terms of:
(a) the total number of adult registered participants in selected activities;
(b) indices of in-depth national rankings in selected competitive sports?
4.   What comparisons may be made between the structures, functions and efficacies of the central administration of amateur sport and physical ; recreation in Great Britain, West Germany and Canada?
5.   Based on the findings and comparisons of the study, what conclusions may be drawn, and what recommendations made for adoption in the proposed development of the central administration of amateur sport * and physical recreation in Canada?

Need for the Study

On March 20th, 1970, the Honourable John Munro, Minister of National Health and Welfare, presented a new Proposed Sports Policy for Canadians, the cornerstone of which is an emphasis on participation in amateur sport and physical recreation by the greatest possible number of Canadians. An incidental aim is the upgrading of the calibre of Canadian participation in international sport.

The primary means of implementing the new policy is to be a strengthening of the administrative core of sports governing bodies at the national level. Thus, the proposed central administration of amateur sport and physical recreation in Canada will have much in common with the present systems in Great Britain and West Germany. It will, however, be at a less advanced stage of development. In comparison with the longer established British and German systems it appears to have distinct limitations in both structure and functions. The governing bodies of amateur sport and physical recreation in the two European countries, in conjunction with their Sports Federations, appear to offer a range of services, at national and subordinate levels, which will be offered either on a reduced scale, or not at all, in Canada.

This study examines the central administration of amateur sport and physical recreation in Great Britain, West Germany and Canada. The structure and functions of the two European systems will be analyzed and their major characteristics will be compared to those proposed for Canada. It is hoped that the findings of the study will contribute to the debate on the proposed Sports Policy for Canadians. At the same time, it is hoped that the outcome of this investigation will be of interest in the United States. In 1964 President Lyndon Johnson commissioned a study of the central administration of amateur sport and physical recreation in the United States by Arthur D. Little, Inc., of Cambridge, Massachusetts. The report, entitled "A Proposed National Amateur Sports Federation" was neither acted upon or released to the public. However, the issue will assuredly be reopened.

Definition of Terms

1. Central administration of amateur sport and physical recreation - The agencies at national and para-national level involved in the control, promotion and servicing of all forms of organized amateur sport and physical recreation.

2. Amateur sport and physical recreation - All forms of amateur competitive and non-competitive physical activity. In the terms of this study, all such activities are organized into groups, and have national or regional associations. However, it is by no means a necessity for individuals to join an organized group in order to participate.

3. Governing body - The national, or regional, parent controlling association of an activity

4. Sports Federation - A federation of governing bodies.

Limitations

In this study the central administration of amateur sport and physical recreation in Canada is compared with that in Great Britain and West Germany. It is recognized that by considering only two European countries certain noteworthy factors may be excluded. However, the two countries selected, Great Britain and West Germany, are widely accepted as leaders in this particular area.

Field work for this study will, of necessity, be limited to a 2-3 month period between November 1970 and January 1971.
The problems of making meaningful comparisons between the two European countries, Great Britain and West Germany, and Canada, which differ in terms of size, topography, climate, and population size and distribution are acknowledged. Cognizance of these differences will be taken before any recommendations are made.

Sources of Data

The historical background to the study will be based on a careful examination of the literature which relates to the organization and administration of amateur sport and physical recreation. As the chapter unfolds the examination will focus on three twentieth century developments the greatly expanded role of the central administration of amateur sport and physical recreation, the evolution of the sports federations, and the role of the central government in the central administration of amateur sport and physical recreation. The primary emphasis in the present century will be directed towards developments in Great Britain, West Germany and Canada.

The main sources of data for the historical background to the study will be the writings of Brailsford, Carl Diem, Liselott Diem, Dixon, Howell and Howell, Lindsay, McIntosh, Staley, and Zeigler.

1. Brailsford, D. *Sport and Society: Elizabeth to Anne*. London: Routledge and Kegan Paul, 1969
2. Diem, C. *Developments and Aims of Physical Education in Germany. JOHPER*, June, 1948
3. Diem, C. *German Sport Movement*. Cologne, Sporthochschule, 1957.
4. Diem, L. "Health, Physical Education and Recreation in the Federal Republic of Germany," in *The World Today in Health, Physical Education and Recreation* (Editors: L. Vendien and J. Nixon). Englewood Cliffs, NJ: Prentice-Hall, 1968.
5. Dixon, J. G. "Prussia, Politics and Physical Education," in *Landmarks in the History of Physical Education*. (Editors Dixon, Mcintosh, Munrow, and Willetts). London: Routledge and Kegan Paul, 1957.
6. Howell, N, and Howell, M. L. *Sports and Games in Canadian Life*. Toronto: Macmillan of Canada, 1969.
7. Lindsay, P. "The Impact of the Military Garrisons on the Development of Sport in British North America." Canadian *Journal of History of Sport and Physical Education*. Vol. I,

No. 1, May, 1970.

8. McIntosh, P. C. "Twentieth Century Attitudes to Sport in Britain," in *The International Review of Sport Sociology*. (Editor Andrzej Wohl). Warsaw: Polish Scientific Publishers, 1966.

9. McIntosh, P. C. *Landmarks in the History of Physical Education*. London: Routledge and Kegan Paul, 1957.

10. McIntosh, P. C. Physical Education in England Since 1800. London: G. Bell and Sons, 1968.

11. McIntosh, P. C. "The British Attitude to Sport," in *Sport in Society*. (Editor Alex Natan). London: Bowes & Bowes, 1958.

12. McIntosh, P. C. *Sport in Society*. London: C. A. Watts and Company, Ltd., 1963.

13. Staley, S. "Physical Training and Sport in Pre-Nazi Germany," in *The Athletic Journal*. January, 1941.

14. Zeigler, E. F. *Problems in the History and Philosophy of Physical Education and Sport*. Englewood Cliffs, New Jersey: Prentice-Hall, Inc., 1968.

Additional sources are listed below:

Arntz, Helmut.
1. Facts About Germany) The Federal Government
2. The Rising Generation) Office, 1968.
3. Youth Affairs and Sport)
Britain in the World of Sport. Physical Education Department, University of *Olympischer Sportverlag* Birmingham. London: The Physical Education Association, 1966.
Dambach, J. *Physical Education in Germany*. New York: Columbia University Press, 1937.
Deutscher Sport. GmbH, Dortmund. Dortmund: Druckerei Friedrich Wilhelm Cruwell, 1967.
Howell, M. L. and Van Vliet, M. L. *Physical Education and Recreation in Europe*. Fitness and Amateur Sport Directorate, Department of National Health and Welfare, Canada, 1965.
Karbe, Wolfgang. "Physical Education and Sports in East and West Germany." *The Physical Educator*. October, 1962.
Molyneux, D. D. "Central Government Aid to Sport and Physical Recreation in Countries of Western Europe." Birmingham, 1962.
(The Honourable) John Munro, Minister, Department of National Health and Welfare. "Canadian Sports Potential." (Speech to AAPERA Conference, Moncton, N. B., November, 1968).

211

Olafson, G. A. "The History of Bill C 131." *Canadian Journal of History of Sport and Physical Education.* May, 1970.

Richter, P. "Physical Education in Germany." *Physical Education Around the World.* Editor W. Johnson. Monograph 1, 1956.

Singer, C., et al. *History of Technology.* London: Oxford University Press, Vols. 2, 3, and 5, 1948-1958.

Sport. A magazine of the Federal Republic of Germany, 1965-1970. Hamburg: Broschek and Co., K. G.

Sport and the Community. Report of the Wolfenden Committee on Sport. London: Central Council of Physical Recreation, 1960.

Sport and Recreation. A magazine of the Central Council of Physical Recreation. London.

Sports Development Bulletin. London: Central Council of Physical Recreation. London. 1967-1970.

Winterbottom, W. "The Pattern of Sport in the United Kingdom." Sports Council. London, 1966.

World Sports. The official magazine of the British Olympic Association, London

Data on the present status of the central administration of amateur sport and physical recreation in Great Britain, West Germany, and Canada will be obtained primarily from personal interviews with officers in the central administration in the three countries. This data will be supplemented and cross-validated by data obtained from documentary analysis of government publications and official reports and records of which the following are examples:

Great Britain
　　Central Council of Physical Recreation. Annual Reports.
　　The Sports Council: A Report. London: H. M. S. O., 1966.
　　Planning for Sport. The Sports Council. London, 1968.
　　The Sports Council: A Review, 1966-1969.
West Germany
　　Deutsche Sportbund. Annual Reports.
　　Deutsche Sportbund. German Sport Manifesto. 1966.
Canada
　　Fitness and Amateur Sport Directorate. *Annual Reports.*
　　Canadian Amateur Sports Federation. *Annual Reports.*
　　Report of the Task Force on Sports for Canadians. Department of National Health and Welfare, 1969.
　　A Proposed Sports Policy for Canada. Presented by the Honourable John Munro, Minister of National Health and Welfare, March 20, 1970.

Data on the total number of adult registered participants in selected activities will be obtained from the official records of the sport and physical recreation associations in each country. In addition, data on the national performance rankings, of both men and women, in track and field and swimming will be obtained from the annual ranking lists of the top 100 performers in the world in each sport.

Research Methodology and Techniques

The survey of literature will place in historical perspective the central administration of organized amateur sport and physical recreation in the last one third of the twentieth century. In order to demonstrate the metamorphosis of the administration to its present stage of development, an examination will be made of amateur sport and physical recreation, and the form of its administrative structure, throughout history.

To facilitate this examination of the promotion and administration of sport and physical recreation, history will be arbitrarily divided into four time periods. This division will enable the examination to focus on the twentieth century, in which the major developments in the central administration of amateur sport and physical recreation have occurred. Throughout the examination developments will be viewed in the political, economic, cultural and social contexts. The first time period will be up to 1750 and, although the examination of sport in early societies will be rather cursory, it will be more detailed in the last 150 years of the period. In this latter part of the period the examination will be centered on Europe.

The second period of history is the century and a half from 1750 to 1900, during which modern sport first became organized, and an embryonic administrative structure was established. It was in the third period, 1900 to 1940, that two major developments in the field of amateur sport's administration occurred. These developments were the evolution of the sports federations, and the beginning of the involvement of the central government in the administration of amateur sport. In the fourth period, from 1940 to 1970, the role of the central administration of amateur sport and physical recreation was greatly expanded. The examination in these three periods, from 1750-1970, will be primarily concerned with developments in the three countries under review, Great Britain, West Germany, and Canada.

The collection of data will be carried out primarily by utilizing survey research techniques. Personal interviews will be arranged with officers in the central administration of amateur sport and physical recreation in Great Britain, West Germany and Canada. The interviewees will be asked to respond to an unstructured questionnaire based on the present structure and functions of the central administration of amateur sport and physical recreation in their country.

Basically, this investigation will employ the descriptive method of research, more specifically the comparative method of descriptive research developed by Bereday. Still more specifically, the following techniques of descriptive research will be employed to gather the data needed: (1) personal interviews which utilize structured and open-ended questions, (2) mailed questionnaires which contain both types of questions, (3) documentary analysis, and (4) check lists.

Development of the Instrument

In this investigation of the central administration of amateur sport and physical recreation in England and Canada, data will be needed in two distinct categories: 1) the major characteristics of the present structure and functions, and 2) an assessment of the present structure and functions. (Note: At this point it was decided to eliminate Germany from the study.) The instrument to be employed in the personal interviews will be made up of questions designed to elicit data for both categories, while the instrument to be used in the mailed questionnaire will seek to secure data only for the second category. In both the personal interview and the mailed questionnaire instruments, the questions in the assessment category will be designed to elicit a response on a five-point scale. Both instruments will contain structured and open-ended questions.

Collection of the Data

Personal interviews will be arranged with the Director and Deputy Director of the Sports Council (S. C.), and the Principal Technical Administrative and Executive Officers of the Central Council of Physical Recreation (CCPR) in England, and the Director and two specialist Consultants of the Fitness and Amateur Sport Directorate (FASD), and a Director and the Secretary of the Canadian Amateur Sports Federation (CASF) in Canada.

The mailed questionnaire will be sent to every governing body of amateur sport and physical recreation in England and Canada, (1) at national level, and (2) in one province and one country selected by the senior officer in each country as an example of a regional sports federation in their country. Documentary analysis will be carried out on Government Publications of both countries, and on official reports and records of the Sports Council and the Central Council of Physical Recreation, and the Fitness and Amateur Sport Directorate and the Canadian Amateur Sports Federation in Canada.

Check lists will be utilized to support the data obtained by the three principal methods outlined above. They will be employed wherever possible.

A 35 mm. still camera will be used to obtain photographic slides of facilities controlled by the central administration of amateur sport and physical recreation in each country. These facilities will primarily consist of sports training and recreation centers.

When travel from city to city, or sports center, is involved, time will be devoted before departure for a careful examination of the accumulated data. In this way, shortcomings or trends may be noted, acted upon, or corrected while the opportunity to do so still exists.

Analysis and Interpretation of Data

In the analysis of the data, four stages–as advocated by Bereday (1964)–will be employed. These stages will involve: (1) description,(2) interpretation, (3) juxtaposition and (4) comparison.

The data obtained from the personal interviews and the documentary analysis will be primarily descriptive and interpretive in nature. Thus, the first stage of the analysis will be a description of the existing structure and functions of the central administration of amateur sport and physical recreation in each country.

In order to facilitate the later stages of comparative analysis, the data obtained from the personal interviews and the documentary analysis will be organized into categories and sub-categories. The main categories will be: (1) Central Government allocation of funds to amateur sport and physical recreation, (2) organizational structure, and (3) functional role, which is subdivided into: (a) external relations, and (b) areas of operation. The 29 sub-categories within the four main categories may be seen in the Horizontal Analysis below.

An interpretation, or explanation, of the developments leading to the existing central administration of amateur sport and physical recreation in the two countries under review, will have been provided in a political, economic, cultural, and social context in the historical background to the studypresented in Chapter II.

The data obtained from the returns to the mailed questionnaire, supported by assessment data from the personal interviews of senior officers, and the documentary analysis, will be analyzed to make an assessment of the existing structure and functions of the central administration of amateur sport and physical recreation in each country. The assessment will be made within a framework of organization structural levels developed by Talcott Parsons. Parsons' model consists of three levels: (1) the Institutional, (2) the Managerial, and (3) the Technical, which, in the case of the central administration of amateur sport and physical recreation, correspond to the advisory committee, national executive, and regional executive levels.

In the third stage of analysis a juxtaposition of data will be carried out.

215

The major characteristics of the central administration of amateur sport and physical recreation in the two countries will be related within the established categories which have determined the criteria for comparability. Through the process of juxtaposition, similarities and differences between the categorized data will be established in preparation for the final stage of comparison.

An examination of the juxtaposed data will be made in search of unifying concepts to confirm the tentative hypotheses. The formulated hypotheses will be tested in the final comparative stage of the analysis.

Reporting of Data

The allocation of government funds for amateur sport and physical recreation in the two countries will be presented in tabular and graphical form for the five year period 1964-1969. To permit the grants to be viewed comparatively, the data will be categorized according to the type of organization, and/or the purpose for which the grants were made. Similar illustrative techniques will be employed wherever possible with other data.

The final comparative analysis of the existing structure and functions of the central administration of amateur sport and physical recreation in England and Canada, and an assessment of the major characteristics of the two systems will be reported within the framework of the existing categories. A comparative analytical report of the two countries will be presented category by category.

The final comparisons will consider the status of each country in terms of size, topography, climate, economy, population size and distribution. Cognizance of differences will be taken before any conclusions are drawn.

Proposed Organization of the Thesis

Chapter I. Introduction

Chapter I will include a brief introduction to the role of the central administration of amateur sport and physical recreation in the countries under review. It will also include a statement of the problem, and sub-problems, a justification of the study, the scope of the study and its limitations, and definitions of pertinent terms.

Chapter II. Related Literature

The purpose of Chapter II will be to place in historical perspective the central administration of organized amateur sport and physical recreation in the last third of the twentieth century. In order to demonstrate the metamorphosis of the administration of sport and physical recreation to its present stage of development a brief examination will be made of sport, and the consequent form of its administration, throughout history.

Chapter III. Methodology

In this chapter will be a detailed outline of the research methods employed in the study. The collection of data will be carried out primarily by means of personal interviews based on an unstructured questionnaire. This data will be supplemented and cross-validated by data obtained from documentary analysis and by measures which reflect overall adult participation and national competitive strengths. In addition, the methods which will be used to categorize, analyze and compare the data will be included.

Chapter IV. Analysis and Interpretation of the Data

The data will be categorized and analyzed in this chapter. In the analysis of the data, four stages of comparative analysis will be employed: (1) description, (2) interpretation, (3) juxtaposition, (4) comparison. Following the third stage, hypotheses will be formulated, and in the comparison stage an attempt will be made to test the hypotheses derived from the juxtaposition.

Chapter V. Summary and Conclusions

The final chapter will contain the summary, findings and conclusions drawn on the basis of the study. A short discussion section will be included. Recommendations for adoption in the proposed development of the central administration of amateur sport and physical recreation in Canada will also be made.

(See horizontal analysis beginning on the next page)

A COMPARATIVE ANALYSIS OF THE CENTRAL ADMINISTRATION OF AMATEUR SPORT AND PHYSICAL RECREATION IN GREAT BRITAIN, WEST GERMANY AND CANADA*

STATEMENT OF THE PROBLEM: The central problem of this study is to identify, categorize, analyze, and compare the major characteristics of the central administration of sport and physical recreation in Great Britain, West Germany and Canada.

SUB-PROBLEMS	WHAT FACTS ARE NEEDED?	WHERE & HOW MAY THE FACTS BE OBTAINED?	HOW WILL THE FACTS BE ORGANIZED AND ANALYZED?	PROBABLE OUTCOMES

1. What influences have resulted in the evolution and development of the central administration of amateur sport and physical recreation.	The role of sport and physical recreation from early civilization to the present.
	
	The political, economic, cultural and social factors which have influenced the status of sport and physical recreation and the form of its administrative structure and function, throughout history
		Survey of the Literature: Library research techniques.
		
		1) Personal Interviews based on an unstructured questionnaire.
		a) Officers of Sports Federations.
		b) Officers of amateur sport and physical recreation governing bodies.
		c) Officers of Government departments which liaise with the agencies involved in the central administration of amateur sport and physical recreation.
			The evolution and development of the central administration of amateur sport and physical recreation will be viewed in the political, economic, cultural, and social context. History will be arbitrarily divided into 4 time periods:
			   1) up to 1750,
			   2) 1750-1900,
			   3) 1900-1940,
			   4) 1940-1970. The existing situation will thus be placed in historical perspective.
				Political, economic, cultural and social differences in the 3 countries under review have resulted in the evolution and development of the central administration of amateur sport and physical recreation occurring at different rates and in different spheres.
				
				The structure of the central administration of amateur sport and physical recreation in both European countries will be integrated, and encompass the whole country. In contrast, the structure in Canada will be more fragmented.

2. What are the key features in the organizational structure of the central administration of amateur sport and physical recreation in Great Britain, West Germany and Canada?	The following facts concerning the agencies involved in the central administration of amateur sport and physical recreation:
	   1) Aims and objectives
	   2) Operating mandate
	   3) Policies and procedures
	   4) Budget
	     a) Sources of operating funds
	     b) Legislation permitting Government grants
	     c) Criteria for Government grants
	     d) Machinery of grant allocation
	     e) Extent of Government grants
	   5) Organizational structure
	   6) Remuneration levels and policies
	   7) Personnel policies
	   8) Facilities controlled by the agency.
		2) Documentary Analysis
		   a) Official reports and records of the Sports Federations and their constituent member associations
		   b) Government publications
			The data relevant to sub-problems 2 and 3 will be organized into the categories listed in column 2. Wherever possible the data will be presented in tabular or graphical form.
			
			Comparative Analysis
			In the analysis of the data, 4 stages-as advocated by Bereday (1964), will be employed. These stages will involve:
			   1) description
			   2) interpretation,
			   3) juxtaposition,
			   4) comparison.
			Stages 1, 2, and 3 will be undertaken in response to sub-problems 2 and 3	

* It was finally decided to eliminate Germany from the study.

SUB-PROBLEMS	WHAT FACTS ARE NEEDED?	WHERE & HOW MAY THE FACTS BE OBTAINED?	HOW WILL THE FACTS BE ORGANIZED AND ANALYZED?	PROBABLE OUTCOMES

3. What are the key features in the functional role of the central administration of amateur sport and physical recreation in Great Britain, West· Germany and Canada?
 	
4. How may the existing structure and functions of the central administration of amateur sport and physical recreation in England and Canada be assessed
	A. External Relations
	  1) National, regional, local government
	  2) Governing bodies of sport and physical recreation
	  3) Education authorities
	  4) Universities and colleges
	  5) Professional organizations
	  6) Commercial sport
	  7) Industry
	  8) Community
	
	B. Areas of Operation
	  1) Administration
	  2) Coordination
	  3) Clerical
	  4) Coaching schemes
	  5) Training of coaches
	  6) Accreditation of coaches
	  7) Sports promotion
	  8) Organization of competition
	  9) Research
	  10) Documentation
	  11) Planning
	  12) Advisory
	  13) Publicity
	
	Opinions of the strengths and weaknesses and functions of the central administration of amateur sport and physical recreation in England and Canada.
		As in Sub-problem 2
		
		1) Personal interviews of senior officers of:
		-Sports Council
		-Central Council of Physical Recreation
		-Canadian Amateur Sports Federation
		-Fitness and Amateur Sport Directorate.
		2) Mailed questionnaire to governing bodies of amateur sport and physical recreation at:
		1) national, and
		2) regional level in England and Canada.
		3) Documentary analysis of Government publications and official reports of governing bodies of sport and physical recreation.
		4) Check lists.
			As in Sub-problem 2
			
			The assessment will will be made within the framework of organization structural levels developed by Parsons. The three levels will be: 1) Institutional,
			  2) Managerial, and
			  3) Technical.
				The external relations of the central administration of amateur sport and physical recreation in Great Britain and West Germany will be comprehensive in nature, whereas those in Canada will tend to be sparse.
				
				The areas of operation of the central administration of amateur sport and physical recreation in the 2 European countries under review will be much more extensive and coordinated than those offered in Canada.

SUB-PROBLEMS	WHAT FACTS ARE NEEDED?	WHERE & HOW MAY THE FACTS BE OBTAINED?	HOW WILL THE FACTS BE ORGANIZED AND ANALYZED?	PROBABLE OUTCOMES
5. What comparisons may be made between the structures, functions, and efficacies of the central administration of amateur sport and physical recreation in Great Britain, West Germany and Canada?	Details of the structure, functions, and efficacies of the central administration of amateur sport and physical recreation in Great Britain, West Germany and Canada.	Through a **comparison** of the categorized data obtained in response to subproblems 1, 2, 3 and 4.	**Following the juxtaposition** stage undertaken with the the categorized data in sub-problems 2, 3 and 4, the fourth stage of **comparative analysis** - namely **comparison** - will be carried out. Throughout the comparison the data will be analyzed in the established categories.	A comparison of the structure, functions and efficacy of the central administration of amateur sport and physical recreation in the 3 countries under review will reveal a uniformly advanced level of development in the 2 European countries, but widespread limitations in Canada.
6. Based on the findings and comparisons of the study, what conclusions may be drawn, and what recommendations made for adoption in the proposed development of the central administration of amateur sport and physical recreation in Canada ?	Limitations in structure, function and efficacy of the central administration of amateur sport and physical recreation in Canada. Knowledge of the methods by which the 2 European countries under review have overcome problems similar to those presently experienced by Canada.	From the **comparative analysis** in response to sub-problem 5.	A brief discussion in which the conclusions drawn from the **comparative analysis** will be presented.	Accept or reject the hypotheses. A list of recommendations for adoption in the proposed development of the central administration of amateur sport and physical recreation in Canada. Recommendations for further study.

Selection #9
The Comparative Approach to Research in Physical Education and Sport

Donald H. Morrison
Canada

Note: This is essentially Chapter 3 of a M. A.
Thesis completed by Mr. Morrison at the
University of Alberta in 1967.

It would be difficult at this time to state exactly what the nature of comparative study in physical education is. * This will become more apparent as the field develops and as attention is given to both theoretical concepts and methodological approaches. It is possible, though, to give consideration to certain factors which will be involved in structuring methods of research.

The Scope of Studies

With each empirical study it is necessary to delimit in some way the scope of the investigation. A common approach in other comparative fields is to select specific geographic areas such as Great Britain or South America. Generally the areas chosen fall within political boundaries. Although many cultural features ignore such boundaries, the organizations associated with physical education and physical recreation tend to be structured so as to operate within the boundaries of political units. Area studies, as these are often called, may focus on a block of countries such as Scandinavia, or on national, provincial, district, or local units. The smaller the area, the more specific and detailed the investigation tends to be.

A second method of limiting the breadth that a study is to cover is to focus on a certain level or on a particular organization. It would be useful to look at physical education at certain school or grade levels, or to survey topics such as national sports organizations, professional preparation programs and public recreation.

Bereday recommends the "problem approach" to provide an even narrower scope and to give beginning researchers an opportunity to employ the techniques of comparative research on a small scale.- One topic or theme is selected and examined in a number of countries. The ICHPER report on the "Status of Teachers of Physical Education,"[2] and Molyneux's study of "Central Government Aid to Sport and Physical Recreation in Countries of Western Europe,"[3] are examples of this approach. The range of topics which can be dealt with by a problem approach is unlimited and such information could be of significant value in solving certain problems in the field. With experience, the researcher can gradually increase the scope of his problem area until he reaches the point where he feels confident in attempting a total analysis of a country. In making the decision as to the scope of the study, the researcher will be influenced by his interests and experience, and by the type of information that he requires to adequately cover his topic.

Stages of Comparative Research

Regardless of its scope or the particular methods that are employed, each comparative study seems to pass through a number of steps or phases. The important first task in comparative research is to provide descriptive data. Some care must be taken to ensure that the data which is collected is relevant to the topic and that all the data required for an adequate analysis has been located, m addition to describing the organizational structures under study and their functions, it is necessary to Identify and describe the relevant factors in the cultural context which interact with them. Kandel refers to descriptive analyses as "valuable provided that they are accurate and written with a knowledge and insight into the forces that give them meaning, and they provide the materials for comparative education without themselves being entitled to be called by that name."4 Although description is essential, the implication here is that it is merely the First step in comparative research.

It is important not only to "learn about" or describe another system, but, also to endeavor to "study into" or explain the reasons for its character and the ways in which it functions.5 This process of explanation involves the interpretation of information and consists of subjecting descriptive data to analyses which use the techniques of other social sciences" such as cultural anthropology, sociology, and social psychology. Without such analyses, true understanding of the structure and function of any aspect of a system can never occur. Even though the preceding steps of description and explanation are carried out, it does not necessarily mean that it is a comparative study

Comparison implies that two or more things are compared, and it is not adequate to merely list the analysis of one country after another. A true comparative approach involves juxtaposition; a process by which materials related to a particular aspect in each of the countries are brought together and viewed simultaneously. Comparison, then, is the final analysis which presents this data in an orderly and interrelated manner, that highlights the similarities and differences, and comments on the reasons for them.7

The Researcher's Background and Interests

Each of the phases in the comparative process is coloured by the researcher's personal background and interests. In the descriptive phase this factor often influences what is s elected as being the relevant data. It also governs the choice of techniques and theoretical concepts which are employed to carry out explanation and analysis. For example, the historian

222

would employ historical techniques and theories in his search back into history to discover and explain how certain events and personalities have been significant In the development of the organizations under study. Similarly, the geographer would pay close attention to the effect of physical environment, the cultural anthropologist to aspects of the cultural context, and the sociologist to the social environment. Each specialist approaches comparative research with certain biases for the type of data he requires and for the way he intends to analyze and present this data. As a result, several different approaches to comparative study are possible and each has particular strengths and weaknesses.

Interdisciplinary Approach

In the past, the various disciplines which make up the behavioral and social sciences have tended to maintain their autonomy. Each established boundaries for its areas of investigation and developed its own approaches to research. In many cases the boundaries overlapped and this compartmentalized approach to research tended to segment complex phenomena into unnatural divisions. This prevented any one discipline from adequately investigating the subject of study. The application of the knowledge and techniques of several of these disciplines is necessary before any significant understanding of social and cultural phenomena occur. Thus, it was a logical step to introduce interdisciplinary research in order to more realistically study complex behavioral and social phenomena. This approach to research has been utilized a great deal more in recent years.

Comparative research is particularly suited to an interdisciplinary approach, either through the cooperative efforts of researchers in several disciplines or the eclectic use of concepts and methods from several fields by a single researcher. The latter is much more difficult to do successfully because of the depth of knowledge that must be mastered in each area before good research can be accomplished. The comparative researcher tends to professional training of teachers. I6 On three occasions, Matthew Arnold was appointed to commissions whose tasks were to study education in selected European countries. He made detailed reports in government "Blue Books" as well as in his personal publications.17 In all cases, these administrators based their reports on their own subjective observations and opinions of the formal educational institutions in the countries visited. Little concern was given to other institutions in the culture which may have had either direct or indirect influences on the educational process. In most cases, the focus of attention was entirely on the educational administration, facilities and programs.

In the past, there have been several examples of administrators journeying to other countries to study the system of physical education or to promote their own system of physical education in those countries. For example, Per Henrik Ling, the prominent leader in Swedish physical education, first became acquainted with Nachtegall's version of Guts Mums' system of gymnastics while he was a student in Copenhagen.18 He also made summer travels to Germany, France and England to further increase his knowledge of physical education in these countries.19 Ling returned to Sweden and over a number of years gradually developed what became known as the "Ling System." This system was, in turn, taken to England by men like Indcbetou, Ehrenhoff and Georgii, and to the United States by Nissen and Posse. This serves to illustrate one of the ways in which administrators played a role in the spread of practices in physical education from one country to another,

The Basis for Modern Methods

Comparative educators are indebted to Sir Michael Sadler for drawing attention to the weaknesses of the traditional approach to comparative study. At the turn of the century, he established certain principles which have been the cornerstone of the theoretical orientation of the field during the twentieth century.[20] Sadler was able to take the studies made by administrators preceding him and "systematize and extend them with sociological insight and scientific accuracy." [21] Sadler stressed the fact that:

> In studying foreign systems of Education we should not
> forget that the things outside the schools matter even
> more than the things inside the schools and govern and
> interpret the things inside. We cannot wander at pleasure
> among the educational systems of the world, like a child
> strolling through a garden, and pick off a flower from one
> bush and some leaves from another and then expect that
> if we stick what we have gathered into the soil at home,
> we shall have a living plant. A national system of
> Education is a living thing, the outcome of forgotten
> struggles and difficulties, and 'of battles long ago'. It has
> in it some of the secret workings of national life. It
> reflects, while it seeks to remedy, the failings of the
> national character.[22]

As a result, he placed emphasis on the concept of national character as a methodological tool to explain educational ideas and practices.[23] Sadler recommended that researchers acquire a sound knowledge of the local educational scene so that they would be able to judge how well successful arrangements employed elsewhere would fit local conditions. He felt that there were often possibilities for adapting points of foreign systems to one's own use if they were "shed of their localizing context. "[24]

In summary, Sadler's main contributions to methodology in comparative education were: (1) to point out the need to pay attention to the natural and socio-cultural factors in the setting surrounding the educational system; (2) to have a sound knowledge of the local situation; and (3) to consider the surrounding contexts when adapting ideas from other systems.

The Historical Approach

Kandel, Hans and Ulich are among the chief proponents of the historical approach to comparative education. Hans captures the essence of this method of research (n the following explanation:

> The historical approach tries to investigate the past
> causes of individual and group variations among
> religious or national communities. The differences of
> denominational attitudes, of national aspirations or of
> so-called 'nation al character' go deep into the past
> and sometimes subconsciously determine the present.
> Only historical investigation **can** bring them to the
> surface, illuminate their potency **in** the cultural lives
> of nations and make Comparative Education really
> educative. [25]

Both Kandel and Hans recommend historical studies of the national background and environmental forces which determine the character of the educational system. [26] Kandel foresees the need for interdisciplinary cooperation to study these underlying sociologic, economic, technologic, political and cultural factors [27] Hans develops certain categories to be considered in the analysis and they are summarized briefly In the following outline:

> 1. Natural conditions. The natural conditions which
> Influence national systems of education include: (a)
> racial factors, whether a pure race or a hybridization of
> two or more races; (b) national language as the medium
> of social intercourse and an outward symbol of
> nationality, and whether the country is unilingual,
> bilingual, or multilingual; and (c) social and physical
> environment including economic conditions and
> occupational activities, and the geographic conditions
> of physiographic features and climate.
>
> 2. Religious traditions. Hans considers the religious
> traditions of humanity under four main groups: (a)
> Christianity, (b) Islam, (c) Hinduism, and (d) Oriental.
>
> 3. Secular movements. Hans recognizes three main
> movements of protest and reform: (a) humanism, the
> attempts to liberate the common people from
> deplorable conditions; (b) socialism, the protest against

the economic exploitation of the masses by the ruling minority; and (c) nationalism, the natural expression of national character.

In summary, then, Hans would consider three definite groups of factors in his analysis: (1) Natural factors; (a) race, (b) language, and (c) environment; (2) Religious factors, (3) Secular movements: (a) humanism, (b) socialism, and (c) nationalism.28

Hans also recognizes the fact that education is a factor in the moulding of national character. Therefore, a cyclical process takes place in which factors of national character affect education, and education, in turn, has an influence on them.29

In covering the historical background upon which several education systems are based, Ulich employees historical analysis to show how education followed different paths as a result of national factors and characteristics. He then attempts to make generalizations to new nations. 30

Lauwerys adopts a slightly different approach to comparative education by emphasizing the importance of understanding "national styles in philosophy." He feels that explanations based on the "national character" approach are too vague and too general.[31] He asserts that the education system and its aims are influenced by the philosophy in favor in the country at the time and so are the other systems which operate in the country. Therefore, an understanding of the basic underlying philosophy assists the researcher to become aware of the ideological climate whic h guides the decisions of educational policy makers. [22]

The historical approach, based on Sadlerian principles, represents one Of the earliest attempts to establish methodology for comparative education in the twentieth century. The ideas surrounding the themes of "national character" and "national philosophy" are recognized today as an important aspect of comparative studies. 33

Although the historical approach has proven adequate for assessing the effects of national character, it fails to distinguish between national characteristics and other group characteristics. Thus, It does not consider all the factors which interact with the education system. 31

Recent Trends in Comparative Education

The modern trends in comparative education represent an attempt to combine the benefits of the historical approach with the scientific advantages of the methods employed by social scientists In a number of fields, On the whole, there has been Increasing emphasis on the need for interdisciplinary cooperation in research. 35 The stress on educational planning has created the need for a conceptual framework for comparative studies which not only assess the historical determinants but also analyze the present functioning of the educational system. With this type of research it may be possible to predict some of the problems which will face education in the future, thus enabling plans to be made in advance. [56]

Bereday establishes four phases for a comparative study; description, explanation, juxtaposition and comparison. [37] In the explanation phase he recommends an analysis of the pedagogical data available by the application of the methods of other social sciences, Bereday does not provide a precise set of categories to identify the relevant factors that should be considered in a social analysis, but he does recommend that attention be paid to history, economics, philosophy, psychology, sociology, anthropology, political science and science. [38]

Moehlman tends to be more specific In outlining categories to guide comparative research. For the analysis of the education system itself he identifies the three major categories of orientation, organization and operation. Under "orientation" he considers the factors of philosophy, law and finance which give direction to the system. The "organization" mirrors the philosophy and is the general structure of the education system with its various levels and departments. The "operation" of the system involves students, teachers, curricula, methods of instruction, instructional materials, evaluation and testing, guidance, supervision and administration. [39] But Moehlman feels is it not enough to compare education systems on the basis of these three categories. He indicates the necessity of considering the interaction as "the long-range factors making up the various sectors of the nation's culture" with the education system. Moehlman sets out the following theoretical model for analysis:

(Please move forward to the next page.)

TABLE I
LONG-RANGE FACTORS AFFECTING THE EDUCATION SYSTEM

FOLK—Ethnic sources, quantity, quality and age structure of population

SPACE—Spatial concepts, territoriality and natural features

TIME—Temporal concepts, historical development and evolution of culture

LANGUAGE—Symbols, message systems and communication of conceptual thought

ART—Aesthetics, search for beauty and play

PHILOSOPHY—Value choices, pursuit of wisdom and the good life

RELIGION—Relation of man and the universe, belief systems

SOCIAL STRUCTURE—Family, kinship, sex, etiquette and social classes

GOVERNMENT—Ordering of human relations, governmental structures and operations

ECONOMICS—Satisfaction of wants, exchange, production and consumption

TECHNOLOGY—Use of natural resources through machines, techniques and power resources

SCIENCE—The sphere of knowledge concerning both natural and human realms

HEALTH—The condition of physical, mental and emotional well-being Including functions of living

EDUCATION—The social process of directed learning, both formative and informal

---

Arthur Moehlman. *Comparative Education Systems*. Washington; Center for Applied Research in Education, 1963, p. 9.

Moehlman states that "The impact of these long-range factors determines the profile of education." These factors tend to interact with each other and determine the efficiency of education, but these are, in turn, affected by the changes that occur in the educational pattern. 40 Moehlman does attempt to provide a conceptual structure and his categories and long-range factors do facilitate the analysis of educational systems.

King and his colleagues in England are presently employing the computer to aid in the analysis of school developments. King recognizes the complicated dynamics of forces in the "ecological" situation (language, religion, race, sociology, economics, politics, psychology and philosophy) which are constantly interacting with the education system to change it and be changed by it. 41 His plan is to feed myriads of observations about the education system and the other relevant systems into the computer which accelerates the calculations between the various factors. The results may reveal certain trends in education. 42 King's work is still in the embryonic stage and may be of greater value as it becomes better developed. The present difficulty is that only certain types of data are amenable to computer treatment and as a result the importance of ideological and behavioral components which cannot yet be quantified is not assessed.

Anderson is a strong supporter for the use of sociology in comparative education. He recognizes that sociology does not have a monopoly role to play but indicates certain directions In which It can be useful. 43 Anderson states that:

> In its broadest sense, comparative education might
> be defined as cross-cultural comparisons of the
> structure, operation, aims, methods and
> achievements of various education systems, and
> the societal correlates of these educational systems
> and their elements, 44

Based on this definition of comparative education, Anderson proposes that sociology can make potential contributions in the following areas: (1) the assessment of the function of education in maintaining societal cohesion such as finding a balance between national unity and the striving for international unity; (2) trying to assess the influence of public opinion in educational policy making; (3) analysis of accelerated change of certain aspects of culture; (4) investigating the relationships between education and the social status system; (5) studying "the molding of personality by social structure to discover the distinctive way in which education transmits selected aspects of culture"; (6) studying education as a profession; and (7) studying education as a bureaucracy. 45 Anderson also feels that sociological techniques such as the Nadel theory of co-variation can assist in the development of "typologies" of educational systems by identifying common fundamental features that are found in them all. 46 As shown earlier, sociology helps display the relationships between various educational characteristics and associated sociological, economic, or other non-educational features. 47

The theme of the expert meeting convened by the UNESCO Institute for Education. Hamburg, in March, 19C3, was "the need to Identify and classify background data as they bear upon the formulation of policy and upon its outcomes. "48 During the conference, the twenty-four participants from fifteen countries presented and discussed a number of frameworks for classifying relevant data in three general areas; (1) description of the institutions of education; (2) causal explanation of educational systems in terms of important background factors; and (3) planning and the evaluation of educational success. "19 The results of the conference are aptly reported by Holmes and Robinsohn in a book which would prove valuable for anyone contemplating comparative studies in physical education. 50 Some of the frameworks, particularly those employed to describe institutions of education, appear to have application for studies in comparative physical education. They are produced in brief form here and will be explained more fully in the final chapter where they are applied to the physical education context.

Hilker presented the following framework for classifying the organization of the school system:

(Please see Table II on the following page.

TABLE II
CLASSIFICATION OF VERTICAL AND HORIZONTAL RELATIONSHIPS3

(a) **Pre-school Education**

(b) **Education at the First Level**

    Stage 1 - Primary schools

(c) **Education at the Second Level**

    Stage 2 - Upper section of elementary schools; intermediate schools; lower section of high schools, grammar schools, gymnasiums,

    Stage 3 - Upper section high schools, grammar schools, gymnasium teacher training, full-time and part-time. vocational schools.

(d) **Education at the Third Level**

    Stage 4 - Undergraduate colleges, advanced technical schools, lower stages of university study, teacher training.

    Stage 5 - Professional schools, higher stages of university study, teacher education.

(c) **Education at the Fourth Level**

    Stage 6 - Postgraduate study.

Holmes and S. B. Robinsohn. *Relevant Data in Comparative Education.* **Hamburg: UNESCO Institute for Education, 19fi3, pp. 51, 57. An adapted version.**

For the comparison of schools, Hoz presented the following framework on the next page:

TABLE III
CLASSIFICATION OF DATA FOR THE COMPARISON OF SCHOOLSa

1. Origin and Evolution of the School
2. Aims and Objectives
3. Personnel
   3:1 Teachers
   3:2 Technicians
   3:3 Pupils
4. Material Elements
   4:1 Buildings
   4:2 Equipment
   4:3 Teaching Materials
       4:3:a Books
       4:3:b Audio-visual aids
5. Organization
   5:1 Plan of work
   5:2 Curriculum and methods of teaching
   5:3 Guidance and counseling
   5:4 Extra-curricular activities
   5:5 Control
6. The School's Social Relations
   6:1 With the parents
   6:2 With community
7. Educational Policy
8. Budget-economic Aspects
9. Pertinent Legislation

B. Holmes and S. B. Robinsohn. *Relevant Data in Comparative Education.* Hamburg: UNESCO Institute for Education, 1963, p. 55.

Holmes lists several out-of-school activities and considers the type of institutions that may be involved in promoting and conducting these. Of particular significance to physical educators Is his first category of "Leisure Time Activities," which includes: (a) sport, and (b) cultural. The types of institutions involved in out-of-school activities that he considers are on the next page:

TABLE IV
INSTITUTIONS PROVIDING OPPORTUNITIES
FOR OUT-OF-SCHOOL ACTIVITIES

A. Social/Cultural
   1. Family
   2. Educational Institutions
   3. Parent Organizations
   4. Youth Movements
   5. Mass Media
   6. Clubs
   7. Former-pupil Organizations
   8. Religious Institutions

B. Economic
   1. Industrial Organizations
   2. Commercial Organizations
   3. Agricultural Organizations

C. Political
   1. Political Institutions

B. Holmes and S. B. Robinsohn. *Relevant Data in Comparative Education.* Hamburg: UNESCO Institute for Education, 1963, p. 55.

Also included in the report is Moehlman's classification of long-range factors which was presented earlier in this section. [51]

The preceding paragraphs present an overview of certain trends in the methods of comparative education. In recent years there has been greater emphasis on the development of classification systems and the application of techniques from related social sciences. [52]

Much of the Information presented here has relevance for comparative studies of physical education, in particular, and physical recreation. Most comparative educators recommend evaluation of the influence of other systems in the cultural and social context in which the education system functions. In addition to the Holmes and Robinsohn report, Bereday, Moehlman, and Hans provide classification schemes to guide analysis. Bereday, Moehlman, King, and Anderson all point to the value of employing the techniques for analysis that are available in the other social sciences. It seems quite probable that information of this nature can prove very helpful in stimulating more rapid development of mature methodology In comparative physical education.

Footnotes

1. George Z. F. Bereday. Comparative Method in Education. New York: Holt, Rinehart and Winston, Inc., 1964, p. 23.
2. Status of Teachers of Physical Education. Washington: ICHPER, 1963.
3. D. D. Molyneux. Central Government Aid to Sport and Physical Recreation in Countries of Western Europe. University of Birmingham: Physical Education Department, 1962.
4. L. K. Kandel. The New Era in Education—A Comparative Study. New York: Houghton-Mifflin Company, 1955, pp. 8-9.
5. L. K. Kandel. "The Methodology of Comparative Education." p. 271.
6. Bereday, *op. cit.*, p. 19.
7. *Ibid.* p. 22.
8. I. K. Kandel, "Problems in Comparative Education," *International Review of Education,* II, 1956, pp. 9-11; and B. Holmes and S/ B. Robinson, *Relevant Data in Comparative Education.* Hamburg: UNESCO Institute for Education, 1963. A report on a meeting of experts.
9. Holmes and Robinson, *op. cit.*
10. Bereday, *op. cit.*, pp. 20, 28; Arthur Moehlman. *Comparative Education Systems.* Washington: Center for Applied Research in Education, 1063, pp. 83-206; and Holmes and Robinsohn, *op. cit*, pp. 42-88.
11. Stewart Fraser. *Julien's Plan for Comparative Education. 1816-1817.* New York: Bureau of Publications, Teachers College, Columbia University, 1964.
12. Paul Monroe (ed*.). A Cyclopedia of Education.* Vol. II, 1919, pp. 224-225.
13. *Ibid.*, Vol III, 1918, p. 184.
14. *Ibid.*, Vol. V, 1919, p. 148
15. Lawrence A. Cremin (ed.). *The Republic and the School.* New York: Bureau of Publications Teachers College, Columbia University, 1960, p. 54; B. A. Hinsdale. *Horace Mann and the Common School Revival in the United States.* New York: Charles Scribner's Sons, 1900, pp. 170-173; and Albert E. Winship. *Horace Mann—The Educatpr.* Boston: New Eng;lanf Publishing Co., 1896. Pp. 50-52.
16. Monroe, *op. cit..* Vol. m. 1918, pp. 587-588.
17. Sir Joshua Fitch. *Thomas and Matthew Arnold—and Their Influence on English Education.* New York: Charles Scribner's Sons, 1897, pp. 128-130.
18. Deobold B. Van Dalen, Elmer D, Mitchell and Bruce L. Bennett. *A_World History of Physical Education; Cultural-Philosophical-Comparative.* Englewood Cliffs, New Jersey: Prentice-Hall, Inc., 1953, p. 245.
19. Emmett A. Rice, John L. Hutchinson and Mabel Lee. *A Brief History of Physical Education.* New York: The Ronald Press Company, 1958, p. 110.
20. Andreas M. Kazamias and G. Byron Massialas. *Tradition and Change in Education—A Comparative Study.* Englewood Cliffs, New Jersey: Prentice-Hall, Inc., 1965, p. 3.
21. J. H. Higginson. "The Centenary of an English Pioneer in Comparative Education." International Review of Education. VII, 1961-1962, p. 287.
22. *Ibid.*, p. 290.

23. Kazamias and Massialas, *op. cit.*, p. 3.
24. Higginson, *op. cit.,* pp. 288. 291.
25. Nicholas Hans. "The Historical Approach to Comparative Education." *International Review of Education.* V, 1959, p. 307.
26. I. K. Kandel. "The Methodology of Comparative Education." p. 271; Nicholas Hans. Comparative Education. London: Routledge and Kegan Paul, Ltd., 1951, pp. 9-16.
27. Kandel, *op. cit..* p. 273.
28. Hans, Comparative Education, pp. 11-16.
29. *Ibid..* p. 10.
30. Kazamias and Massialis, *op. cit.*, p. 2.
31. Joseph A. Lauwerys. "The Philosophical Approach to Comparative Education.*" International Review of Education.* V, 1959, pp. 283-290.
32. *Ibid..* pp. 293-294.
33. Holmes and Robinsohn, *op. cit.*, pp. 14-15.
34. Kazamias and Massialis, *op. cit.*, pp. 6-8.
35. Holmes and Robinsohn, *op. cit.*, p. 22.
36. *Ibid..* pp. 15-17.
37. Bereday, *op. cit..* pp. 11-23,
38. *Ibid..* pp. 19-21.
39. Moehlman, *op. cit..* pp. 82-91.
40. *Ibid*, p. 9.
41. Edmund J. King. "The Purpose of Comparative Education." *Comparative Education*, 1:3, June, 1965, pp. 150-151.
42. *Ibid..* p. 152.
43. C. Arnold Anderson. "Sociology in the Service of Comparative Education." *International Review of Education.* V, 1959, p. 310.
44. C. Arnold Anderson. "Methodology of Comparative Education.*" International Review of Education.* VI, 1961-1962, p. 4.
45. Anderson. "Sociology," pp. 301-18.
46. Anderson. "Methodology."
47. Holmes and Robinsohn, op. cit., pp 11-19.
48. *Ibid.*, p 11.
49. *Ibid.*, pp. 20-21.
50. *Ibid.*, complete text.
51. *Ibid.*, pp. 75-76.
52. *Ibid.*, p. 12.

-

Selection #10
Professional Preparation in Physical Education in the United States and Canada (1960-1985): A Comparative Analysis

Earle F. Zeigler
Canada

Purpose of the Study

In this study, a comparative analysis was made of undergraduate professional preparation in physical education in the United States and Canada. I hypothesized that there have been significant changes, some similar and others different, in the undergraduate professional preparation programs of both countries. I further hypothesized that, if changes occurred, they typically tended to come about in the U.S. first. Lipset (1973) pointed out that there has been reluctance on the part of Canadians "to be overly optimistic, assertive, or experimentally inclined." Finally, it should be recognized that it is difficult, if not impossible, to obtain true historical perspective on at least the latter half of this 25-year period.

I was concerned with both the theoretical and the practical aspects of this historical development of professional development (having spent equal time on an alternating basis in the United States and Canada at both the undergraduate and graduate levels during this period). In addition, I had carried out historical research on the topic of professional preparation and disciplinary scholarship commencing with doctoral dissertation work in the 1940s. These experiences may have equipped me uniquely to make this comparative analysis; nevertheless, highly competent men and women–people who have lived through these 25 years in both countries–were called upon to buttress and expand upon the facts and opinions that are provided.

Most people in my generation thought that progress in life, and accordingly that in professional preparation in physical education, would be mostly an unhindered upward growth after World War I. However, such has not been the case, and many changes (some good and some bad) have undoubtedly occurred because of prevailing social forces or influences that developed in each country (e.g., the influence of values, nationalism, economics) (Zeigler, 1975).

In addition, a number of professional concerns (e.g., approach to professional preparation, curriculum content, instructional methodology) have been precipitated by these social forces. Therefore, I decided in 1984 to investigate developments in the United States since 1960 using descriptive methodology and a questionnaire technique (Good & Scates, 1954). The instrument was sent to a small group comprising 10 members of the American Academy of Physical Education, each person selected primarily because of geographical location and because of a deep interest in undergraduate professional preparation. The results of this survey about developments in physical education in the U.S. were reported at the 100th Anniversary Convention of the American Alliance for Health, Physical Education, Recreation, and Dance in 1985 (Zeigler, 1986).

Here the results of a similar investigation for Canada are reported. Selected leaders from across Canada, professors who were involved in professional preparation during the 1960s, 1970s, and 1980s were asked to describe what they believe took place in Canada during the same 25-year period (see Paton, 1975 and Canadian Association for Health, Physical Education and Recreation, 1966). The results of the U.S. survey carried out first were shown to the Canadians just before they made their own analysis of the situation north of the Border.

Methodology

The investigation employed broad descriptive methodology together with the following techniques to gather and analyze data: (1) a questionnaire distributed to approximately 10 authorities in each country; (2) a comparative approach (recommended by Bereday, 1964, 1969) that included four steps explained as description, interpretation, juxtaposition, and comparison; and (3) selected documentary analysis.

Five problems, phrased as questions, were included in the questionnaire. They were: (1) What have been the strongest social influences during each decade? (2) What changes were made in the professional curriculum? (3) What developments took place in instructional methodology? (4) What other interesting or significant developments occurred (typically in higher education)? and (5) What are the greatest problems in professional preparation currently? In addition, respondents were asked to make any additional comments that they wished.

Description and Interpretation

The questionnaires distributed to respondents in the United States and Canada were identical, both asking the five questions relative to each of the three decades. The results of the first two steps of the Bereday technique (description and interpretation) within broad descriptive methodology were assembled according to the various categories of answers. So much detailed material was obtained form the responses to add to the data uncovered by the investigator that it was decided to describe the results in the form of tables. For the first four questions, a table for each decade presents the results from the United States and Canada, respectively. Separate tables were required to list "the greatest problems in professional preparation." Based on these findings, tentative hypotheses were then postulated in the third step (juxtaposition) of the Bereday comparative technique.

Juxtaposition. The third and fourth steps of this approach are juxtaposition and comparison. In 1969, Bereday introduced two possible approaches for each of these steps: either tabular or textual juxtaposition or balanced or illustrative comparison. In juxtaposition, the preliminary matching of data textually after a degree of systematization presented an opportunity for the orderly establishment of comparable topics. At this point one or more hypotheses are made "in terms of what the assembled data are likely to permit one to prove" (Bereday, 1969, p. 5).

Thinking of this investigation as preliminary because of its extent and complexity, I decided to carry out an illustrative rather than a balanced comparison. Rather than matching each of the many items from one country to the other, a few similar and dissimilar practices or occurrences in each category in each country were selected randomly to illustrate comparative aspects of the two developments. Such an approach obviously has limited effectiveness because no subsequent principles can be reliably established. With this limitation in mind, the data were (1) assembled and juxtaposed textually, (2) 11 broad hypotheses were established, and (3) the data from both countries were compared illustratively in an effort to confirm, disconfirm, or refine the hypotheses established. An analysis of the related literature was helpful at this point.

Based on the textual juxtaposition and analysis of the data obtained for each country, the following 11 tentative hypotheses were made from the categories examined:

Category #1 (Social influences)

1.1 The federal government has had much more influence on physical education and sport in Canada than in the United States.
1.2 Politics influence public higher education more in the United States than in Canada.

Category #2 (Curriculum)

2.1 Canada has developed a greater sub disciplinary orientation in its curriculum than has the United States.
2.2 Non-teaching, alternative-career options in degree programs have developed more rapidly in the United States.
2.3 Enrollment levels in physical education/kinesiology programs have held up better in Canada.

Category #3 (Instructional methodology)

3.1 Development in instructional methodology has been comparable and concurrent in both countries.

3.2 Pressure for improvement in the teaching act arrived somewhat earlier in the United States.

Category #4 (Other campus developments)

4.1 The pattern of rotation for administrators in Canada has tended to preserve their scholarly competence, contrary to the situation in the United States.

4.2 A smaller percentage of women in Canada have been acculturated to become university physical education and kinesiology professors and scholars.

Category #5 (Greatest problem/need)

5.1 The need to control or lessen the impact of highly competitive athletics within the college and university structure is much greater in the United States.

5.2 Different emphases are needed for the development of improved professional training for teacher/coaches in the two countries.

Comparison

The decision to carry out an illustrative rather than a balanced comparison of the data assembled in Bereday's Step #4 was made in an effort to tentatively confirm, disconfirm, or refine the broad hypotheses established as the final phase of Step #3 (juxtaposition).

The following similar and dissimilar practices, occurrences, or stated problems were selected randomly to illustrate the broad hypotheses designated above. (See Table 9.)

Discussion and Preliminary Conclusions

This comparative analysis of undergraduate professional preparation in physical education in the United States and Canada from 1960-1985 should be recognized as preliminary. I hypothesized generally at the outset that significant changes have occurred in undergraduate programs in the previous 25 years. Secondly, I hypothesized that similarities and differences between the two countries exist both because of and despite their contiguity. In addition, earlier studies have shown Canadians to be generally more conservative than Americans toward change.

After carrying out the juxtaposition phase (Step #3) of Bereday's comparative technique, I established 11 tentative hypotheses involving the five different categories. Each is based on textual matching of comparable data. When illustrative comparisons were made in Step #4, the tentative hypotheses established were justified preliminarily by the data presented. Although more in-depth comparative analysis of these developments is called for, this investigative technique has provided a good basis for further study.

Table 1: The United States of America--the 1960s

THE 1960S: Undoubtedly a period where there was considerable social unrest; in higher education, the field was being criticized for the lack of academic rigor in its programs (Conant, et al, 1963.).

a. Strongest Social Influences

- Aftermath of Sputnik
- Call for fitness for "Soft American"
- JFK's plans for America; then LBJ's "Great Society"
    came on the scene
- Civil Rights Movement
- Vietnam involvement
- Hippie Movement (a minority "opted out")
- Students prioritized values; eschewed materialism
- Carnegie Study states that teachers do not relate
    subjects to ongoing living

b. The Professional Curriculum

- Many undergraduate requirements opposed
- Beginnings of sub-disciplines (scientific base!)
- Many disciplinary models & names proposed
- Generalist concept challenged
- Academic rigor of programs under question
- Beginnings of individualized, specialized programs

c. Instructional Methodology

-Effort made to improve laboratory experiences
-Token student involvement typically did not result
    in intelligent modifications; faculty still reticent
    about allowing basic student contributions
- Improved instructional materials (A-V, etc.)
- Decreased funding beginning to create specter of
    overly large lecture classes
- Mosston's recommendations regarding teaching
    styles (from "command to discovery")

d. Other Campus Developments

- Student demand for input in decision-making

240

- Greater use of mainframe computers
- Beginnings of sub disciplinary societies
- A variety of inputs into proposed disciplinary models
- Increasing demand for academic integrity begins to
    open rift between researchers/scholars & people
    involved with teacher training primarily
- Physical education faculty members judged by same
    standards as other disciplines
- Excesses in gate-receipt sports continue
- Assessment of joint arrangements with intercollegiate
    athletics units on campuses
- Spiraling costs of intercollegiate programs
- Many faculty unprepared for new standards of
    accountability (including research output)
- Faculty on campuses beginning to organize unions

Table 2: The United States of America--the 1970s

THE 1970S: Aftermath of the 1960s; a Ph.D. glut; the job market slackens generally; "stagflation"; financial cutbacks in education, etc.

a. Strongest Social Influences

- Lingering effect of Vietnam
- Adding of Watergate guilt to scene; increasing
    distrust of politicians
- Taxpayers' revolt against increasing burden
- Slowing down of economy (stagflation)
- Influence of oil cartel
- Carter's leadership style deplored by some; the
    Iranian hostage incident
- Concern about falling birthrate
- Women's Movement (role expectations of men and
women tended to blend together)
- Professionals began to break away from tradition in
    terms of dress, behavior, and educational values
- Continuing threat of legal suits against teachers
- Enforced busing to promote "racial mix"
- Affirmative action hiring
- Legislation regarding education of handicapped
- Promotion of idea of "competency-based curricula"
- Variety of analyses appearing about most notable
    improvements in U.S. undergraduate teaching
    (Change)

b. The Professional Curriculum

- Curriculum becomes more "scientifically" oriented; effect of physical fitness thrust
- Growth of opportunities for specialization
  elective sequences or emerging tracks such as athletic training, fitness specialist, sport management, special physical education recommended as alternate careers)
- Concern for a core program in physical education theory & practice (basic requirements)
- Sub-disciplinary areas continue to expand within Departments (biosciences, social sciences, And humanities)

c. Instructional Methodology

- More fieldwork opportunities
- Independent course experiences
- Demand for teacher evaluation grows with possible improvement in instruction resulting
- Impact at several educational levels of Mosston's work on teaching styles
- Courses taught by specialists to greater extent
- Computer-assisted instruction (e.g., PLATO)
- The sport pedagogy thrust in Federal Republic of Germany with some later influence in U.S.A.

d. Other Campus Developments

- Merging of men's and women's departments by administrative fiat
- Title IX legislation (women in sport)
- Improvement shown re faculty professionalism; younger faculty definitely a "new breed"--but without a definite interest in the broad picture of developmental physical activity in the schools
- Increase in number of graduate students (few jobs!)
- Splintering of departmental faculty, all "doing their own thing"
- Changing departmental titles reflecting disciplinary emphases & continued growth of allied professions
- Concern for licensing & certification (action?)
- Job market grim in higher education; faculty faced with few opportunities to move except in highly specialized areas

- Opportunity for faculty grievances increases
- Pressure to "publish or perish" in PE too!
- Grant moneys less available
- Re-tooling of faculty a definite concern
- Excesses in gate-receipt sports seem to increase
- Emergence of the "female jock"--a Catch 22 situation!

Table 3: The United States of America--the 1980s

THE 1980S: Financial recovery of a sort; job market still tight in higher education, but shortages are predicted at other levels; federal government influences education, research funding, etc.

a. Strongest Social Influences

- Conflicting world ideologies; how to combat spreading
  communism without invoking its methodology & techniques
- Worldwide communication via satellites
- Impact of Reagan's administration at high level;
  many people, including the young, like the leader-
  ship style ("proud to be American," etc.)
- Rise of fundamentalist religious phenomenon (TV)
- Urban population soaring in desirable parts of the
  country; other cities suffering and crime rates
  increase, thus enhancing the problems of cities
- Demographic surveys indicate increasing number of
  elderly in the nation
- Enormous increase in health care costs
- Federal government establishes Health Objectives,
  1990 (for all five stages of life)
- Impact of high technology (e.g., computers, software)
  -the "knowledge industry"
- Certain large industries suffering greatly; recovery
  of automobile industry
- Enrollment decline beginning to have an effect in
  many colleges & universiti
- Funding from federal level for education decreasing
- Cost of education soaring at all levels
- Presidential Task Force on Education proclaims
  the prevalence of mediocrity in the secondary
  schools
- Continuing concern that "teacher can't teach"
- Demand for accountability at very high level
- Steady call for "back to basics" in education
- Concept of 'mastery teaching' is "catching on"
- Greater cooperation between the public schools and
  higher education

- Competition for top students
- Federal Government eases off on Title IX
  enforcement
- Less than one-third of the school population (10-17)
  receive daily physical education

b. The Professional Curriculum

- Concern for greater teacher effectiveness
- Continued expansion of non-teaching programs;
  importance of job orientation; decline of
  liberal education
- Continued concern for improved standards (regular
  certification or voluntary accreditation?)
- Stressing of need for improved scholarship
- Need to eliminate superfluous courses
- How to generate increased revenue
- Declining enrollment in professional curriculum
- Faculty positions being lost due to inadequate funds
- Intra-institutional research funding drying up

c. Instructional Methodology

- Larger lecture groups/combining of sections
- Need to somehow streamline learning experiences
- Introduction of microcomputer into curriculum
- Continued concern for teacher/coach effectiveness
- Continued retooling of faculty to improve level of
  instruction
- Some stress for education for "human fulfillment"
  with teacher as facilitator

d. Other Campus Developments

- Salary schedules still at low ebb at all levels
- Get the grants whether there is time to complete the
  research or not
- Creative "early semi-retirement" schemes are needed
- Faculty members often find outside means to
  increase substandard salary levels- The
  environment is definitely too stressful
- Faculty sub disciplinary specialization increases in
  the large universities; in smaller institutions--
  perhaps because of heavy workloads—faculty
  members are still broadly based (i.e. less
  research and publication; heavier
  teaching/coaching loads)

- NASPE Task Force working on revision of NCATE
accreditation standards for undergraduate
physical education teacher preparation

Table 4
The Greatest Problems in
United States' Professional Preparation

- Need to develop consensus about a disciplinary
definition from which should evolve a more
unified, much less fractionated curriculum (i.e.,
a greater balance among the bio-scientific
aspects, the social-science & humanities aspects,
and the "professional aspects" of our field).
- Need to develop a sound body of retrievable
knowledge in all phases of the profession's
work.
- Need to implement the educational possibilities of a
"competency approach" within the professional
preparation curriculum.
- Need to develop a variety of sound options for
specialization within a unified curriculum
extending to a 5th year of offerings. This
should involve the expansion of alternate-career
options in keeping with the profession's goal of
serving people of all ages and all abilities.
- Need to develop a format whereby regular "future
planning" between staff and students occurs.
- Need to graduate competent, well educated, fully
professional physical educator/coaches who have
well-considered personal philosophies
embodying an understanding of professional
ethics.
- Need to seek recognition of our professional
endeavors in public, semi-public, and private
agency work through certification at the state
level and voluntary accreditation at the national
level.
- Need to help control or lessen the impact of highly
competitive athletics within the college and
university structure so that a finer type of
professional preparation program is fostered.
- Need to recognize the worth of intramural
recreational sports in our programs, and to make
every effort to encourage those administering
these programs to maintain professional
identification with the National Association for

Sport and Physical Education.
- Need to continue the implementation of patterns of
    administrative control in educational
    institutions that are fully consonant with
    individual freedom within the society.
- Need to work for maintenance of collegiality among
    faculty members despite inroads of factors
    tending to destroy such a state: -i.e., inadequate
    funding, faculty unionization, pressure for
    publication and the obtaining of grants, and
    extensive intra-profession "splintering."
- Need to develop an attitude that will permit us to
    "let go of obsolescence." In some way, we will
    have to learn to apply new knowledge creatively
    in the face of an often discouraging political
    environment.
- Need to work to dispel any malaise present within our
    professional preparation programs as to
    the future of the profession. If we prepare our
    students to be certified and accredited
    professionals within their respective options in
    the broad curriculum, we will undoubtedly bring
    about a service profession of the highest type

Table 5   Canada--the 1960s

THE 1960S. Undoubtedly a period when there was some unrest, but rarely as much as in the U.S.A. (except possibly for Quebec). There was considerable expansion within education at several levels in Canada.

a. Strongest Social Influences

- Era of economic "sufficiency"
- Evidence of Canadian nationalism (e.g., concern
    for independence from the U.S.A.)
- Social unrest due to world situation
- Beginning of women's "liberation"
- Education more highly valued
- Continued faith in government to solve societal
    ills; resulting governmental expansion and
    involvement in education
- Developing rift in Canada--a "quiet revolution"
    leading toward "Western separatism"
- Growing concern with the use of leisure, including

    significant improvement in municipal recreation
    offerings

246

- Lack of fitness of Canadians indicated; poor showing
     in international competition decried; Bill C.
        131 enacted (Fitness and Amateur Sport Act)
- Growth of professional sport

b. The Professional Curriculum

- Aftermath of 1966 Physical Education & Athletics
     Conference in Toronto
- Largely oriented to producing high school teacher/
     coaches
- Gradual expansion of curriculum offerings in the
     late 1960s
- Emergence of the social-science aspects of physical
     education and sport
- More electives; fewer requirements in curriculum
- Significant growth of the number of professional
     programs
- Division of task in Ontario: physical education
     units adopt a disciplinary approach, while
     Teacher education is allotted to professional
     education schools or departments; the
     arrangement in Western provinces is a combined
     one similar in nature to that offered in the U.S.
- Outdoor education and orienteering added to
     curriculum

c. Instructional Methodology
- Quality of teaching mediocre; little effort to
     evaluate performance as faculty members "do
     their own thing"
- Increased use of seminars and laboratories
- Introduction of texts with "readings"
- Audiovisual aids stressed more

d. Other Campus Developments

- Expansive development of universities, community
     colleges, and secondary education
- Student unrest on campuses; but phys. educ.
     students' demands for greater involvement are
     limited
- Governing boards subjected to variety of pressures
     to which they often submitted
- Only "strongest" top administrators survived
- Physical education develops somewhat higher profile
     in Canadian universities

247

- Concern for "academic respectability" begins to
    drive wedge between researcher/scholars and
    those concerned mainly with preparation of the
    teacher/coach
- Gradual entry into graduate education in physical
    education/kinesiology in the late 1960s
- Prospective faculty members work toward
    specialized programs for their doctoral degrees
- Very few well-qualified faculty to cope with newer
    disciplinary approach
- Beginning of federal funding to competitive sport--
    and to a lesser extent to physical education
    (e.g., undergraduate scholarships)
- Job market for graduates is open; very difficult to
    predict future developments
- Team sports grow in popularity; gymnastics declines
- Continued struggle to make the Canadian Association
    for Health, Physical Education and Recreation a
    fully viable professional society
- Expansion of facilities (e.g., swimming pools,
    racquet courts)

Table 6   Canada--the 1970s

THE 1970S. Aftermath of the 1960s; beginnings of the Ph.D. glut in higher education (not with physical education initially, however); the job market declines at the secondary level; the beginning of financial cutbacks in education at all levels, etc.

a. Strongest Social Influences

- Faith in the "just and rational" society (early
    impact of Trudeau)
- Economic downturn ("stagflation")
- Further development of "The Cold War";
    proliferation of the hydrogen bomb
- Impact of oil shortage (OPEC)
- Sharp increase in Women's Movement
- Separatist Movement in Quebec (FLQ)
- Falling birth rate; predictions of enrollment slump
    at university & community college level
- Developing Western Canada "isolation"
- Physical activity promoted by federal government
    (e.g., Participaction, a crown corporation);
    designed to ultimately reduce health costs
- Federal government's decision to promote elite
    sport nationally and internationally as an aid to

248

the promotion of national unity and world status
- Continued struggle between provincial and federal
  governments threatens federal support to higher
  education
- Professionals begin to break away from traditional
  values & behavior patterns (e.g., dress, grooming)

b. The Professional Curriculum

- Opportunities for greater specialization (including
  fitness options because of governmental
  influence)
- Concern for a core program in physical education/
  kinesiology theory and practice
- Gradually increasing interest in administrative
  theory as a sub-discipline within the field
  (along with accompanying recognition of the
  importance of the "mother disciplines")
- A significant increase in the sophistication of the
  field's knowledge base
- Federal government's attention to elite sport
  brings a demand for training programs for
  coaches and a national certification plan
- Universities feeling pressure to develop high
  performance\athletes (including testing centers
  and various types of laboratories)
- De-emphasis on teacher training per se as
  disciplinary based curriculum receives steadily
  increasing emphasis (with courses often
  seemingly designed to meet the teachers' needs)
- De-emphasis of the activity-based aspect of the
  total curricular offerings
- A steady increase in female enrollment in programs
- Departments, schools, and faculties called a
  variety of names (e.g., kinesiology, human
  kinetics)

c. Instructional Methodology

- Larger classes resulting in fewer seminars and
  fewer essays to correct (i.e. less individual
  attention)
- Audiovisual emphasis has a big impact on activity
  teaching
- Play increasingly recognized as learning
- Greater opportunity for laboratory experiences
  (including individual help from teaching/research

249

assistants)
- Field work opportunities (e.g., internships) are
    greater
- Significant decrease in the use of ever more
    expensive textbooks as professors increasingly
    develop their own texts and study guides
- Demand for teacher evaluation grows with seemingly
    greater emphasis on the teaching process
- Courses are being taught typically by professors
    with greater specialization (at the upper
    undergraduate level at least); typically use a
    greater theoretical orientation
- Attempts were often made to use new technologies in
    the teaching act, but the profession seems slow to
    adopt them

d. Other Campus Developments

- Faculty members gradually developing a larger
    number of areas for research and scholarly
    investigation
- Earlier altruism and professional dedication
    declines significantly
- Some faculty disillusionment due to aging, outmoded
    equipment
- Growth typically comes to a halt in the mid-1970s
    due to the increasingly stringent financial
    situation
- A decrease occurs in the emphasis on health and
    safety education within many curricula
- The Sport Administration Centre in Ottawa continues
    to grow in size, scope, and influence
- Participaction, as a crown corporation, increases
    in influence through sound marketing approach
- Increase in the number of students enrolled in
    graduate study; this is due to the job market
- Significant change did not occur rapidly enough
    when the climate was right for such innovation
- Grantsmanship develops increasingly because of the
    need for external funding

Table 7   Canada--the 1980s

The 1980s. Financial recovery of a sort takes place; nevertheless, education continues to be underfunded (especially at the university and community college level); job market still tight; decline of the Canadian dollar, etc.

a. Strongest Social Influences

- Constitution Act becomes law in 1982; includes
    Canadian Charter of Rights & Freedoms; will
    Have tremendous influence in all areas of living
- Heating up of the Cold War (terrorists, Central
    America, Middle East conflict, Afghanistan,
    Libya, etc.)
- Satellite communication becomes a boon, but
    incipient problems for the world loom large
- Impact of high technology (the "knowledge
    industry")
- Conservative political control at the national
    level, and also in certain provinces as well
- Gradually increasing financial crises at both the
    federal and provincial levels despite recovery
    from recession of the early 1980s
- Unemployment problem (especially with the young);
    fewer government jobs available
- The "haves" and the "have-nots" grow further apart
- Enormous increase in health care costs
- Increased awareness of the need for preventive
    medicine
- University and community college enrollments do not
    drop off as predicted; some actually increase
- The "Computer Age" is upon us

b. The Professional Curriculum

- Curriculum aims and objectives are lacking
- A back-to-basics emphasis (the core courses)
- Concern over which courses should be required and
    which should be elective
- Continued expansion of non-teaching options and
    concentrations with curricula (e.g., sport
    management, athletic training, fitness testing &
    aerobics, coaching)
- Continuing decline of teacher education
- Concern for improved program standards and
    scholarship

251

- Some recognition that each university can't "be all
    things to all people" with its program offerings
- Inability to predict what curricular changes should
    be made to best equip our graduates for job
    placement
- Students are typically more serious and
    goal-oriented
- Increased number of students with poor physical
    skills in the professional program
- Beginning of a new emphasis on special physical
    education
- Call for lengthening of curricular program in some
    universities

c. Instructional Methodology

- Computer instruction is slowly being incorporated
    into pattern of instruction
- Larger lecture groups/combining of sections
- Instruction based more on research findings and
    improved theory
- Improved research/teaching facilities & equipment
    available
- Continued concern for teacher/coach effectiveness;
    many faculty members taking teaching
    responsibilities more seriously; improved level of
    creativity & innovation
- Some retooling of certain faculty members to
    improve instruction, thereby making them more
    valuable
- Increased use of videotaping
- More Canadian educational materials become
    available

d. Other Campus Developments

- Physical education/kinesiology has achieved greater
    respectability on most campuses
- Some faculty pessimism and cynicism present
- Salary schedules have not kept pace with other
    professions and occupations; pension schemes
    leave something to be desired
- Sharp increase in faculty unionization (more than
    50% of faculty members in country unionized)
- Early retirements schemes appearing, but they are
    not sufficiently creative to encourage faculty
    departure; also, mandatory retirement illegal in

certain of the provinces
- Requirements for promotion and tenure are ever more stringent; moreover, faculty positions are threatened because of continued economic pressures
- Circumstances have created managers rather than "old style" department heads
- Dedication to the established profession is sorely lacking
- Increased number of students going on for degrees in other fields

Table 8
The Greatest Problems in
Canadian Professional Preparation

- Need regular turnover in faculty to change the "collective staleness" that has developed.
- Need to find more money to carry out an improved level of professional preparation.
- Need to provide a sharper focus to professional preparation programs to counter present "aimless wandering."
- Need to zero in on the best ways of preparing teachers and coaches (i.e., improve the teaching/learning process)
- Need to provide meaningful, relevant, challenging professional preparation for those seeking alternative careers employing purposeful physical activity in sport, exercise, dance, and play.
- Need to graduate competent, well-educated, fully professional physical educator/coaches who have sound personal philosophies and professional ethics.
- Need to develop a more selective admission process for the undergraduate programs in physical education and sport.
- Need to achieve a consensus as to what constitutes the core of the curricular sub-disciplines.
- Need to convince qualified women that there is a place for them at the university level--and then find it!

Table 9
Comparisons Between the United States and Canada

Note: The illustrative comparisons relate directly to the 11 hypotheses established above.

United States	Canada

Category #1: Findings about Social Influences:

1.1 The federal government has had much more influence on physical education and sport in Canada than in the United States.

United States	Canada
Federal government has Typically been involved Financially more Directly with higher Education	Education has been clearly established as belonging to the provinces; influence of federal government More indirect, because Funding must be granted by each province

1.2 Politics influence public higher education more in the United States than in Canada.

United States	Canada
State legislatures often become directly involved established with the state university operations and programs	A "hands-off relationship has been traditional at the provincial level

Category #2: Findings about the Curriculum)

2.1 Canada has developed a greater sub disciplinary orientation in its curriculum than has the United States.

United States	Canada
Teacher education occurs typically within the four-year bachelor's degree program in a school of education	In much of Canada teacher education begins after the "disciplinary" degree has been granted

2.2 Non-teaching, alternative-career options in degree programs have developed more rapidly in the United States.

The teacher surplus developed sooner in the U.S., thus creating pressure for alternative-career options; more difficult for U,S. students to gain admission to degree programs in other fields

Pressure for alternative-career options came somewhat later in Canada; difficult to implement within present degree program because of stronger arts and science and disciplinary orientation

2.3 Enrollment levels in physical education/kinesiology programs have held up better in Canada

The slumping job market caused a sharp drop in enrollment in many colleges and universities;- the financial outlook caused retrenchment- that affected physical education, also

Despite slumping job market, and forecasts of statisticians, the enrollment figures held up; this may be because of the liberal arts & science nature of the programs (i.e., many students could switch to other fields more easily)

Category #3: Findings about Instructional Methodology

3.1 Responses to the survey in both countries indicated that developments and improvements in instructional methodology have been comparable and concurrent

This finding seems reasonable in that politics and other factors do not appear to have been a consideration here (with the possible exception of inadequate funding for physical education at the local level).

3.2 Social unrest influenced higher education sooner in the U.S.A. (except for Quebec) resulting in a demand for greater emphasis on the teaching act.

The evidence is that the social unrest of the 1960s impacted higher education sooner in the U.S. with resultant

Social unrest in Canada was evident in Quebec largely with fewer demands for teacher account-

demands for more
      attention to the teaching
act on the part of
professors

ability elsewhere

Category #4: Findings about Other Campus Developments

4.1 Administrative roles are typically defined differently in several ways in the two countries.

In the United States, deans, directors, heads, and chairpersons were rarely appointed for specified periods of time; study or administrative leave was a rarity

In Canada there is typically a specified-number of years associated with each category of appointment; study leave was usually available

4.2 The role and status of women in the field at the university level differed historically.

In the United States graduate study was established during the first 25 years of the century; women typically had separate departments and earned professorial rank at all levels

In Canada, graduate study began in the 1960s; women were not acculturated to carry on to the doctoral level in physical education; as a result there are very few full professors in the country

Category #5: Findings about "Greatest Problems"

5.1 The nature of intercollegiate athletics differs greatly among the various universities and colleges in the United States, whereas it appears to be more consistent in Canada.

Gate receipts in athletics and the extra-curricular nature of highly competitive sport brought many evils that influenced teacher

The universities and colleges are still in control of their own own destinies in inter-university athletics; it has been fully education in physical education negatively; in many cases it has become necessary to separate athletics from the educational unit

possible to maintain unified departments & schools including a division of interuniversity athletics

5.2 Significant differences are evident between the United States and Canada in regard to the overall nature of the academic program.

Teacher/coach education in the U.S. requires more more selective admission along with a stronger arts and social science background; often more professional theory & practice is needed as well

Canadian students have a longer period of training that includes considerable arts and science work; also, in Canada there is an additional year of training required for certification

Concluding Statement

A great deal of progress has been made in physical education and sport on many countries located in all parts of the world during the twentieth century. Obviously, much of this progress has resulted from the leadership of the many programs involved. In North America, as might have been expected, there are many similarities between the historical development of professional preparation in physical education in the United States of America and Canada. Both countries have developed well in the field of physical education, each in its own way, but the findings indicate that the United States has several significant concerns not evident on the Canadian scene.

Concurrently, the national interest in all kinds of sport has continued to grow unabated. There has been an ever-present demand, admittedly with limited success, for an improved level of physical fitness for citizens of all ages. Despite financial stringencies and overemphasis in certain areas, there is evidence for reasonable optimism while we trust that continuing, sincere efforts will be made by politicians in many countries to strive for healthy, fit populations along with efforts toward world peace.

There is obviously a continuing value struggle going on in the United States that results in distinct swings of the educational pendulum back and forth. It seems most important that there be a continuing search for consensus. Fortunately, the theoretical struggle or "confrontation" fades a bit when actual educational practice takes place. If this were not so, possibly less progress would be possible. If we continue to strive for higher educational standards for all, this should result in the future in greater understanding and wisdom on the part of the majority of North American citizenry.

To bring this about, science and philosophy should make ever-greater contributions. All concerned members of the allied professions of health, physical education recreation, sport, and dance in both the United States and Canada need to be fully informed as they strive for a voice in shaping the future development of their respective countries and professions. It is essential that there be careful and continuing study and analysis of the question of societal values as they relate to sport, exercise, dance, and play. The implications that societal values and norms hold for the allied fields demand ongoing investigation as well.

Acknowledgments

I wish to express my deep appreciation to the following members of the American Academy of Physical Education for their assistance: Anita Aldrich (Indiana), Ted Baumgartner (Georgia), Jan Broekhoff (Oregon), Charles Corbin (Arizona State), Marvin Eyler (Maryland), M. Dorothy Massey (Rhode Island), and George Sage (Northern Colorado).

In Canada the following colleagues were equally helpful in giving time and knowledge to this undertaking: P.J. Galasso (Windsor), Patricia Lawson (Saskatchewan), Donald Macintosh (Queen's), Fred L. Martens (Victoria), John Meagher (New Brunswick), William Orban (Ottawa), and Garth A. Paton (New Brunswick).

Note:

1. Because of the difficulty of obtaining true historical perspective from 1960 on, at this point the reader will find below the results of an investigation employing a comparative technique of broad descriptive method that was presented in to the Fifth International Symposium on Comparative Physical Education and Sport held at The University of British Columbia, Vancouver, Canada, May 26-31, 1986. The proceedings were edited by E. Broom, R. Clumpner, B. Pendleton, and C. Pooley and published as *Comparative physical education and sport,* Volume 5. Champaign, IL: Human Kinetics Publishers, 1988.

References and Bibliography

American Alliance for Health, Physical Education, Recreation and Dance (1962). *Professional preparation in health education, physical education, recreation education.* Report of national conference. Washington, DC: Author.

American Alliance for Health, Physical Education, Recreation and Dance. (1974). *Professional preparation in dance, physical education, recreation education, safety education, and school health education.* Report on national conference. Washington, DC: Author.

Bereday, G.Z.F. (1964). *Comparative method in education.* New York: Holt, Rinehart and Winston.

Bereday, G.Z.F. (1969). Reflections on comparative methodology in education, 1964-1966. In M.A. Eckstein & H.J. Noah (Eds.), *Scientific investigations in comparative education* (pp. 3-24). New York: Macmillan.

Bookwalter, K.W., & Bookwalter, C.W. (1980). *A review of thirty years of selected research on undergraduate professional preparation physical education programs in the United States.* Unionville, IN: Author.

Canadian Association for Health, Physical Education and Recreation. (1966). *Physical education and athletics in Canadian universities and colleges* (pp. 14-21). Ottawa: Author.

Good, C.F., & Scates, D.E. (1954). *Methods of research.* New York: Appleton-Century-Crofts.

Lauwerys, J.A. (1959) The philosophical approach to comparative education. *International Review of Education,* V, 283-290.

Meagher, J.W. (1965). Professional preparation. In M.L. Van Vliet (Ed.), *Physical Education in Canada* (pp. 64-81). Scarborough, ON: Prentice-Hall of Canada.

Paton, G.A. (1975). The historical background and present status of Canadian physical education. In E.F. Zeigler (Ed.), *A history of physical education and sport in the United States and Canada* (pp. 441-443). Champaign, IL: Stipes.

Proceedings of the 6th Commonwealth Conference. (1978). *Sport, Physical education, recreation proceedings* (Vols. 1 and 2). Edmonton, Alberta: University of Alberta.

Van Vliet, M.L. (Ed.). (1965). *Physical education in Canada.* Scarborough, Ontario: Prentice-Hall.

Zeigler, E.F. (1962). A history of professional preparation for physical education in the United States (1861-1961). In *Professional preparation in health education, physical education, and recreation education* (pp. 116-133). Washington,, DC: The American Association for Health, Physical Education, and Recreation.

Zeigler, E.F. (1975). Historical perspective on contrasting

philosophies of professional preparation for physical education in the United States. In *Personalizing physical education and sport philosophy* (pp. 325-347).Champaign, IL: Stipes.

Zeigler, E.F. (Ed. & author). (1975). *A history of physical education and sport in the United States and Canada.* Champaign, IL: Stipes.

Zeigler, E.F. (1980). An evolving Canadian tradition in the new world of physical education and sport. In S.A. Davidson & P. Blackstock (Eds.), *The R. Tait McKenzie Addresses* (pp. 53-62). Ottawa, Canada: Canadian Association for Health, Physical Education and Recreation.

Zeigler, E.F. (1986). Undergraduate professional preparation in Physical education, 1960-1985. *The Physical Educator,* 43(1), 2-6.

Zeigler, E.F. (1988). A comparative analysis of undergraduate professional preparation in physical education in the United States and Canada. In Broom, E., Clumpner, R., Pendleton, B., & Pooley, C. (Eds.), *Comparative physical education and sport, Volume 5.* Champaign, IL: Human Kinetics.

Selection #11
Assessment of Cross-Cultural Comparison
and International Relations in the Mid-1980s

Earle F. Zeigler
Canada

More than a decade ago I began to recommend the promotion of an awareness of three fundamental concepts that would in the long run greatly improve international relations: the concepts of 'communication,' 'diversity,' and 'cooperation' (Zeigler, 1975).1 First, the concept of 'communication' has now become vitally important because a "fourth revolution" has been occurring within this aspect of life. The world has moved from (1) the invention of speech, to (2) writing, to (3) mechanical reproduction of the printed word, and now (4) to relay stations in space creating a blanketing communications network that are making possible a type of international personal relationship hitherto undreamed of by men and women (Asimov, 1970).

In other words, technological advancement in the area of communications has brought us to the point where we are being well informed about the world's tragic happenings before we have created a situation in sharing has become the operative mode of existence. This development has fantastic implications for the profession of sport and physical education which make it mandatory that we view this aspect of our present and future task in a new light. Basically, the world must "win this race"--that is, a race between the fostering of international goodwill on the one hand through this means and, on the other hand, the tendency of the superpowers or some radical fanatic with nuclear capability to pull the trigger that will blow us all up more effectively than was possible previously.

Second, the concept of 'diversity'--the state of being different, unlike, or diverse--must be fostered and fully understood as well, while at the same time we help people to understand the many likenesses and similarities that human being have. It is at this point that the struggle between the world's leading ideologies come into focus. Communist ideologues argue that human societies must pass through four stages--from agrarianism to capitalism, and from there to social and eventual (ideal) communism. Having already reached the third stage in their opinion, we can observe that communists have completely stifled the concept of 'diversity' in their culture. Can we indeed hope for a world where significant diversity is permitted? Must we have a type of *operant conditioning* at work as recommended by Skinner (1971). In such a world we would find various types of behavior modification being implemented so that people's action would be regulated more stringently than ever before. For example, it would be necessary to modify behavior because of over-population in the world and many other problems that are besetting humanity.

Third, the concept of 'cooperation' must be paramount in our planning for the future along with the two concepts recommended immediately above. Cooperation implies working together for mutual benefit, and there are innumerable opportunities for such planning and cooperation to take place. As the world "grows smaller," so to speak, we simply must pay ever so much more attention to international relations. This will be vital within society generally, as well as in the field of education. Consequently, both within education and in society at large, we in sport and physical education should do our part and more as we develop new plans and extend the horizons for cooperation in the various aspects of our field among individuals, groups, and societies on earth (and soon perhaps in space).

"Third Wave" World

As we approach this "new world," this world of the twenty-first century, we must ask ourselves what this "Third Wave" world is going to mean to us in the profession of sport and physical education. We are people who are interested in human motor performance in sport, exercise, dance, and play primarily within our own countries, but also to a lesser degree within our own continents, our own hemispheres, and on a worldwide basis.

We are not looking at this topic only from the standpoint of comparative *education* at some level of the educational system, but even more broadly in the sense that our profession has a responsibility to serve people of all ages in all cultures on a lifelong basis (i.e., from pre-school to school, college or university, and adult life from the twenties through the eighties or longer).

Our role is to so guide general education that all people, whether in accelerated, normal, or special populations, will truly comprehend the need for rigorous and yet enjoyable physical activity to promote: (1) circulo-respiratory efficiency, (2) joint flexibility, (3) adequate muscular strength, and (4) the development and maintenance of correct and functional segmental alignment of bodily parts to foster health, functional efficiency, and aesthetic movement.

Those of us in the profession who are concerned in a scholarly way with the comparative and international aspects of sport and physical education have, therefore, a challenging problem to resolve: how to devise and execute a step-by-step approach for the description, interpretation, comparison, and evaluation of prevailing patterns of human movement from a cross-cultural standpoint. As matters stand now, many travelers' tales have been told, but very little educational borrowing has been carried out in our field, for example, in a country that tends to think the best answers to problems are found right here at home in the United States. Canadians are much more cosmopolitan in this regards, as have been a number of other countries. Thus their progress in certain areas has ofteen been significant. It is true, of course, that a certain amount of international educational cooperation has occurred, but language barriers, economic shortages, new variations of nationalism, and other barriers have hampered such development. For example, many have come to North America to learn, but very few of us have the desire or opportunity to go elsewhere, much less the language capability or necessary funding.

I certainly do not wish to convey the impression that progress has not been made in the area of international relations within the International Council for Health, Physical Education, and Recreation within the Western world, far from it. Many solid interrelationships and friendships have been developed and maintained over the decades since World War II. However, so-called <u>comparative</u> physical education and sport--the scholarly study of specific programs of ours in various countries and continents of the world and their comparison on a social scientific basis has unfortunately not yet reached a stage of "early maturity" even in the early 21st century. This point becomes immediately apparent as we observe what comparativists in the field of professional education were able to accomplish between 1960 and the present day.

In this selection, it will not be my task to trace the history of the comparative and international aspects of our field's endeavor. Of course, we are too close to the present to gain true historical perspective about the past ten or fifteen years either. I will attempt to carry out an analysis proceeding from the underlying thesis that the area of comparative sport and physical education should approach its task "using bifocal eyeglasses," so to speak.

Such an analogy may be made, in my opinion, because there is a need to view our *specialized* endeavor is ever-greater detail through the employment of highly refined research methodology. At the same time, there is a concurrent need to place the field and its research and scholarly endeavor in a broader perspective within the individual cultures that are increasingly resembling what might be called an embryonic world culture. Thus, to continue with the eyeglasses analogy, the need is "to see both near and far with our bifocals" as the world moves into the twenty-first century.

This chapter will, therefore, be divided into eight sections as follows: (1) social considerations viewed globally; (2) recent trends in the area of comparative education; (3) a proposal for a consensual definition of the profession; (4) the two basic questions to resolve; (5) question #1--what shall we compare?; (6) question #2--how shall we make such comparisons?; (7) the need for "data, knowledge, and wisdom"; and (8) a concluding statement.

Social Considerations Viewed Broadly

We in the profession of sport and physical education should attach ever so much greater significance to international relations than we do at the present. This opinion can be substantiated in several ways, but no more importantly than the argument that it is through efforts such as this that we in this profession may be able to assist civilization to move a bit faster toward what Glasser (1972) has postulated as "Civilized Identity Society" in which the concerns of humans will *again* focus on such concepts as 'self-identity,' 'self-expression,' and 'cooperation.' Postulating that so-called "Primitive Identity" societies ended in many parts of the world several thousand years ago as the population increased sharply. When some countries then found it necessary to take essential resources from neighboring societies, Glasser argued that a "Civilized Survival Society" ensued. Now for the continuation of life on this planet as we know it, he believes that it should be possible for the world's peoples to enter a phase that could be called "Civilized Identity Society."

Support for possible progression into such a fourth stage of development as proposed by Glasser comes from the findings of Kaplan who found certain "recurring elements" bas on his analysis of an emerging world culture. Despite the variety of "hot and cold" wars of the present, Kaplan (1961) theorizes that there are indeed four recurring themes present in the leading world philosophies that he examined (with the exception of Christianity--which everybody knows--and that of Islam that was not available for his firsthand inspection. These recurring themes he characterized as (1) evidence that people were employing *rationality* to a greater degree in the solution of their problems, (2) belief that *activism* was necessary to effect desirable change, (3) a position of *humanism* indicating that people themselves were going to have to assume responsibility for improvement of their lives, and (4) a concern with *values* and their realization in their societies and cultures. In his opinion organizations working to improve international relations offer great hope to people as they plan for the future.

Recent Trends in the Area of Comparative Education

Wisdom suggests that we take a brief look at what has transpired in the area of comparative education during the past few decades. Fortunately, we can call on the *Comparative Education Review* (1977) where a special issue entitled "The State of the Art" appeared. Most helpful here is a paper entitled "Intellectual and Ideological Perspectives in Comparative Education: An Interpretation" by Kazamias and Schwartz *(Ibid.)*. Specifically, these scholars reviewed the past 20 years in regards to its definitional orientation and the research methodology and techniques employed in analysis. First, they inquired as to whether comparative education was an art, a science, or a combination of both. Then they asked whether it was a discipline or an area of study on which several disciplines are brought to bear, whether it was a theoretical or an applied activity, and whether its techniques of analysis should be "empirico-statistical, historical, or philosophical." Finally, in regard to the determination of appropriate subject-matter for study, they pondered over the focus for investigation--that is, should they emphasize school-centered problems or on school-society relationships (*Ibid.*, 153). Obviously, those of us in sport and physical education who have been around since the late 1950s at least are hearing questions that have a most familiar ring!

Summarizing their historical analysis, it can be reported that significant change in subject-matter focus and research methodology began to occur within comparative education in the late 1950s. The newer lines of thought at that time placed emphasis on (1) structural-functionalism from the field of sociology, (2) development education because of renewed concern for the so-called Third World, and (3) empirico-statistical research techniques that were also in the ascendancy in the socio-cultural and behavioral sciences generally *(Ibid., 157).*

Also interesting to us in sport and physical education is the observation by Kazamias and Schwartz that, when this heavy disciplinary orientation became the vogue in comparative education, it seemed that the results of the investigations being carried out became increasingly useless to teachers as they sought to carry out their professional assignments. Bennett, Howell, and Simri (1983) sensed this deficiency too when they stated that "comparative educators need to be careful not to study just those issues and cases that lend themselves to scientific inquiry." They lament a further deficiency also--the fact that "unfortunately, writers of comparative education have had little interest in physical education and sport," and that "references to our subject-matter are virtually non-existent" (p. 18).

The thrust for scholarly investigation in comparative education in the 1960s was toward development education and modernization based on instrumental means of bringing about such desired change. Possible strategies for change were viewed from the standpoints of economics, political science, sociology, and psychology *(Ibid.,, 169-173).* In the 1970s there has been continuing use of methodological empiricism as it can be applied to problems that have been emerging steadily and increasingly since the late 1950s. Nevertheless, there has been continued concern with the social order and consensus, as well as theories of development and modernization, but such concern has been based almost exclusively on the employment of value-free investigation to develop findings and subsequent generalizations. This period was characterized by more constructive dialogue among those concerned, less "cannibalistic poaching" on other disciplines in favor of *greater identity for comparative education,* and an improved relationship with the work of the practicing professional--the teacher--was recommended (*Ibid.*, 175-176). This represent an interesting parallel for the profession of sport and physical education, and it can only be hoped that a similar development will take place within out field.

Proposal for a Consensual Definition of Our Field

Proceeding from the premise that we in this field need "to see both near and far with our bifocal eyeglasses" as we move toward an uncertain future, I have been proposing that the profession adopt a consensual definition on a worldwide basis to the effect that our domain includes "developmental physical activity in sport, exercise, dance, and play," or as some prefer "sport, exercise, and related expressive activities." As part of an effort to consolidate our profession's endeavor by bringing it into better focus and possibly reversing the direction of present movement within the total field, Dr. Laura J. Huelster, Professor-Emerita, University of Illinois (C-U), and I have developed a taxonomical table to explain proposed areas of scholarly study and research using *our own* nomenclature as follows (1983):

(Please proceed to the following page.)

Table 1
DEVELOPMENTAL PHYSICAL ACTIVITY IN SPORT, EXERCISE, AND RELATED EXPRESSIVE MOVEMENT

Areas of Scholarly Study & Research	Subdisciplinary Aspects	Subprofessional Aspects
I. BACKGROUND, MEANING, & SIGNFICANCE	-History -Philosophy -International & Comparative Study	-International Relations -Professional Ethics
II. FUNCTIONAL EFFECTS OF PHYSICAL ACTIVITY	-Exercise Physiology -Anthropometry & Body Composition	-Fitness & Health Appraisal -Exercise Therapy
III.SOCIO-CULTURAL & BEHAVIORAL ASPECTS	-Sociology -Economics -Psychology (individ. & social) -Anthropology -Political Science -Geography	-Application of Theory to Practice
IV. MOTOR LEARNING & CONTROL	-Psycho-motor Learning -Physical Growth & Development	-Application of Theory to Practice
V. MECHANICAL & MUSCULAR ANALYSIS OF MOTOR SKILLS	-Biomechanics -Neuro-skeletal Musculature	-Application of Theory to Practice
VI. MANAGEMENT THEORY & PRACTICE	-Management Science -Business Administration	-Application of Theory to Practice
VII.PROGRAM DEVELOPMENT	-Curriculum Studies	-Application of Theory to Practice

(General education; professional preparation; intramural sports and physical recreation; intercollegiate athletics; programs for special populations--e.g., handicapped--including both curriculum and instructional methodology)

VIII.EVALUATION & MEASUREMENT	-Measurement Theory	-Application of Theory to Practice

Admittedly, you, the reader, may regard this recommendation as controversial. This doesn't worry us (Dr. Huelster and I) at all, and it shouldn't worry you either. We most certainly do not regard the specific of this proposed taxonomy as being etched in stone! As a matter of fact, we have made a number of minor alterations in the table ourselves during the past several years based on advice from specialists in the various sub disciplinary and sub professional areas. We are anxious to receive sound, constructive criticism from a variety of sources. The point to be made is that we will all be developing *together* a consensual definition that can change over time--but may well stand the test of time!

In Table 1 we have therefore *tentatively* agreed upon eight areas of scholarly study and research that are correlated with their respective sub disciplinary and sub professional aspects as follows:

(1) Background, Meaning, and Significance
(2) Functional Effects of Physical Activity
(3) Socio-cultural and Behavioral Aspects
(4) Motor Development and Control
(5) Mechanical and Muscular Analysis
    of Motor Skills
(6) Management/Administration
(7) Program Development
(8) Measurement and Evaluation

You will notice immediately that there is a (relatively) balanced approach between what we have identified as the sub disciplinary aspects of our field (#1 through #5) and what we have called the sub professional or concurrent sub professional components. By this we wish to convey the idea that what many have called--often in a semi-derogatory tone--*professional* writing (e.g., curriculum studies or investigation into the teaching-learning process) is to be regarded as scholarly--*if and only if* the best available research methodology and accompanying techniques have been employed. Similarly, what many have regarded as more scholarly, scientific endeavor (e.g., exercise science investigation or the "functional effects of physical activity" as we have called it here) is only to be regarded as such if it is well done. Further, we want to stress that the latter is itself also professional writing in the sense that it should ultimately serve the best interests of the profession.

Most importantly, note that the name selected for the eight areas do not include terms that are currently part of the names, or the actual names, of other recognized disciplines and that are therefore usually identified by the public--and also by professors on campus--with these other related disciplines. Our position is simply that *we must promote our own discipline of developmental physical activity in sport, exercise, and related expressive activities, while at the same time working cooperatively to the extent that our scholarly interests overlap.* If we continue to permit scholars with degrees in our field, and who are employed for the greatest percentage of their time with our units, to continue to claim primarily that--for example--they are *sociologists* of sport or *physiologists* of exercise, we are simply hastening the day when our field will be permanently assigned to second-class status--or perhaps even eliminated! The end result, if this were to continue to prevail, would inevitably not be in our best interest.

The Two Basic Questions to Resolve

Granting that we may in time be able to achieve a modicum, or "irreducible minimum," of agreement on a worldwide basis as to a definition for our quasi-discipline-profession, there are two basic questions that should be answered to the best of our ability: (1) *what* shall be compared, and (2) *how* shall it be done? In regard to the first question (the <u>what</u>), ongoing scholarly endeavor should provide us with accurate descriptions of (1) what is actually occurring in the eight areas of scholarly study and research, and (2) what social forces are influencing the development of the field, and (3) what recurring professional concerns and problems are confronting the profession.

Moving from the "what" or the *content* aspect of our endeavor, we are confronted with the "how" or the research methodologies and techniques to be employed. Here it seems logical that comparative sport and physical education should not be limited *solely* to Bereday's recommended approach (1964; to be explained below). Also, I hasten to assert that his recommended technique is just that, a very fine and useful *technique*. It is *one* technique of broad descriptive *method* of research--but somewhat more about this too shortly.

Here it seems logical that comparative sport and physical education should not be limited *solely* to Bereday's recommended research approach within broad descriptive method (1964; to be explained below). Also, I hasten to assert that his recommended technique is just that, a very fine and useful *technique*. It is *one* technique of broad descriptive <u>method</u>--but somewhat more about this too will be offered shortly.

Question #1--What Shall We Compare?

The first question to be answered here was indicated above as "What Is Occurring?" Here I want to reemphasize what was said above about our field should elevating its sights far beyond what happens under our aegis within some level of the educational system on this continent and elsewhere in the world. By this I meant that we should be extending our consideration so that they include an age range with a "womb to tomb" orientation! This is one of the reasons why Dr. Huelster and I have urged the broadening of the name to be applied to our field to "developmental physical activity" or

269

"human motor performance" in sport, exercise, and related expressive activities. We are urging further that our profession should have concern for the so-called normal individual, the accelerated person, and also the individual who for some reason or other may need special physical education (i.e., a specifically designed program of developmental physical activity) temporarily or permanently as part of his or her lifestyle.

Broadening our scope in this manner means that we should assume both "disciplinary concern" and "professional concern" for the type of developmental physical activity provided for the pre-school child, and then follow through all the way on to what type of physical activity is desirable for older citizens. Obviously, there is a need for attention to all age groups and, if we in this profession don't get fully involved, some other less-qualified group will take over. In fact, because of our "sins of omission," this has already taken place to a degree. Assuming this responsibility means that the best available knowledge from all of the eight areas of scholarly study and research should be available for this purpose (e.g., functional effects of physical activity or management/administration).

A second consideration under "what shall be compared?" should be the ongoing analysis of the various social forces and influences that impact upon the type of developmental physical activity provided--or perhaps even urged upon--citizens of all ages. Under this heading I have postulated that we should be considering the following forces or influences in our country, culture, and other cultures of the world:

1. Societal values and norms
2. The type of political state in existence
3. The level of nationalism present in a country
4. The approach taken to economic theory and practice
5. The impact of organized religion in the culture
6. The level of ecological awareness in the country
7. The level of science and technology present
8. The concern for a peaceful world
9. The concept of 'progress' that is present

All of these forces or influences exert a greater or lesser amount of impact upon the type and level of developmental physical activity in sport, exercise, and related expressive activities present.

Third, under the category of "content for comparison," I have identified over the years a number of professional concerns or issues that make up a second set of persistent historical problems. These are perennial problems with which our profession has been faced, and which give every indication of being with us for the foreseeable future. (These professional concerns have been reported in the literature for many years; see, for example, Zeigler, 1964, 1968, 1975, 1977, 1979.) These are now time-tested concerns for the profession in the sense that a substantive body of literature has accrued relative to each of them.) The following, then, is a list of them:

1. Program development (i.e., what shall be included and/or taught?)
2. Instructional methodology (i.e., how shall it be presented?)
3. Professional preparation or training (i.e.,what overall approach)
4. The concept of 'the healthy body' (i.e., what constitutes sound health?)
5. The place of women, handicapped people, and ethnic minorities in sport, exercise, and related expressive activities (i.e., what opportunities shall they have?)
6. The role of dance and music in developmental physical activity (i.e., to what extent shall each be employed in the process?)
7. The use of leisure (i.e., to what extent physical activity--and what type of activity--may be conceived as worthy use of leisure?)
8. The delineation of amateurism, semiprofessionalism, and professionalism in sport, exercise, and related expressive activities (i.e., to what extent is such delineation necessary or desirable?)
9. The approach to management or administration (i.e., how shall programs of developmental physical activity be administered?)
10. The concept of 'progress' (i.e., what constitutes professional progress?)

   (Note: In connection with these two listing of persistent problems, the concept of 'progress' is viewed as both a social force *and* a professional concern.)

Over and above this three-pronged approach to "what shall be compared" that has just been recommended, there is an excellent source available for the conceptualizing of the area of comparative and international physical education and sport. Here I am referring to Donald Morrison's "Towards a Conceptual Framework for Comparative Physical Education" (1967) as presented in *Methodology in Comparative Physical Education and*

271

Sport by Howell, Howell, Toohey, and Toohey (1979). Here the broad headings recommended for the analysis of a system of physical education are as follows:

1. Ecological setting
2. Socio-cultural system
3. Development and change of systems of physical education
4. The system of physical education itself from socio-cultural, economic, political, school system, and coordinating organizations' standpoints
5. Structures and functions of physical education organizations

Here, indeed, is a fine taxonomy from which to proceed as to "what shall we compare?" The format I have recommended above and this taxonomy complement each other very well.

Question #2--How Shall We Make Such Comparison?

The response to the second main question to be answered in this chapter ("How Shall We Make Such Comparison?") directs our attention to the question of research methodologies and techniques that might be applicable to this area of scholarly study and research in sport and physical education (or in developmental physical activity in sport, exercise, and related expressive activities as I have been recommending). As we seek to answer this question, please keep in mind what was being urged upon the field of comparative education in the two decades between 1950 and 1970 (i.e., first, more systematic and less impressionistic investigation; second, more empirical and analytical and less speculative and descriptive analysis; third, a more microcosmic than macrocosmic approach to problems; and, four, a more scientific as opposed to philosophical or historical type of research. The presumption here, of course, was that much more reliable data would be forthcoming if these criteria were applied to just about all investigations carried out (Kazmias and Schwartz, 1977). This criteria have a most familiar ring to us in this field, and it is my guess that these criteria will steadily and increasingly be urged upon us in the field of sport and physical education.

However, whatever criticisms the comparative education scholars may have had for the type of scholarly endeavor that had been carried out in the past--or for that matter that which we ourselves may have for it in our field--I don't believe it would serve any good purpose to assume an overly negative or critical role at this point. This is water over the dam, and there is every reason for us now to be positive and prospective in this regard as we look forward to the possibility of the 'global village' concept becoming a reality for us all because of the steady technological advancement in the area of communications.

Thus I can only recommend that the presently very small number of comparative scholars in sport and physical education should employ <u>all</u> of the research methods and techniques available to men and women who have an interest in developmental physical activity in sport, exercise, and related expressive *activities that extends beyond the borders of their respective countries*. Also, of course, this should perhaps *be the only criterion* that should be employed when we issue invitations to scholars to attend our meetings and take part in our ongoing professional affairs. Further, as a matter of fact, we need many more scholarly people with this type of interest which takes their concerns beyond the borders of their respective countries.

What this recommendation adds up to, therefore, is simply that there is an urgent need for comparative studies of all types that could, and should, be involving scholars who employ historical method, descriptive method, experimental group method of research, and philosophical analysis and interpretation, respectively, as they seek answers to the problems and concerns that our field has all over the world. Immediately, we must recognize that there are a number of different approaches to each of the research methods available. For example, a number of different historical interpretations are being employed as we near the end of the 20th century (e.g., that objectivity is an unattainable ideal), not to mention the many new techniques developed to aid the historian in his or her work (e.g., use of computers for analysis, development of demography, availability of sociological theory). Such new techniques contribute, of course, to the microcosmic nature of present-day historical investigation.

Most of the studies that are carried out in the name of comparative physical education and sport fall into the category typically known as *descriptive* research method--that is, the investigator uses one or more techniques of what used to be called *survey* research (a term that has been largely abandoned in educational research because it was too narrow and limited in most people's opinions). Today any and all techniques of descriptive (method) research are employed to discover one or more facts that are presumably related to the problem(s) under investigation. A good way to understand just when and where *historical* research leaves off and *descriptive* research begins is for the researcher, perhaps with the advice of associates, to ask himself or herself when attempts at historical analysis become blurred. At this point, try as our researcher may, it is quite impossible to evaluate the findings truly and clearly within an appropriate perspective. However, I don't believe this matter can be determined arbitrarily and categorically.

The above statements notwithstanding, the "research waters often become muddied" by careless use of terminology and an inability on the part of some investigators to understand that there are at least twelve to fifteen different techniques employed by social science researchers that fall under the category of descriptive method of research. For example, Bereday's so-called *comparative* method is nothing other than a combination of several of the useful techniques of descriptive method. Thus, I believe it is very confusing when we read or hear such terms as anthropological research, behavioral research, educational research, psychological research, methodological research, scientific research, social scientific research, and sociological research, to name some of the terms that we hear most often daily. Assuredly what is meant in almost every instance--but it is almost never made clear--is that *research* in a specific subject-matter, group of subject-matters, or discipline(s) is being discussed. The point to be made here, I believe, is simply that there are three broad methods of research-- historical, descriptive, and experimental group method using a control group mechanism--which contain within them a vast array of techniques often involving some type of statistical analysis. (A separate chapter could be written about the vague wanderings displayed in statistical discussions that take place at many meetings of thesis committees; this is why I always urge graduate students to special out their research design and appropriate statistical techniques to be employed most carefully--after they have been checked out with an authority in measurement and evaluation.) Finally, it should be obvious that descriptive method of research has to be a strong ally of scholars interested in comparative physical education and sport.

The third broad method of research extant is typically called *experimental* research, but I think it is better and more accurate to designate it as *experimental group method* of research. I see such careful definition as being most important, because it is quite possible and desirable to use an experimental *technique* with descriptive research *method* to determine the status of some measure or condition (e.g., testing a class to see how many sit- ups each member can do in sixty seconds). By using the word in two or more different ways, we are making the concept 'experiment' carries too much weight. It is *control* that is the most important factor for the researcher to keep in mind with the broad category of experimental (group method of) research. Here the investigator has the opportunity to manipulate factors and variables *before* the study or experiment is carried out. There can be randomization, and there can be a control group. The researcher can strive to control all the variables save one. In such a case, the monitoring and delimitation of the investigation is obviously greater, and therefore the probability that such-and-such may be truly related to this-and-that is greater as well.

Obviously, the problem that one faces when consideration is given to the use of some variation of experimental group method of research in the area of comparative and international sport and physical education is obtaining acceptance for the type of study to be undertaken. Nowadays any study that involves individuals or people (collectively) must be approved by a qualified, disinterested committee within a university. Further, leaders and members of organizations are very busy and are simply not ready social or psychologically to permit themselves or their group to be used as guinea pigs experimentally or in a control group. There is typically great concern about the time necessary to carry out such a study and/or the possible effect of negative findings that may result from the study. This negative feeling is enhanced greatly when one is dealing with a profit-making organization in North American culture, and the feeling is probably similar elsewhere as well.

Notwithstanding the difficulty of using this method when you enter the area of "behavioral research"--that is, those research methods and techniques applicable to investigations where people are involved in social (interpersonal) situations--at this point in the development of comparative and international physical education and sport we have not yet been able to even describe accurately those investigations that have been carried out in the past. By that I mean that we have not yet developed an acceptable, embryonic taxonomic classification to describe the area. Accordingly, it has not been possible to employ an integrative technique that would result in a synthesis of published findings and some reasonably tenable theory from which testable assumptions would undoubtedly emanate. Thus, what occurs typically is that a scholarly person wishing to undertake an investigation almost of necessity plans and executes some sort of an ad hoc, descriptive study, one that is only rarely elevated to the point where something akin to Bereday's comparative technique may be applied. (Here I hasten to add that there have been some fine studies employing one or more techniques of descriptive method, but rarely have there been investigations where appropriate sampling and statistical techniques were used to provide an acceptable means of testing a theoretical proposition.

Well, then, if we are indeed *not* able to employ experimental group method of research based on a fool-proof research paradigm because of a variety of difficulties with which we are confronted at this point (i.e., random sampling of subjects and the random assignment of both subjects and treatments to groups--including even the assignment of people and/or groups as control groups), what can be done to improve the situation? One approach that we shouldn't use, of course, is to blithely proceed with erroneous, cause-and-effect assumptions based on the application of historical methods and elementary descriptive method only, followed by a strongly declarative conclusion. If we persist in doing this, we are simply perpetuating the "after this, therefore caused by this" approach--the famous *post hoc, ergo propter hoc fallacy. Thus, if we do decide that we must* employ what have been called ex post facto research techniques (as part of what is really descriptive method), we have to most careful not to gloss over the fact that we haven't been able to control the independent variables, and that therefore our investigation has an inherent weakness.

Before concluding this all-too-brief discussion of research methodologies and techniques as they might apply to comparative and international physical education and sport, I must say some good words about *ex post facto* research despite its inherent limitations (i.e., inability to manipulate independent variables, inability to randomize subjects, and relative inability to interpret directly). This approach to research can at least cope to a degree with investigations that do not readily lend themselves to the institution of these desirable characteristics. In fact, at any time some important variables simply cannot be manipulated (e.g., personality factors), and therefore this approach is probably the only way that any type of semi-controlled inquiry is possible. In conclusion, we need well-executed studies of both types, and we will have to be satisfied with what is available to us at a given time and do the best that we can with it (Kerlinger, 1973).

Finally, in response to the question as to how comparison may be carried out, a few words should be said about what has often (perhaps mistakenly) designated as philosophic <u>research</u>. Let me say right away that I am now completely convinced that there is no such thing as philosophic research in the sense that news facts or knowledge can be uncovered. Philosophy was not always regarded in this way. Early philosophers believed that philosophy should (and could) serve a function not unlike that which we attribute to contemporary science today. However, present-day science and its exacting methods and techniques have ultimately forced the large majority of British and North American philosophers steadily and increasingly to challenge the fundamental basis of philosophic activity. (Those remaining with an existentialistic-phenomenological orientation would challenge the underlying premise of this assertion.)

By this admission I do not mean to imply that I personally do not see an important place for both *speculative* and *normative* philosophizing about our work. Nevertheless, I do recognize that what has been called <u>philosophic analysis</u>--the analytic tradition, if you will--dominates the discipline in the western world at present. This means that philosophy can be regarded as a sort of handmaiden to science through the use of techniques designated as conceptual analysis and language analysis, not to mention a variety of other approaches all involved with some form of critical analysis. As a matter of fact, I believe that most approaches to the doing of philosophy can be helpful to those scholars in our field who are interested in the comparative and international area--if they are well executed. This is why I have been arguing strongly that a more well-balanced approach to philosophizing would be most helpful at present and in the foreseeable future. By this I mean that philosophic endeavor should be more macroscopic as well as microscopic in its outlook. This is not to say that a given scholar concerned with the meaning and significance of developmental physical activity would necessarily be obligated to follow both approaches. It does confirm the position, however, that professionals in our field and the general public both need advice at a time when the societal values and norms are being challenged so mightily on all fronts in a highly troubled world.

The Need for Data, Information, Knowledge, and Wisdom

Earlier in this selection, I outlined what we hope might become a consensual definition of our entire discipline by suggesting that we might call it "Developmental Physical Activity in Sport, Exercise, and Related Expressive Movement." Whatever we eventually decide to call the field, and however we may classify it taxonomically, our professional practitioners are "drowning in data, struggling with information, starving for knowledge, and probably typically lacking in a sufficient amount of wisdom." Lest you think that I am being too harsh in describing our field, let me say quickly that all professions are facing a similar to a greater or lesser degree. That is their problem, of course, but I have been attempting to devise a plan that might work for us.

The terms that I just used are data, information, knowledge, and wisdom. The term "data" refers to facts, while "information" can be described as "facts placed in context so that the information changes the receiver's perceptions, beliefs or knowledge base" (Haggerty, 1985). Knowledge can be conceived of as the next step, so to speak, or "facts, truths, or principles resulting from study or scientific investigation. Finally, wisdom is the quality of being wise--that is, the faculty to discern right or truth and to judge or act accordingly.

Interestingly, we know that the data and information are "out there somewhere," but I challenge you to find the results of the specific study that you need *at the very time that you want to put it to use*! We could reason further that the term "knowledge" refers to data and information that are inventoried in the form of ordered principles or generalizations that represent tenable theory. Such theory can be employed by professional practitioners, and it also contains testable assumptions upon which further research can be based. Where, may I inquire, are these data and information inventoried as principles of knowledge and immediately available to the members of our profession?

By use of the concept of 'wisdom' above, I meant that attribute or competency that mature professionals should employ when making decisions as to what should or should not be done--that is, <u>wise</u> decisions such as are based on tenable theory but considered carefully in keeping with societal values and norms. Here too I don't believe that at the present our professionals in the field have an ever-present opportunity to relate to outstanding people in the various sub disciplinary and sub professional aspects of our profession for advice and guidance. If these statements are accurate, and I believe strongly that they are, this is why I felt constrained above to also make the "drowning, struggling, starving and lacking in wisdom" statement about the members of our field. Keeping in mind that the area of comparative and international physical education and sport is infinitely broader than the provision of the scholarly and scientific findings within just one country--our geographical area of concern is the entire world! Ours is a worldwide task and responsibility as we strive to bring the benefits of the finest type of developmental physical activity to all people everywhere.

Concluding Statement

Finally, based on what has preceded in this chapter on the socio-cultural and international relations aspects of our profession, I offer several suggestions, recommendations, and what I feel are reasonable conclusions as follows:

1. The profession should work for increased recognition for the area of comparative and international sport and physical education in all countries of the world.

2. In carrying out professional and scholarly endeavor in this area, we should encourage outstanding people from all sub disciplinary and sub professional aspects of our field to consider research designs in their work that broaden the perspective to include comparative and international aspects.

3. There is also a need for scholarly people in the field who will identify primarily with the comparative technique of descriptive method in order to develop and make available the necessary data, information, and ordered knowledge about sport, exercise, and related expressive activities on a global scale.

4. Scholarly people in the field with some interest in the comparative and international aspects of our work should be urged to become full or associate members of the International Society for Comparative Physical Education and Sport.

5. There is a great challenge for the profession to meet in this area of our field's work. We should ensure that our task and our responsibility are defined both <u>broadly</u> from the standpoint of breadth of outlook and *narrowly* from the standpoint of specializations of research interests. This subject should be approached both macroscopically and microscopically.

Actually, we need two types of professionals working in comparative investigation and international relations: *professional leaders* with vision in the area of international relations, people who can comprehend the long range goals and lead us down the correct paths to international cooperation and world peace, and *scholars* who will carry out both broadly based and narrowly defined investigations that will provide us with sound knowledge and tenable theory upon which to base our professional endeavors. Now is the time to adjust our bifocal eyeglasses so that we will have the wisdom and dedication to carry out this most important part of our professional task.

Note

1. The inauguration of the International Society for Comparative Physical Education and Sport, ISCPES, quite obviously marked the beginning of a new era within the profession. This was true even though a great many know next to nothing about the society even today. I, as a person who left the United States temporarily in 1949 to teach and coach in Canada, had the feeling that I was going to a foreign country. Accordingly, I made efforts to identify myself immediately with what was called the Foreign Relations Committee of the former College Physical Education Association, a professional grouping of men within the field who subsequently joined with the National Association of Physical Education for College Women, NAPECW, to form the present National Association for Physical Education in Higher Education. Also, from 1949 to 1968, it was my privilege to observe and work closely *on the North American continent only* with what was called the International Relations Council of the American Association for Health, Physical Education, and Recreation (within AAHPER) that was promoted by Dorothy Ainsworth and many others who were most encouraging to people like me who during the early 1950s were true neophytes.

If it weren't for these early experiences , a continuing series of international experiences in many parts of the world starting in 1968 with a trip to Israel and Greece, and a return to Canada as a landed immigrant in 1971, it is quite possible that I would presently be numbered among that vast majority of physical educator/coaches in the United States who feel that "if anything worthwhile is going to happen, it will take place here" and, if something does by chance happen elsewhere, "it had better be made available in the English language if I am to be expected to pay any attention to it." This may sound like harsh, unfair criticism, but it is my considered opinion based on long experience that far too much of this attitude still prevails.

For reasons such as this, it is important that the international society (ISCPES) was inaugurated at the 1978 conference in Israel at the Wingate Institute where so many fine innovations along this line have taken place; that the second (biennial) conference was held in Canada at Dalhousie University in 1980; that the third biennial meeting was carried out at the University of Minnesota, Minneapolis in 1982, the fourth meeting occurred at Malente/Kiel, Federal Republic of Germany in 1984; and the fifth at The University of British Columbia in Vancouver, Canada in 1986. (A sixth conference was held in Hong Kong in 1988, and a seventh conference was held in England in 1990.) What appears is this chapter is based, therefore, on ideas which I presented in several papers presented at Minneapolis and Malente/Kiel.)

References

Asimov, F.. (1970). The fourth revolution. *Saturday Review*, October 24, 17-20.

Bennett, B.L., Howell, M.L. & Simri, U. (1983). *Comparative Physical Education and Sport*. (Second edition). Philadelphia: Lea & Febiger.

Bereday, G.Z.F. (1964). *Comparative method in education*. New York: Holt, Rinehart and Winston, pp. 11-27.

Glasser, W. (1972). *The identity society*. New York: Harper & Row.

Haggerty, T. (1985). Personal conversation in July.

Kaplan, A. (1961). *The new world of philosophy*. Boston: Houghton Mifflin.

Kazamias, A.M., & Schwartz, K. (1977). Intellectual and ideological perspectives in comparative education: An interpretation. *Comparative Education Review* 21, 2/3, 153-176.

Kerlinger, F. (1973). *Foundations of behavioral research*. New York: Holt, Rinehart & Winston.

Morrison, D. (1979). Towards a conceptual framework for comparative physical education. In M.L. Howell, R. Howell, M. Toohey, & D. Toohey (Eds.), *Methodology in comparative physical education and sport* (pp. 89-119). Champaign, IL: Stipes.

Noah, H.J. & Eckstein, M.A. (1969). *Toward a science of comparative education*. New York: Macmillan.

Skinner, B.F. (1971). *Beyond freedom and dignity*. New York: Knopf.

Zeigler, E.F. (1975). *Personalizing physical education and sport philosophy*. Champaign, IL: Stipes.

Zeigler, E.F. (1977). *Physical education and sport philosophy*. Englewood Cliffs, NJ: Prentice-Hall.

Zeigler, E.F. (Ed.). (1988). *A history of physical education and sport* (Revised edition). . (This includes sections written by R.K. Barney, R.G. Glassford & G. Redmond, M.L. Howell & R. Howell, G.A. Paton, & two by E.F. Zeigler.)

Zeigler, E.F. (1983). Relating a proposed taxonomy of sport and developmental physical activity to a planned inventory of sport and developmental physical activity. *Quest*, 35 (1) 54-65.

Selection #12
Assessment of the International Scene
in Physical Education and Sport in 1994

Earle F. Zeigler

An Exploratory Study of Status

Looking at the international scene specifically, as it applies to the profession of physical (activity) education and (educational) sport, was an interesting assignment for me just before the turn of the 21st century. The organizers of the 10th International Scientific Congress of the University of Victoria, British Columbia, Canada, invited me to make a report on the status of our field internationally. My hypothesis prior to some detailed investigation was that physical activity education and educational sport in educational institutions worldwide had deteriorated and would continue to do so in the years immediately ahead. This opinion was based on my professional involvement of various types (including attendance at international conferences), the reading of many journals, and an extensive international correspondence carried on for many years.

This preliminary conclusion was made because all of education has been literally reeling for some time now because of increases in certain negative social forces (e.g., values, economics, religion) caused by a changing social environment. Because of what is now known scientifically about the potential beneficial effects that properly conceived developmental physical activity could have on people of all ages and conditions, we dare not as a profession become pessimistic about the wisdom of striving to create an "improved" social situation. The salutary effects of appropriate developmental physical activity need to be introduced into all people's lives. However, we must be fully aware of the fact that humankind's needs for developmental physical activity will be met IF--*and only if*-- (1) public support for our efforts is earned and (2) highly trained leadership is made available to earn such public support and then to bring about these desirable educational and developmental outcomes.

As professionals, we already have a good understanding of the effects of physical activity as demonstrated by the steadily improving quantitative and qualitative, natural-science type of investigation that has been carried out over the past 50 years. However, I firmly believe, also, that a full understanding of our endeavor as developmental physical activity professionals can only become possible through an ever-greater and stronger understanding of how the social sciences and the humanities can also influence our work. Obviously, the bioscience aspects of developmental physical activity are highly important, but people need to understand also that in the final analysis a more balanced, across-the-board approach to scholarly investigation is required to help us achieve the field's true potential in the service of humankind. For example, the concept of "growth and development" has been well understood and applied for decades in the field of physical education and sport. This perception is accordingly transferable to the process of growth and development that usually occurs throughout the life of a person working in the field as well.

My generation of physical educator/coaches was typically optimistic about the future despite the strong social forces and accompanying persistent professional problems that have influenced physical education and educational sport from decade to decade down through the 20th century. As I see it, my generation, and the "baby boomer" generation too, have an obligation to pass on as much as that optimism as possible to "Generation X" as men and women in this age group strive to become legitimate partners and leaders in our profession looking to the first quarter of the 21st century.

To determine to what degree optimism is, or is not, possible, my preliminary 1994 investigation about the status of our field in the world today was, therefore, an exploratory effort to discover something of what our professionals "out there" are experiencing firsthand in certain countries on the various continents of the world. One could theorize tentatively that current social forces (e.g., (1) the 28 ongoing wars throughout the world in 1993, (2) the recent economic downturn with its inevitable influence on education at all levels; and (3) the "return to essentials" in much of the educational thought we were hearing) were effecting often-debatable curricular changes in programs worldwide. However, in truth, how accurate was such conjecture? To get some feel for what was happening, I decided to contact individuals in the 33 countries represented in the 1993 membership list of the International Society for Comparative Physical Education and Sport.1

In essence, this investigation had two broad, main purposes: (1) to carry out a preliminary analysis of global trends in physical education and (educational) sport and (2) to make some recommendations regarding what the field should do in the immediate future. I developed a listing of sub-problems to investigate as follows:

(1) To set the stage with a brief, general assessment of the international situation,

(2) To obtain some specific reactions about what was happening about physical education and educational sport in each of the 33 countries represented in the 1993 membership list of the ISCPES,

(3) To consider the topic of futurology by offering one futuristic approach that has been

recommended to cope with the "great transition" that the world has been undergoing,

(4) (To offer my personal observations and understanding about how the greatly strengthened under girding knowledge available to the profession of physical education and educational sport around the world might help in addressing the field's future,

(5) To make some recommendations to cope with the "modifications" that the field has been undergoing during the past 30 years to effect improved professional development as the field looks somewhat hesitatingly looks to an indeterminate future, and

(6) To delineate the basic considerations and strategy required meeting the professional task ahead.

The investigation employed both historical method and broad descriptive methodology, as well as what may be called "philosophical assessment" as to field's current direction and immediate future. The broad-based historical analysis of the emerging international situation, based on second-hand literature, was followed by the employment of a descriptive questionnaire technique to gather the required data about the status of physical education and sport internationally. (A pre-tested questionnaire was especially designed for, and distributed to, one member selected from each of the 33 countries represented in the ISCPES membership.) Next, the greatly enlarged, under girding body of knowledge available to the profession was reviewed to assess the field's "current strength" through a statement of 13 "principal principles" that support the field's professional endeavor. Then one futuristic approach to the "world situation" was used as a guide available to the profession for consideration as it faces an uncertain future. Next, a type of historical analysis was then carried out about the numerous "modifications" that the profession has undergone in the past 30 years. Finally, by employing one type of "philosophical analysis," the necessary steps required to accomplish the professional task immediately were delineated and offered as recommendations for strategic professional action in the first quarter of the 21st century.

The difficulty of developing scientific hypotheses for an analysis of this type was recognized. Strictly speaking, hypotheses are statements about the relationship between variables. They also embody an understanding as to how such a relationship may be established (i.e., substantive hypotheses are transposed to [null] hypotheses for statistical testing, for example). I had to be satisfied with a 60% response (20 out of 33 questionnaires sent were returned). Thus, "what I had" was quite simply the opinion about the status of physical education (4) (To offer my personal observations and understanding about how the greatly strengthened under girding knowledge available to the profession of physical education and educational sport around the world might help in addressing the field's future,

(5) To make some recommendations to cope with the "modifications" that the field has been undergoing during the past 30 years to effect improved professional development as the field looks somewhat hesitatingly looks to an indeterminate future, and

(6) To delineate the basic considerations and strategy required meeting the professional task ahead.

The investigation employed both historical method and broad descriptive methodology, as well as what may be called "philosophical assessment" as to field's current direction and immediate future. The broad-based historical analysis of the emerging international situation, based on second-hand literature, was followed by the employment of a descriptive questionnaire technique to gather the required data about the status of physical education and sport internationally. (A pre-tested questionnaire was especially designed for, and distributed to, one member selected from each of the 33 countries represented in the ISCPES membership.) Next, the greatly enlarged, under girding body of knowledge available to the profession was reviewed to assess the field's "current strength" through a statement of 13 "principal principles" that support the field's professional endeavor. Then one futuristic approach to the "world situation" was used as a guide available to the profession for consideration as it faces an uncertain future. Next, a type of historical analysis was then carried out about the numerous "modifications" that the profession has undergone in the past 30 years. Finally, by employing one type of "philosophical analysis," the necessary steps required to accomplish the professional task immediately were delineated and offered as recommendations for strategic professional action in the first quarter of the 21st century.

The difficulty of developing scientific hypotheses for an analysis of this type was recognized. Strictly speaking, hypotheses are statements about the relationship between variables. They also embody an understanding as to how such a relationship may be established (i.e., substantive hypotheses are transposed to [null] hypotheses for statistical testing, for example). I had to be satisfied with a 60% response (20 out of 33 questionnaires sent were returned). Thus, "what I had" was quite simply the opinion about the status of physical education and educational sport from one professionally minded person in 20 of the 33 countries surveyed. Fortunately, the people who responded were representative of countries widely dispersed in all parts of the world, and they obviously had made a sincere effort to respond to the questions raised. Those who responded were representative of countries widely dispersed in all parts of the world, and they obviously had made a sincere effort to respond to the questions raised.

Study Findings and Discussion

Note: Simple descriptive statistics were used. The results were expressed in categories relating to percentage values determined. The data gathered were numerically tabulated, and the responses were summarized by percentage values based on the predetermined questions. The results from each question asked were followed immediately by related discussion to each question asked. With certain questions, because of the type and information sought, agreement was arbitrarily indicated as follows: SUBSTANTIAL MAJORITY (75%-100%), MAJORITY (50%-75%), SUBSTANTIAL MINORITY (25%-50%), and UNSUBSTANTIAL MINORITY (0%-25%)

First, interestingly, a MAJORITY (see "agreement" definition above, i.e., 13 or 65% of the total of 33 respondents) believed that the physical education program, generally speaking, had improved in the recent decade. (This was a surprising but encouraging finding to the investigator whose thinking was undoubtedly influenced by the North American scene. Of course, in some instances the status may have been quite low, and the status had simply improved to some degree.)

Second, a SUBSTANTIAL MINORITY (8 or 40% fits in the 25%-50% grouping above) believed the level of physical fitness had declined. Five or 25% believed that the level of physical fitness had improved, whereas 5 or 25% felt that it had stayed about the same. Two respondents were not able to form a judgment.

Third, a SUBSTANTIAL MAJORITY (20 or 100% = 75%-100% grouping) uses the name physical education at the school level. In addition, a MAJORITY has not made a name change at the university (13 or 65% = 60%-75% grouping). Name changes have been made at the university level during the past decade in those institutions where the units are striving for academic status in a competitive environment. In the U.S.A., at last count, approximately two hundred different names have been introduced at the college & university level.

Fourth, physical education is required in a SUBSTANTIAL MAJORITY of countries (17 or 85% = 75%-100% grouping). The requirement ranges from a low of three (3) years to a high of 14 yrs. Only four (of the 20) countries that responded have no national requirement in physical education: Canada, India, Malawi, and the United States of America.

Fifth, competitive sport of varying "intensity" is considered part of the overall physical education program in a MAJORITY of the schools (11 or 55% = 50%-75% grouping). It is considered extra-curricular in a SUBSTANTIAL MINORITY of countries (9 or 45% = 25%-50% grouping). It is not clear to what extent competitive sport is regarded as an "educational experience" in the same way as what is typically called physical education. At any rate, this matter has not been resolved yet for a variety of reasons. It is certain, also, that in all countries competitive sport is available outside of school through private, semi-public, and public agencies.

Sixth, physical education comes under the jurisdiction of a national ministry in a MAJORITY of the countries surveyed (14 or 70% = 50%-75% grouping). Organized sport is considered sufficiently important in a MAJORITY of the countries to report to a national ministry (12 or 60% = 50%-75% grouping). In six countries, physical education is considered an aspect of education, education being the responsibility of a state or province within a country. The location of organized sport within governmental frameworks does not appear to follow any definite pattern. Physical education, on the other hand, is always located within the governmental bureau concerned with education of the populace.

Seventh, physical education does count for academic credit in a MAJORITY of the countries surveyed (14 or 70% = 50%-75% grouping). The results here are not clear, because there is a great range in the academic credit granted (i.e., from no credit in 7 countries to full acceptance as a tertiary entrance subject in a number of Australian states). Underlying this whole issue, of course, is the question of whether the physical education course experience and subsequent grade awarded--especially in those instances when there is no theoretical component included in the grade allotted for the course experience--should be averaged in with other course grades to determine a GPA (overall grade-point average).

Eighth, since the basic areas or activities generally included (e.g. fitness activities, sport skills, rhythmic activities) in this subject matter at the ELEMENTARY, MIDDLE SCHOOL, HIGH SCHOOL, and UNIVERSITY levels, it was not possible to classify the responses given to this question by each of the 20 respondents. However, the following generalizations are possible:

(a) Generally speaking, the curriculum and instructional methodology are standardized from country to country.
   (Note: It is not possible without first-hand study to make any comparative assessment between or among countries.)

b) Fundamental movement skills and games of low organization are standard at the elementary-school level

c) Sports skills instruction and fitness activities are introduced gradually at the middle-school level and continued on through the high school level on either a required or elective basis

d) A theoretical component in instructional programs is almost completely lacking (except in a few countries in specific states or provinces)

e) Lifetime sport and physical recreation instruction is often offered in the upper high-school years

f) Extramural competitive sport within education is offered only in Canada, Japan, Nigeria, and the U.S.A.

g) University programs, where offered, are largely elective and typically include voluntary sport and physical recreation and fitness-oriented activities. (A few countries [Israel, Philippines, Slovakia, and a relatively few universities in the U.S.A.] have a one- or two-year requirement.)

Ninth, as to whether there was any highly unusual or unique aspect in a particular country's physical education curriculum or instructional methodology, the respondents were almost unanimous in affirming that there was nothing "highly unusual or unique" in their countries' physical education curriculum or instructional methodology. This was a disturbing finding. For greater recognition within general education, it seems evident that the introduction of increasingly sound theoretical material is necessary to provide under girding for the skills instructional program. Australia and Canada report that in certain states or provinces highly sophisticated theory courses using texts have been introduced in the upper-level, high school courses, the results of which are fully credited for university entrance. In addition, Japan has been making extensive use of video cameras to provide sport-skill feedback to students at the high-school level.

Tenth, concerning the assessment of the present, overall STATUS of the subject of physical education *in relation to* other curricular subjects within the field of education in their country (i.e., higher, lower, about the same level), the (present) status of physical education was rated lower than other subjects in the curriculum by a SUBSTANTIAL MAJORITY (i.e., almost unanimously–18 or 90% = 75%-100% grouping). In two countries (Nigeria, Taiwan), the respondents believed that physical education's status was equal.

Finally, in response to a request for open-ended comments, selected responses to the survey instrument were as follows:

(1) In six countries, the respondents believed that physical activity's contribution to health status would eventually help the field to gain more recognition for its contribution.
(2) In three countries, the respondent felt that improved teacher preparation was needed.
(3) In two countries (Canada and the U.S.A.), legislation had served to improve the level of adapted physical education significantly.
(4) In one country (Australia) a recent national conference report about the prevailing situation has tended to bring improvement to the field.

Recent Interesting Developments

The results of the above survey carried out did not produce many "open-ended comments." Thus, I decided to look for some interesting informational developments in four internationally oriented journals (the *International Journal of Physical Education*, the *Journal of Comparative Physical Education and Sport*, the *European Physical Education Review*, and the *Journal of the International Council for Health, Physical Education, Recreation, Sport, and Dance*). As usual, there is some "good news" and some "bad news." I begin with the latter and conclude on a more positive note.

First, an excellent source for present trends globally in physical education has been provided by Ken Hardman (1995), now past-president of the International Society for Comparative Physical Education and Sport. The picture presented by Professor Hardman is well documented and overall a bit depressing. While granting that his "various 'snap-shot' national scenarios presented may provide a somewhat distorted picture of physical education in schools," Hardman does nevertheless makes a solid case for the urgent need "for redefining the parameters for 21st century conditions and needs, and for reshaping the physical education system to meet those needs" (p. 23).

Hardman's report includes brief statements about the status of physical education in Scandinavia (Sweden, Norway, and Finland), the Netherlands, Greece, Germany, Czech and Slovak Republics, Scotland, England & Wales, a number of African countries (e.g., Kenya), Malaysia, the United States, Canada, and Australia. "The news is not good," colloquially speaking again, even in England and Wales where a "government-sponsored national curriculum was imposed in 1989 with physical education introduced as a statutorily required school subject for children aged 5-16" (pp. 19-20). The problem here was that physical educators had no input into the deliberations before its announcement, and thus "economic viability" and not "educational desirability" appeared to determine the time allotment for physical education. As Hardman implied, the day for problem solving, persuasion, and bargaining may have ended, and the "era of politicking" should begin.

Second, although not exactly on the same topic, a statement by John C. Andrews (1995), the World President of the International Federation of Physical Education (FIEP), asks the question, "Is there a need for a continuing differentiation between the terms physical education and sport?" In response to this query, President Andrews comes down strongly for the umbrella term "physical education and sport" (p. 26). (I personally couldn't agree more with his stand and note also that the usage of this longer term [i.e., rather than either sport or physical education] is still widely understood and used worldwide based on the findings of the limited survey reported above. In addition, in the United States especially, I would be inclined to call it "physical activity education and educational sport" to differentiate from overly stressed commercialized sport in both the public sector and a significant portion of higher education.)

In addition, Andrews repeated an excellent series of concerns stressed by AAHPERD and CAHPERD concerning (1) decreasing curriculum time for physical education in schools, (2) "confusion of multiple aims and directions," (3) a growing gap between the researcher and the practitioner, (4) inadequate public awareness and support, (5) a murky relationship among the so-called allied professions, and, finally, (6) a widening gap between physical educational and sport opportunities available in developed and underdeveloped nations (p. 28).

Third, a further statement by Cheffers (1996) titled "Sport versus education: The jury is still out" raised a highly interesting point (paraphrased loosely here): Required physical education has seemed more like work, while voluntary sport is more like play. Therefore, sport is more alluring, while physical education is viewed as "dour" and "funereal" (p. 107). With this as an introductory thought, Cheffers raises 19 penetrating "sport-education statements" and concludes with 10 excellent hypotheses for serious consideration by all who are concerned with the future of physical education and sport. For example, Sport-Education Statement No. 5 states that, "Sports invite the short-cut, cheating drugs, gross egos. Education invites the same, but celebrates less" (p. 107). One seemingly increasingly important hypothesis (No. 6 of the 10 hypotheses suggested) is that "The essential periphery (parents, press, business associates, and spectators) need also take responsibility for their part in the total enterprise" (p. 109).

Despite the utmost serious nature of the alarming state of school physical education worldwide stressed in the above articles by Hardman, Andrews, and Cheffers, several encouraging notes were sounded in a variety of other articles in the four above-noted journals. For example, Roberts wrote about "the success of school and community sport provisions in Britain." He reported:

(1) that "in the years up to 1994 Britain's schools were improving their sports facilities,
(2) that young people were playing more sports in and out of school than in the past,
(3) that the drop-out rate on completion of statutory schooling had fallen dramatically,
(4) that social class and gender differences had narrowed, and
(5) that by the mid-1990s sports had higher youth participation and retention rates than any other structured forms of leisure" (1996, p. 105).

He concluded with a plea that authorities not return to the earlier male-dominated, "traditional games regime" that never held much attraction for young women.

Moving to the east, Krawczyk (1996) explains that the "image of sport" in Eastern Europe had changed radically since the influence of communism has waned. There was still significant concern for a responsible system of physical activity and sport for children and young people. Interestingly, however, it was predicted that the promotion of elite sport would emerge again as a problem. In doing so, however, Krawcyzk believes that the money expended would be more in line with a depressed economy (p. 9). Overall, because the situation was in a state of constant flux, he did not feel that evidence confirming a future "strong recovery" overall in the entire region was yet present.

Once again moving eastward, but also in a southerly direction to Australia, Saffici (1996) wrote interestingly about a successful initiative in physical education there called "Aussie Sport." The two main philosophic stances of this program for both boys and girls are "sport for all" and "fair play." "The hope is that people who find sport attractive will continue to have active lifestyles, and thus be able to decrease likelihood of suffering from cardiovascular disease and/or low back problems" (p. 52). A further objective of this program is to involve also an increasing number of elementary school teachers over and above the physical education specialist.

Julian Stein (1996), who as editor of the *Journal of the International Council for Health, Physical Education, Recreation, Sport, and Dance*, has strengthened this widely distributed publication immeasurably, offered an uplifting report of the (post-Olympic Games) Third Paralympic Congress and the Atlanta Declaration of People with Disabilities. The Declaration itself (p. 43) expresses a grand vision for the rights of "people with disabilities" in the future and should be enlarged and framed in the office of every physical educator worldwide. Programs of physical education and educational sport for normal, accelerated, and special populations must be ever cognizant of the need to strike a balance that recognizes the inborn rights of all.

In concluding this section, Penny and Kirk (1996) showed serious concern in their article comparing recent national curriculum developments in Australia and Britain. They explained that the evident trends in curriculum development appearing in "a climate of low morale among some sections of the physical education profession in the face of public criticism and amidst constrained and pressured contexts appear to be encouraging a tendency toward backward-looking conservatism rather than forward- looking experimentation and risk taking" (pp. 35-36).

Finally, physical (activity) education and (educational) sport within educational boundaries as a subject-matter is confronted today with a paradox: At the very time when the evidence is available to make the case for a sound program of required and voluntary developmental physical activity, economic restraints and public criticism of many prevailing programs are making progress extremely difficult.

North America

North Americans, generally speaking, still do not fully comprehend that their seemingly unique position in the history of the world's development may well change radically in the 21st century. The years ahead could really be difficult ones. Indeed, although it is probably truer of the United States than Canada, history is going against them in several ways.

This means that previous optimism must be tempered to shake people loose from delusions, some of which they may still have.

These are hard words, but they must be stated to help assess status of a diverse collectivity called the profession of sport and physical education in the United States. Then we need to place our status in broader perspective as well. Norman Cousins sounded just the right note when he stated a generation ago (1974) that perhaps "the most important factor in the complex equation of the future is the way the human mind responds to crisis" (pp. 6-7). The world culture as we know it must respond adequately to the many challenges with which it is being confronted. The various societies and nations must individually and collectively respond positively, intelligently, and strongly if humanity as we have known it is to survive.

Approaching the situation from a somewhat less broad perspective, I wish to argue that much of the current problem stems from the fact that education is faced with almost insurmountable problems because other basic societal institutions (e.g., the church, the family) are floundering to a considerable degree. Consequently, the school's burden is being increased to fill the gaps--to remedy deficiencies that could be made up largely if we had the funds *and the attitudinal support* to implement a competency-based approach to the needed knowledge and skills required for adequacy in life mastery in the late twentieth century.

Of course, it is at this point that we in the profession should persist strongly with the idea that developmental physical activity in exercise, sport, and related expressive activities can make a vital contribution to the lives of all people everywhere through the improvement of both the "quantity and quality" of life. With a quality product and greatly improved marketing techniques, we should be able to make a sound case for inclusion of our subject matter as *an integral part of any educational curriculum.*

We have tended to let others browbeat us intellectually in what has been typically a theoretical, subject-matter curriculum in the schools. Resultantly, the general education curriculum at all levels has been characterized by grossly inadequate attention to the *entire* body. The stress has been traditionally on the transmission of "knowledge" in a vague entity characteristically known as mind. (Also, legislation passed has insured that the development of "spirit"--to the extent that such can be defined--belongs to the church as a private agency.)

Teachers of physical activity education and educational sport designed for either normal, accelerated, or special populations simply have to become more "offensive" in their approach. The approach that has been characterized in the past by often inarticulate *defensive* posturing has no place in the 21st-century world. People in many other subject matters (e.g., in the language skills and the computational skills) "know" that they are important--but even they are being criticized sharply. Why is this so? It is occurring because the necessary attitudinal development is not sufficiently strong for students to overcome often-inadequate instructional methodology and techniques (not to mention often insufficient content). Johnny cannot read; Jane cannot do math; Jimmy's grammar is atrocious, and Rose does not care whether she learns anything or not. We haven't seen any evidence that a "return to basics" is going to teach our children how to think and reason logically, how to develop a set of ethical values, or how to take care of their bodies—all presumably vital to the educational process and throughout people's lives.

The Situation in Physical Activity Education and Educational Sport

There is every evidence that the next ten to fifteen years will be crucial ones for the field of physical activity education and educational sport. This is true because the profession is not growing and developing as rapidly and strongly as it should be in a society where the idea of change must now become our watchword. View it as you will, it is impossible to refute the thought that change, like death and taxes, is here to stay.

Diagnosis of the present situation leads to the belief that the field of physical (activity) education and (educational) sport--as it has been known and promoted--is structurally deficient in what may be called the field's architecture. Many people recognize that something is wrong, but most of them do not appear to understand the extent of the malady that has gradually infected a still embryonic profession.

Fortunately, the American *Association* for Health, Physical Education, and Recreation earlier substituted the word "Alliance" in recognition of the fact that health education (and safety education) and recreation (and park administration) are *separate* but *allied* professions. In addition, it was indeed timely that dance received similar recognition, and that its name was added to the overall title as well. Further, and this is especially important to physical educators/coaches, the emerging profession has witnessed the steady development of an entity called the National Association for Sport and Physical Education (NASPE) within the AAHPERD as presently constituted. In addition, of course, within AAHPERD we now have the American Association for Physical Activity and Recreation--that is, "physical education's" one-two punch!

Use of the term "sport and physical education" as our profession's official name in NASPE may need a bit of discussion. It could be argued that this should be a "holding-pattern" term, since the profession of sport and physical education--or whatever it may eventually be called--is still searching for an appropriate name well over 100 years after the founding of the Association for the Advancement of Physical Education. Of course, as explained immediately above, it is now the American Alliance for Health, Physical Education, Recreation, and Dance in the United States (although there have been "rumblings" urging a name change). (And the Canadian Association for HPERD in Canada changed its name to Physical and Health Education Canada in 2008). What has happened "along the way," of course, is that the parent field of physical education spawned a number of newer professions, and now they are all typically called the *allied* professions. (In Canada only physical & health education and parks & recreation have separate identities used in this context.)

Here, however, the term "physical activity education and educational sport" will be used primarily to describe the *professional* entity in the United States. Yet, it is true that the terms "physical education and sport" and "sport" [alone!] are now more popular in certain other countries that identify with the Western world including the European continent, respectively. However, "developmental physical activity in exercise, sport, and related expressive movement" will be used here typically when the field's *disciplinary* aspects are being discussed. In the latter instance, even more technically, the reference is to *the underlying theory of developmental physical activity* that is based increasingly on scholarly and research endeavor of a high order. People, both professionals *and* the public, need to understand such linguistic usage. (Note, also, that the term kinesiology [i.e., the study of human movement] is used increasingly in higher education.)

These terms too may change in the course of time, but for now they seem to be acceptable ones for those people specifically concerned. Interestingly, many other disciplines and professions seem to be able to "divide and subdivide" and still (somehow!) call themselves by one name basically (e.g., anthropology, medicine), but unfortunately the field of physical education cannot boast of a similar achievement. Whether it is called human kinetics, kinesiology, ergonomics, exercise science, sport studies, sport science, movement arts and sciences, etc., no euphemism is going to protect the field if it isn't doing the job that is needed "out there" in the public domain! (As Shakespeare stated in *Romeo and Juliet*, "that which we call a rose by any other name would smell as sweet.")

A Call for Reunification

The placing of increased emphasis on *their own* profession is an important point for physical educators/coaches today, because it is symptomatic of the many divisions that have developed in the past fifty or sixty years. Physical educators now recognize that there are indeed allied professions represented to a greater or lesser extent in the Alliance. It is not a question of attempting to bring these other professions back into the physical education fold again--they are gone forever. However, in interest of these "allied" professions, and that of physical activity education, they must be kept as closely allied as possible.

What is crucial now is that physical educators seek to bring about a recognizable state of *REUNIFICATION within* what is here called the physical activity education and educational sport. If the present splintering process taking place is not reversed, both in the United States and in Canada, prospects for the future may be bleak indeed. The profession that "exists both within a profession [education!] and also in the public domain as one purporting to serve humanity from 'womb to tomb'" must figure out the ways and means of unifying the various aspects of its *overall* profession to at least the degree that full public recognition results. Here the reference is to human movement, human motor performance, or developmental physical activity--*however it is eventually defined*--in exercise, sport, and related expressive movement for those who are qualified *and* officially recognized *and officially certified* in the theory and practice of such human movement--be they performers, teachers/coaches/teachers of teachers/coaches. scholars and researchers, practitioners in alternative careers, or other professional practitioners not yet envisioned.

So, to this point my argument is that "we are not dead or even dying," because death implies complete inactivity and cessation of all vital functions. It could be argued that the field is presently quiescent, in that many seem to be following a "business as usual" approach characterized by (1) unimaginative programs, (2) routine drill with inadequate motivation, (3) too much free play even though inadequate skill levels prevail, and (4) teacher pedantry. With fifty states and commonwealths and ten provinces and three territories (excluding Mexico as we are prone to do typically) to consider on a continental basis, we simply cannot speak with authority as to the present state of what is called physical education generally, much less offer a specific, detailed analysis on a state-by-state or province-by-province basis.

Therefore, I suggest that we take a different tack and listen for a moment to one of our severest critics, Harold VanderZwaag of The University of Massachusetts, Amherst. He argued vigorously that physical education has become an anachronism, that what it's all about is sport, dance, play, and exercise, all functioning quite separately within education and in society at large. What he suggested is "elimination of the field as such" (VanderZwaag, in Zeigler, 1982, p. 54). Where "it's at," he said, is "sport management!"

> (**Note:** Interestingly since Dr. VanderZwaag made that statement, there are now more than 200 academic programs in sport management in North America. However, as significant as this development has been in the provision of management personnel for competitive, commercialized sport, the emphasis accordingly has not been on

developmental physical activity for normal and special populations. This is where the profession of physical activity education and educational sport should retain its place and identity!)

VanderZwaag's argument challenges physical activity education and educational sport to redefine the very core of what it is all about when it requests space and time in the general education curriculum. Frankly, this is more than just a debate about terminology (e.g., the Germans have substituted the terms "sport" and "sport science" *(Sport* und *Sportwissenschaft)* for the former "physical education" (or *koerperlicher Erziehung*). What knowledge, competencies, and skills are achieved through the medium of what has been called the physical education program for more than a century? It is useless to argue that other subject matters have not been this precise in making their case for inclusion in the curriculum. That is their problem; physical education and educational sport has its own plight that should be resolved very soon.

VanderZwaag's criticism and recommendation is not a completely isolated case. For example, consider the hypothetical case of a program called the department of kinesiology (or human kinetics) that was eliminated from the leading university in a particular state or province (this has already happened, of course). For at least the past thirty years, higher education has been in unusual difficulty financially. The extent of this hardship has varied greatly from state to state and region to region. (The same problem came to Canada, a bit later as it has turned out. Professionals in educational institutions often buy their own paperclips, staples, and stamps.)

When university administrators have their backs to the wall financially, they obviously begin to look around for places to cut back arguing that only those programs central to the university mission can remain. If their glance happens to fall (1) on a department, unit, or division called "human kinetics," "kinesiology," or "sport studies" (formerly known as the physical education department), and (2) the undergraduate enrollment of this unit has been falling off, and (3) the many other arguments that can be mustered typically prevail, it is understandable that the rather desperate president or vice-president (academic) is going to think that the department of kinesiology is one place where a considerable saving can be effected. "After all," he or she may argue, "there are six–or eight or 10 or 36–other colleges and universities in the state turning out physical educators and coaches." In addition, the quality of research in such units has often been questioned because they have been located within schools or colleges of education.

Further, this newly named department may also be "easy pickings" since it has relatively few tenured members, being completely separate from intercollegiate athletics and (possibly) intramural and recreational sports as well. With these extra-curricular activities (as they are unfortunately designated typically), it is now often the case that they are usually self supporting and can't be expected to provide a great amount of backing for an academic unit that has not regarded them as being part of the department's basic structure.

Let us follow this hypothetical situation along a bit further because it gets to the heart of the problem of physical education and educational sport in a college or university setting. The profession should be able to present a strong case for the support of a *discipline* that purports to examine "developmental physical activity in sport, exercise, and related expressive activities" within the academic program of the leading university in *every* state or province on the continent. It can be argued, also, that the field is unique, and that no other unit purports to have as its primary aim doing what it claims to do.

Further, since men and women must move in a great variety of ways in order to survive and to experience a desirable quality of life, it can be argued that it is essential to study this phenomenon in order to help people of all ages. This should be the case whether they are normal, accelerated, or special–population individuals. All should be moving with the greatest possible efficiency and with the maximum amount of pleasure and reward that comes from any movement of which they are capable. Additionally, it can now be argued successfully that lifetime involvement in developmental physical activity will actually help people live longer!

Steps to Take

Problem situations such as those described above remind us that, first, if it is decided to change the name of a department (at whatever level of education), the basic terms offered for use should be fully understandable to people. (For example, there is the tale of a physics professor's reply to a plan to change a departmental name to "human kinetics." He stated, "Well, I suppose I shouldn't object too much if you want to call yourself by a term that is a subdivision of my field.") Interestingly, however, the word "kinesiology" has been in the dictionary for many years--but it never seemed to be used very much. However, the word "kinesiology" relates to *all* human movement, and there are many applied kinesiologists today in alternative medicine. As a result, the term requires delimitation for the purpose of physical education and educational sport.

Second, the disciplinary unit in college and university circles is certainly best advised to strive for independent status (i.e., not under a school of education, perhaps under an arts and science division, but most desirably as a completely separate, multi-purpose division or unit within higher education. This is definitely better than following the "splintering pattern" that seems to be occurring so frequently. In such cases "small splinters are easier to excise," whereas units with basic physical education instructional programs, professional education, and disciplinary-based programs, intramurals and recreational sports programs, intercollegiate programs, and programs in allied fields (e.g., health education) are harder to get at typically. There are so many *functional* cross-appointments.

Third, the field is unwise to fight the idea that it has a hybrid status within higher education. By that is meant that it is not only a professional unit such as law is. The argument can be made that it is a basic general education unit for all on campus (such as the subject-matter English). Further, it is a department or division that can be regarded as a discipline because faculty members are seeking to add to the body of knowledge about human motor performance in developmental physical activity in exercise, sport, and related expressive activities. Because of this last very important point, the field must continue to insist that all teachers/coaches in higher education be *scholarly* people. A university professor should generate and disseminate knowledge uncovered in *either* so-called scholarly and/or professional journals (or clinics, textbooks, and monographs).

Fourth, this brings up another important point touched on briefly above: professors of physical education and--say--kinesiology in universities would be well advised to *use their own terms* to describe what it is they are offering in our courses for students. If they persist in using course names like sociology of sport and exercise physiology, they are simply asking for future problems. Additionally, they have on their rosters typically a substantive block of professors who do not possess advanced degrees in these other disciplines, but who persist in identifying themselves as psychologists, physiologists, sociologists, historians, etc. If they *must* use the names of other disciplines, why not put words like "sport" or "exercise" first. Better yet, use phrases like "functional effects of physical exercise" or "socio-cultural aspects of sport and exercise."

(See Table 1 on the nest page for a description of recommended terms for what we argue should be called the discipline of developmental physical activity. With each sub disciplinary subject matter, both the sub disciplinary and the sub professional aspects that relate to it are included.)

Table 1

DEVELOPMENTAL PHYSICAL ACTIVITY IN SPORT, EXERCISE, AND RELATED EXPRESSIVE MOVEMENT

Areas of Scholarly Study & Research	Subdisciplinary Aspects	Subprofessional Aspects
I. BACKGROUND, MEANING, & SIGNFICANCE	-History -Philosophy -International & Comparative Study	-International Relations -Professional Ethics
II. FUNCTIONAL EFFECTS OF PHYSICAL ACTIVITY	-Exercise Physiology -Anthropometry & Body Composition	-Fitness & Health Appraisal -Exercise Therapy
III. SOCIO-CULTURAL & BEHAVIORAL ASPECTS	-Sociology -Economics -Psychology (individ. & social) -Anthropology -Political Science -Geography	-Application of Theory to Practice
IV. MOTOR LEARNING & CONTROL	-Psycho-motor Learning -Physical Growth & Development	-Application of Theory to Practice
V. MECHANICAL & MUSCULAR ANALYSIS OF MOTOR SKILLS	-Biomechanics -Neuro-skeletal Musculature	-Application of Theory to Practice
VI. MANAGEMENT THEORY & PRACTICE	-Management Science -Business Administration	-Application of Theory to Practice
VII. PROGRAM DEVELOPMENT	-Curriculum Studies	-Application of Theory to Practice

(General education; professional preparation; intramural sports and physical recreation; intercollegiate athletics; programs for special populations--e.g., handicapped--including both curriculum and instructional methodology)

VIII. EVALUATION & MEASUREMENT	-Measurement Theory	-Application of Theory to Practice

Five, the field should stress and publicize its willingness to serve the total community, including citizens of all ages within the political constituency that it has a responsibility for jurisdictionally. (In this connection, reflect on the incident of a track and field coach who was denied tenure by his dean because his numerous "professional" publications were not refereed. However, the outcry from the community and surrounding counties can still be heard. He received his tenure from a "higher level"!)

Finally, on this important point of status, as true professionals in a field that has the potential to become an important profession (or series of allied professions), the field of physical activity education and educational sport has a duty and responsibility to press for statewide or province-wide rationalization of its various program offerings. This is needed so that equal opportunity will prevail for qualified citizens of all ages, abilities, colors, and creeds (Zeigler, 1990, pp. 9-10). To accomplish this, the field will have to join with colleagues and like-minded people wherever they may be to implement lobbying techniques with legislators and other groups at all levels of society.

References

Aburdene, P. & Naisbitt, J. (1992). *Megatrends for women*. NY: Villard Books.

Andrews, J.C. (1995). Physical education and sports of children and youth: F.I.E.P. policy and action. *IJPE*, 32, 4:26-30.

Asimov, I. (1970). The fourth revolution. *Saturday Review*, Pct. 24, pp. 17-20.

Brubacher, J.S. (1961). Higher education and the pursuit of excellence. *Marshall University Bulletin*, 3:3.

Cheffers, J. (1996). Sport versus education: The jury is still out. *IJPE*, 33, 3: 106-109.

Glasser, W. (1972). *The identity society*. NY: Harper & Row.

Hardman, K. (1995). Present trends in the state and status of physical education. *IJPE*, 32, 4:17-25.

Hess, F.A. (1959). American objectives of physical education from 1900 to 1957 assessed in light of certain historical events. Ph.D. dissertation, New York University.

Huntington, S.P. (1993). *New York Times, The*, June 6, p. E19.

Kaplan, A. (1961). The new world of philosophy. Boston: Houghton Mifflin.

Krawczyk, Z. (1996). Image of sport in Eastern Europe. *JCPES*, 18, 1:2-11.

March, J.G. & H.A. Simon. (1958). *Organizations*. New York: Wiley.

Northrop, F. S. C. (1946). *The meeting of east and west*. NY: Macmillan.

Naisbitt, J. (1982). *Megatrends.* NY: Warner

New York Times, The. (1970). Report by the Commission on Tests of the College Entrance Examination Board, Nov. 2.

Penney, D. & Kirk, D. (1996). National curriculum developments in physical education in Australia and Britain: A comparative analysis. JCPES, 18, 2:30-38.

Rand, A. (1960). The romantic manifesto. New York: World Publishing.

Roberts, G. (1996). Youth cultures and sport: The success of school and community sport provisions in Britain. *EPER*, 2, 2:105-115.

Saffici, C.L. (1996). Aussie Sport: A physical education initiative. *JICHPERSD*, 32, 4:50-53.

Shea, E. J. (1978). *Ethical decisions in physical education and sport.* Springfield, IL: C. C. Thomas.

Skinner, B. F. (1971. *Beyond freedom and dignity*. NY: Alfred A. Knopf.

Sparks, W. (1992). Physical education for the 21st Century: Integration, not specialization. *NAPEHE: The Chronicle of Physical Education in Higher Education*, 4, 1:1, 10-11.

Stein, J.U. (1996). Third Paralympic Congress and the Atlanta Declaration of People with Disabilities. *JICHPERSD*, 33, 1:41-44.

Steinhaus, A.H. (1952). Principal principles of physical education. In *Proceedings of the College Physical Education Association*. Washington, DC: AAHPER, pp. 5-11.

Ten events that shook the world between 1984 and 1994. (Special Report). *Utne Reader*, 62 (March/April 1994):58-74.

Zeigler, E.F. (1977). Philosophical perspective on the future of physical education and sport. In R. Welsh (Ed.). *Physical education: A view toward the future* (pp. 36-61). St. Louis: C.V. Mosby.

Zeigler, E.F. (1989) *Sport and physical education philosophy*. Carmel, IN: Benchmark.

Zeigler, E.F. (1990). *Sport and physical education: Past, present, future*. Champaign, IL: Stipes.

Zeigler, E.F. (1994). Physical education's 13 principal principles. *JOPERD*, 65, 7:4-5.

Zeigler, E.F. (Late Winter, 1997). From one image to a sharper one. *The Physical Educator*, 54:1-6.

Part Five
Looking to the Future in Physical Activity Education and Sport

Selection 13
How the Field of Sport and Physical Activity Education
Might Provide Experiences Basic to World Peace

Earle F. Zeigler
Canada

Dedication

To the memory of Laura J. Huelster
University of Illinois, Champaign-Urbana,
friend, colleague, and professional leader,
who fervently believed and worked for
the theme underlying this article.

Introduction

This paper is based on the underlying premise that the world situation has become so threatening on a continuing basis that all professions should now work assiduously to make a contribution toward the goal of world peace.1

Keeping in mind that bona fide professions have historically developed codes of ethics which included an obligation to work for both the public good and that of the profession, this clearly means that the sport and physical education profession has an obligation to foster and maintain societal values. There is an accompanying duty and responsibility on this continent for us to preserve and enhance the role of the sport and physical education profession as represented by the National Association for Sport and Physical Education in the United States, for example, and the Canadian Association for Health, Physical Education and Recreation.

We believe that this profession has been highly traditional and has typically *reacted* to prevailing social conditions and pressures while rarely *anticipating* desired change in the culture. However, the world situation in relation to strategic nuclear power and other means of conducting warfare is such that the public good <u>demands</u> that we as the established sport and physical education profession join the fray in the struggle required to achieve lasting peace and international good will.

The late Laura J. Huelster (1982, p. 1) pointed out that, the survival of our society is threatened unless there is fitness to live the quality of life that deemphasizes war and promotes peaceful solutions to national and international social, economic, and political conflicts. She argued further that general education should include knowledge about the conditions of human societies that are conducive to minimizing wars and maximizing peace. Huelster stressed additionally that a willingness to accept and act upon that knowledge depends not only upon convincing evidence, but also upon having attitudes and ideologies that are compatible with it.

What should be included in general education should undoubtedly be reflected in professional education as well. This is apparent because the highly threatening world situation makes us aware of the urgent need for a practical response so that future generations will possess both the knowledge and the accompanying attitudes to bring about a peaceful, productive state in the world.

How can we as one profession, therefore, a field often known as physical and health education in Canada, and sport and physical education in the United States, proceed to join in with any trend leading to such a future state? This question becomes poignantly vital when we appreciate that we were warned a half century ago about the need for worldwide "social-self-realization" (Brameld, 1956, p. 272), and yet this is fully appreciated by a small minority of the world population. When Naisbitt (1982) in his *Megatrends* explained that he and his colleagues had determined through research that 10 "new directions were transforming the lives" of people in the United States, for example, the urgency of a vigorous quest for peace was seemingly not evident. The research technique employed by Naisbitt was that of monitoring selected publications carefully throughout the world to determine future trends. For example, this research pointed out that the United States was moving rapidly from an industrial society to an information society (pp. 11-38). Interestingly, however, as he postulated future trends for living, *there is no mention made of a trend toward the pursuit of world peace* so that this wonderful dream of an even better future *can* indeed be realized! Even in *Megatrends 2000* (1990), Naisbitt and Aburdene didn't find sufficient evidence of a strong quest for peace on the part of humankind. They do state, however that,

> The 1990's present a new world view. The cold war ended in the last years of the 1980's, and the arms race has been slowed, perhaps even halted. The postwar period of nationalism and ideological cold war is over, and a new era of globalization has begun. . . . (p. 14). These were optimistic sentiments, of course, but keep in mind that this book appeared before the almost unbelievable developments in eastern Europe, not to mention the crisis caused by Iraq's harsh conquest of Kuwait. Therefore, certain "reasonable" assumptions formulated by Huelster and others leading to a tenable theory are postulated for the

profession to consider. These assumptions lead to
a set of tentative principles and recommendations
for use in the implementation of a *social relevance
perspective f*or the profession of sport and physical
education in all phases of its program in sport,
exercise, and related expressive activities.

We must understand, of course, that the sport and physical education profession would assuredly not be alone if it were to move forthrightly in this direction both within the educational system and in the larger society where public and private programs of sport and exercise, and physical recreation are sponsored. For example, there exists already a group called "Concerned Philosophers for Peace" within the American Philosophical Association that in April, 1988 sponsored a joint meeting with another group named International Philosophers for the Prevention of Nuclear Omnicide in Cincinnati, Ohio. In a paper made available earlier (1983), Allen explained the situation as "Either/Or: How Should Philosophers Respond to the Threat of Nuclear War and the Arms Race?" He was quite correct with his question to his colleagues, and we in the sport and physical education profession also face an either/or situation. Either we accept the challenge to respond to this unique, potentially devastating world situation, or we continue as usual with our programs of promoting physical fitness and presumably positive aggression in highly competitive sport (which somehow often emerges as negative aggression).

Interrelated Assumptions Forming the Theory

Based on the assumptions, therefore, (1) that unrestrained aggression in the world and potential nuclear devastation is forcing us to reconstruct our social environment, (2) that rational plans for peaceful resolution of conflicts are available that can move nations from ongoing wars to peaceful resolution of disputes, (3) that societies have before and can presently change their values, institutions and systems, and (4) that a will for peace will depend on the people's desire for it because of the attitudes, ideologies, and behaviors inculcated as they mature, Huelster (1982, p. 2) has provided us with a logical, sequential rationale that, if adopted, could lead or guide the profession toward a considerable re-orientation of its recommended program. By this we mean that the knowledge, competencies, and skills promoted in developmental physical activity in sport, exercise, and related expressive activities could well be re-arranged to offer quite different input, thruput, and output resulting in a markedly different product at the delivery stage.

In regard to Assumption #2 immediately above--that rational plans for peaceful resolution of conflicts are available--one example was recommended in the Special Session on Disarmament held by the United Nations in the late 1970s. Representatives of 149 nations adopted a set of principles for international disarmament strategy. There were recommendations for balanced and gradual reductions of armaments with the recommendation that the money saved be directed to the establishment of an international peace force and for the promotion of the well-being of people everywhere. In retrospect, we ask, "Why did this plan fail?" The answer is that leaders from the USSR and the USA were elsewhere at that very moment agreeing to a three percent increase in armaments! Today we can breathe a slight sigh of relief because these two superpowers are indeed involved in negotiations leading to massive disarmament. Of course, a cynic would argue that the underlying reason for such moves is more economic than ideological.

We appreciate that significant social changes do not come about overnight (Assumption #3 immediately above). For example, for thousands of years, slavery had been an accepted social practice throughout the world. When ancient Athens was in its so-called Golden Age, the population of the city was about 300,000--260,000 slaves and 40,000 freemen. And it was only a little more than 100 years ago that the U.S.A. had its Civil War, and even today racial prejudice still prevails in many quarters. Look further at the improving, but still terrible, situation in South Africa right now. However, overall changes have been made, and we must continue to work for a more wholesome world culture in all regards--although we do understand that progress has never been a straight-line affair.

Assumption #4 above is a truly difficult one to bring about--the assumption that a will for peace will depend on the people's desire for it because of the attitudes, ideologies, and behaviors inculcated as they mature. In his investigations on this subject, Eckhardt (1972) measured personality traits and social attitudes with the finding that dominant factors were compassion (loving, merciful drives) and compulsion (cruel, merciless drives). Love appears to be the fundamental ingredient of compassion, whereas hate is the feeling basic to compulsion. Building on Eckhardt's research, Alcock (1976) discovered that most of his subjects highly desired happiness and a world at peace, and further that honesty and courage would be needed to attain these goals. Huelster (1982, p. 10) summarized what this all adds up to as follows:

Those among us who want to promote peace apparently need to confront and correct imbalances and inconsistencies in our compassionate attitudes and behaviors. We would need to promote conditions to minimize war by the nonviolent means of knowing the conditions for peace, and taking stands on them through petitions, demonstrations, and supporting legislation on disarmament and economic and political justice. We would also need to commit ourselves to the related problems of reducing populations, improving the welfare of the poor and the oppressed, and improving our ecology. Increased people-power is needed to pressure political leaders to take national and foreign actions in support of enduring peace.

This is obviously going to be extremely difficult to bring to pass in the United States and Canada at this time, not to mention in other sections of the planet. Further, we in the profession of sport and physical education-- especially the men--are going to "swallow mighty hard" before we put ourselves on the line for a futuristic, non-combative orientation such as this statement implies is necessary. Yet, does this fact mean that we shouldn't try to bring about change?

General Education for Peace

One would think that a *fifth assumption* (#5), the idea of 'general education for peace,' would be relatively simple to introduce into the educational system. However, such will probably not be the case. There has been a tradition of keeping organized religion out of public institutions, and this separation of church and state is undoubtedly a good thing. However, the end result has been unfortunate from one standpoint: we have resultantly and concurrently kept discussions of ethics and moral values out of the schools and universities as well. We worship the god of value-free science that provides knowledge in the form of scientific facts that presumably adds up to improved living and a higher level of technology. But, we might ask, what good is all of this value-free knowledge going to do us if we end up with a desolate planet characterized overwhelmingly by radiation and nuclear fall-out? Thus, it would appear that we need both, what we call *value-free knowledge* and also what might be called *value-prone knowledge*. The former will give us the knowledge upon which we can call prior to the making of value-oriented decisions--decisions that some day may provide a high quality of life for all people everywhere!

What this adds up to is that a steady, strong theme will have to be injected into our entire general education program right up through the second year of university at least. This will be difficult to bring about right now when the hue and cry is for higher test scores, ratings that designate achievement levels in language, reasoning, conceptual, and mathematical skills. Also, there is no doubt but that the concept of 'general education' is in the doldrums because of the overriding demand for professional knowledge, competencies, and skills to be used in a high-paying position. As I see it, advocates of liberal arts and science curricula would be well advised to stress, and then measure the attainment of, the general and specific life competencies that their general education programs produce.

Experiences Basic to Peace
in the Sport and Physical Education Program

The Present Situation. A sixth assumption (#6) should be consideration of our role both (1) within our general education program and (2) within our professional preparation efforts for people who will subsequently "profess"

306

developmental physical activity in sport, exercise, and related expressive activities for all people of all ages and conditions both within schools and universities and in the society at large. Providing experiences basic to peace in the sport and physical activity program--here is really where the "going will really get rough." (Once again, we believe that this will be more difficult with the men than with the women in our field.) How indeed are we going to promote personal and social traits leading more in the direction of compassion and considerably less in the direction of compulsion as explained by Eckhardt and Alcock above? This will be especially difficult in highly competitive sport for men, and now will also be quite difficult for women too. It may be a bit easier in Canada than in the United States--with the exception of Canada's national sport, ice hockey. In that instance the name of the game has been INTIMIDATION and VIOLENCE (with all letters capitalized)! To make matters worse, it is so obvious that even a recent beer advertisement (Karlsberg) jokes about the fact that we have exported this violent North American style of play to the rest of the world!

Our problem appears to be that we have let so much of this get out of hand. Highly competitive sport, as now practiced at all levels in North America, amateur, semiprofessional, and professional, has increasingly become our momentary substitute activity as we seemingly move ahead to eventual warfare on a grand scale. We are presently functioning in competitive sport with an operational philosophy that daily promotes and rewards the following type of statements, questions, and actions: "get him before he gets you"; "the watchword is *intimidation;* "call on the good foul when you need it to win"; "isn't it thrilling to watch the 'black gladiators' in the basketball arena and on the gridiron?"; "the hell with the spirit of the rules"; "drugs and doping are necessary to achieve superior performance and *win*; "it is okay to cheat so long as you are not caught"; "winning may not be the only thing, but it beats the hell out of whatever comes next"; and so on *ad infinitum.*

As a former athlete and a coach of three sports, the author wants to win just as much as the next fellow, and perhaps a bit more. He doesn't like "good losers" in sport or in the rest of life--that is, people who give every evidence of not much caring about the struggle of the quest for 'the good life', one way or the other. However, even this professional person is finding himself increasingly turned off by what occurs so often in competitive sport. Yet one can become extremely happy, almost ecstatic, because there is a Wayne Gretzky in professional hockey and an Isiah Thomas in professional basketball, for example. As Metheny (1965, pp. 41-42) sought to explain, what we should be promoting above all is the concept of 'the good strife' rather than the 'bad strife' examples we see around us every day.

Paradoxically, the word "competition" literally means to strive <u>with</u> rather than <u>against</u> according to the established letter and spirit of the rules. Even the word "contest" has a similar implication. It means to <u>testify with</u>

another rather than against him or her. We need to arrange our competitions so that both the winners and the losers in a "good strife" gain from the experience. They have tested "themselves within the rules by doing their best against opponents who also did their best" (Huelster, 1982, p. 17). Competition characterized by 'good strife' remains the ideal for which we should be striving.

And so we can still argue idealistically that highly competitive intercollegiate and interscholastic athletics can be justified inside the realm of sport and physical education if--and this is a very big IF!--positive educational goals characterize the good strife. The late Laura Huelster reluctantly disagreed with this position (1982, p. 17). She agreed that it might still be possible in Canadian inter-university sport, but that it is much less so in the United States--and particularly so in the top 100-150 universities who rely so heavily on gate receipts to maintain their enterprises. As she stated:

Pressures from alumni and university communities to have winning teams is at the point at which success in recruitment of super-athletes determines the amount of financial support in grants-in-aid funds, and there is little freedom for recruited athletes to make curricular choices. It is increasingly being realized by universities that their athletic systems have little to do with their educational systems.

She even recalled an earlier statement (p. 17) where Zeigler had argued that, "in the classification of athletics in the continuum of *players*, from amateurs to semiprofessionals to professional athletic *workers*, it is undoubtedly true that intercollegiate athletes in football and basketball [in the U.S.] can be classified as semiprofessionals" (1979, p. 204). Thus, we are forced to ask rhetorically, "What *should* we do?" What <u>must</u> we do in light of the world situation?" "What *can* we do in the final analysis?"

The Possible Future Situation. What <u>can</u> we do "in the final analysis." Some are moving in Dr. Huelster's direction on this point, but are not yet ready to concur with her that, "except for the basic sport skills in SPE programs, highly competitive athletics should be outside the realm of SPE . . ." (p. 17). Perhaps it is inevitable that it will end up that way in our educational system, but there are many who still feel that <u>we should and must work for</u> 'the good strife' in competitive sport at all levels from children's competitions to the Olympic Games and even professional sport (is there a still difference here between the last two named?). However, time is running out on the United States, and Canada seems to be "inclining" similarly because the trend toward <u>compulsive</u> attitudes and behaviors is outstripping any efforts in the direction of promoting what Eckhardt and Alcock called <u>compassionate</u> attitudes and behaviors in the world social structure--and this appears to be especially true in highly competitive sport.

As members of the established profession (NASPE) in the United States, we should not continue to "run away" from highly competitive sport. When the issue was raised at an international meeting recently, the writer was told, "We don't have any problem with intercollegiate sport on our campus; they're over there!" The immediate reaction was to ask, "What are *we* doing over there? Isn't sport is an integral part of the "life blood" of our field?." However, this splintering is what has happened on what may be called the "worst" campuses. The sport and physical education unit, now employing a variety of presumably academically sounding titles (e.g., kinesiology, human kinetics, sport and exercise science), has completely disassociated itself from competitive sport--and that's the way they both like it but for different reasons.

One approach that an honorable, courageous profession could employ to reverse the prevailing situation, including the trend toward separate educational units and facilities, is to meet the matter directly by "declaring itself in" on the struggle to improve the quality of experience that is taking place in all parts of the program that we are offering in developmental physical activity. We should state boldly--when and where such a condition exists--that highly competitive sport has become so excessive and corrupt that it is actually perverting society. We should be joining forces with others on campus and in the community who want competitive sport to help us achieve true educational goals--not pervert them and society in the bargain. When the time has arrived that intercollegiate sport can topple university presidents and governors--<u>and it has!</u>--we know that the time has come for the people to speak--if it isn't already too late.

And now, to move this argument up a notch to the level of Olympic sport, the appointment by Olympic officials of George Steinbrenner of the New York Yankees to straighten out some of their troublesome problems relative to drug issues and human relations is evidence of the lack of solid, constructive leadership at the upper levels of this phase of competitive sport in the United States. Steinbrenner unfortunately has set a continuing example of how not to administer sport and how not to deal with athletes and coaches at any level! (See "Playboy Interview: George Steinbrenner," *Playboy,* 38. 5 (May 1991), 63-80, 171 for an enlightening discussion of Mr. Steinbrenner's philosophy of life and sport.)

We all understand that the compulsive-competitive elements in sport and physical education have steadily assumed a more primary role in the program, whereas it is the compassionate-cooperative qualities that need development if we hope to have an influence and perhaps bring about a change in people's attitudes and behavior leading to less social strife at home and enduring peace on an international level. Unfortunately, however, this would typically be *a new social approach* for our profession. There has been an effort by some to adapt older games so that they become newer, more cooperative contests with no losers and games where collective scores are kept (Orlick, 1978, pp. 159-175). However, we can readily understand that making activities such as this popular will be an uphill struggle with both members of the profession and most of our students or clients.

There seems to be no other way to get at this problem, however, other than by (1) selecting a wider body of activities of an individual and dual nature where *cooperative effort* is stressed more than *competition*, and (2) doing everything in our power to lessen the *aggressive behaviors* so evident in many of our team sports, while at the same time rewarding behavior that evidences fair play, sportsmanship, and living up to the spirit (as well as the letter) of the rules. In other words, we need lesson and coaching plans and teaching strategies that will emphasize and possibly heighten the compassionate attitudes and behaviors toward oneself and the people with whom one is playing. For example, even in Canadian hockey the teams line up after a game and shake hands and exchange a few words with members of the other team. Why couldn't that become a common practice in all competitive sport starting with the "collision" sports such as football, wrestling, and (now even) basketball?

Our North American (primarily U.S.A.) "mentality" and attitudes in competitive sport could well be compared with some of the non-aggressive attitudes and behaviors displayed in selected other countries from an international standpoint (e.g., the "friendship approach" evident in China). On the other hand, not so very long ago the ex-British Prime Minister Margaret Thatcher felt constrained to call for an urgent report on ongoing weekend violence by British soccer fans in Stuttgart, Federal Republic of Germany, amid a new wave of anger and shame at the notorious behavior of the country's soccer fans abroad" (*The London [Ontario] Free Press*, June 14, 1988, p. C2). The important idea to keep in mind, of course, is that we *don't continue to export our aggressiveness* as happened, for example, with our forcing European countries and the USSR to employ violenece and intimidation when they played hockey against us. There are some hopeful signs even here, however, as evidenced by the 1988 action taken by the Ontario Minor Hockey Association toward eliminating violent checking into the boards in hockey, a practice that has too often resulted in very serious neck and spinal injuries to young players (*The London [Ontario] Free Press*, June 14, 1988, p. A1).

**Specific Program Recommendations
for Physical Education and Sport.**

Keeping in mind (1) that our program should be directed to developmental physical activity in sport, exercise, and related expressive activities for people of all ages and conditions, and (2) that there is an urgent need to elevate compassionate-cooperative behavior to a level never deemed necessary before while discouraging and downplaying excessive violence, intimidation, unsportsmanlike conduct, and ignoring the spirit of the rules, what specific recommendations can be made at this time? Building on and adapting the tentative "principles," recommended by Huelster (1982, p. 19), the following recommendations are offered for serious consideration:

1. We should stress continually the cooperative elements and the need for more cooperative play in competitive games and sports.

2. We should reward through a variety of forms of recognition those who epitomize the qualities of fair play and sportsmanship that we wish to encourage.

3. We should make every effort to cope with overly aggressive competitive behaviors by redirecting them into more responsible cooperative ones. (In this regard, the profession should be exerting direct pressure on rules-making bodies to make sincere efforts to eliminate undue violence and aggression from their sports.)

4. We should insert the concept of 'individual freedom' to a much greater extent in sport and physical education programs by encouraging students to select freely the motor skills and play forms they want to learn. (Understand that this recommendation does not apply to the student who seemingly doesn't want to be involved and possibly thereby improve his/her quality of life by developing such knowledge and competency.)

5. We should broaden program offerings to include more basic and exploratory motor skills such as (a) exercise patterns for physiological and/or psychological benefits, (b) body mechanics and relaxation techniques, (c) swimming and water safety knowledge and techniques, (d) lifetime individual and dual sports, (e) risk sports, and (f) expressive movement activities including folk, social, and modern dance.

6. We should, while developing such program offerings as in #5 above, use teaching and coaching strategies involving task-setting and problem-solving whenever appropriate. In the process, we should help students and clients to set performance-attainment goals beyond their expectations so as to promote the development of self-confidence.

Concluding Statement

There are many social forces or influences which have become persistent historical problems that impact upon society and education directly (Zeigler, 1988, pp. 255-292). These problems are identified as (1) the influence of values and norms, (2) the type of political state, (3) the influence of nationalism, (4) the influence of economics, (5) the impact of organized religion, and (6) the need for ecological awareness. Two additional social forces have now been added to the growing list of persistent problems: (7) the impact of science and technology, and (8) the need for a search for world peace (Zeigler, 2002, p. 52).

It will be inordinately difficult to convince the sport and physical education profession to follow enthusiastically the recommendations that have been made here. It will be especially difficult to persuade the many sport coaches who do not identify primarily with the organized sport and physical education profession. Nevertheless, the goal of improved international understanding and eventual world peace is so vital, so all-compassing as we think of present trends and what may happen in the twenty-first century, that we should all think this subject through for ourselves with great care. As so often seems to be the case, we cannot simply leave it to the other fellow to do this for us. We must work and strive freely, consciously, and openly as true professionals to employ sport and related physical activity serve humankind. Any other choice is unthinkable.

Note

1. This is a condensed summary of a paper presented at the Peace and Understanding Through Sport Seminar, Institute for International Sport, The University of Rhode Island, Kingston, R.I., June 18, 1988.

References

Alcock, N.Z. (1976). The logic of love. Oakville, ON: Canadian Peace Research Institute Press.

Allen, Paul III. (1983). Either/or: How should philosophers respond to the threat of nuclear war and the arms race? Unpublished paper made available at the annual meeting of the American Philosophical Association, Boston, MA, Dec. 28-29.

American Philosophical Association. (1988). Proceedings and addresses of The American Philosophical Association, D.A. Hoekema, (Ed.). Newark, DE: Univ. of Delaware for the APA.

Brameld, T. (1956). Toward a reconstructed philosophy of education. NY: Dryden Press.

Cressman, J. (1988, June 14). Minor hockey gets tough on boarding. The London Free Press, p. 1.

Violence alarms Thatcher. (1988, June 14). The London Free Press, p. C2.

Eckhardt, W. (1972). Compassion: Toward a science of value. Oakville, ON: Canadian Peace Research Institute Press.

Huelster, L.J. (1982). Social relevance perspective for sport and physical education. In E.F. Zeigler (Ed. & Au.), *Physical education and sport: An introduction.*(pp. 1-22). Philadelphia, PA: Lea & Febiger.

Huelster, L.J. (1982). Social relevance perspective for sport and physical education. In <u>Physical education and sport: An introduction</u> **(Ed. & Au.). (pp. 1-22). Philadelphia, PA: Lea & Febiger.**

Metheny, E. (1965). <u>Connotations of movement in sport and dance</u>. Dubuque, IA: W. C. Brown.

Naisbitt, J. (1982). <u>Megatrends: Ten new directions transforming our lives</u>. NY: Warner Books.

Naisbitt, J. & Aburdene, P. (1990) <u>Megatrends 2000: Ten new directions for the 1990's</u>. NY: Wm. Morrow.

Orlick, T. (1978). <u>Winning through cooperation: Competitive insanity-- cooperative alternative</u>. Washington, DC: Acropolis Books.

Playboy interview: George Steinbrenner, <u>Playboy</u>, 38, 5 (May 1991), 63-80, 171.

Zeigler, E.F. (1979). <u>Issues in North American sport and physical education</u>. Washington, DC: American Alliance for Health, Physical Education, Recreation, and Dance.

Zeigler, E.F. (1988). <u>History of physical education and sport</u> (Rev. ed.). Champaign, IL: Stipes Publishing Co.

Zeigler, E. F. (2002). *Socio-cultural foundations of physical education and educational sport.* Aachen, Germany: Meyer & Meyer Sport.

Selection #14

A Proposed Creed and Code of Ethics
for an International Sport Coaching Society

Earle F. Zeigler & Darwin Semotiuk

Brief Historical Resume

As an aftermath of the Ethics and Sportsmanship Seminar held by the University of Rhode Island Institute for International Sport on June 21-24, 1989, a Sport Ethics Committee was established with the approval of Daniel E. Doyle, Jr., Executive Director of the Institute. Prof. Earle F. Zeigler, The University of Western Ontario, agreed to assume the post of committee chairperson. Collaborating with his colleague at the University of Western Ontario, Prof. Darwin Semotiuk, a proposed creed and code of ethics was developed.

> Note: This creed and code was originally developed for a national sport coaching society. For the purposes of this volume, it was adapted to that of an international sport coaching society.

The following is a listing of the Committee's membership who were individually consulted in the process:

1. Dr. Joy DeSensi, Dept. of Human Performance and Sport Studies, The University of Tennessee, 1914 Andy Holt Avenue, Knoxville, TN 37996-2700
2. Dr. Richard Fox, Dept. of Philosophy, Cleveland State University, 1983 East 24th (Euclid), Cleveland, OH 44115
3. Dr. Darwin Semotiuk, Chairman, Intercollegiate Athletics, Thames Hall, The University of Western Ontario, London, Ont., Canada N6A 3K7
4. Dr. Kenneth Ravizza, Dept. of Health, Physical Education, and Recreation, California State University, Fullerton, Fullerton, CA 92634-4080
5. Dr. Earle F. Zeigler, Faculty of Kinesiology, The University of Western Ontario, London, Ont., Canada N6A 3K7, <u>Committee Chairperson</u>
6. Mr. Dan Doyle, Jr., Director, Institute for International Sport, The Univ. of Rhode Island, 306 Adams Hall, Kingston, RI 02881, <u>ex officio</u>
7. Dr. Richard Polidoro, Department of Health, Physical Education, Recreation, and Dance, The Univ. of Rhode Island, Kingston, RI 02881 <u>ex officio</u>

The committee chairperson initially developed a proposed creed for sport coaches. These brief statements were forwarded to members of the committee for reaction. Simultaneously, the chairperson and Dr. Semotiuk, started work on the development of a draft code of ethics to be recommended for employment *both nationally and internationally*.

Next, based on a paper presented by Prof. Zeigler at the Commonwealth Conference in Scotland in 1986, a recommended, tentative framework for use with a code for sport coaches was prepared for distribution to committee members. Additionally, a meeting was held at the Institute for International Sport, Kingston, Rhode Island in November of 1989 to keep officials there apprised of progress being made.

In December, 1989, Zeigler, as chairperson, informed committee members about reactions received concerning the draft creed statement for coaches that he had prepared. Additionally, he offered some examples of values basic to the subject matter of ethics, as well as some examples of categories that could be used in developing a code of ethics for any profession. Examples of standards, principles, and rules were offered under each category, along with an example amplifying the application of each proposed category. In February, 1990, the chairperson forwarded another memorandum to committee members that built on the previously sent material (December 1989). Subsequently, with advice from Dr. Semotiuk, along with reactions from the other members of the IIS Sport Ethics Committee, a more complete proposal was developed.

Introductory Statement

Initially, it should be understood that there are values and norms that are basic to life in democratic societies that, accordingly, also relate to the subject matter of ethics. (The term norm here refers to one of a series of standards of virtue that are expected to prevail in this type of society or culture as explained below.) Persons in a responsible world culture can also be expected to be honest, fair, truthful, etc. These are ordinary norms that inevitably have a relationship to professional norms.

Additionally, over time certain rights and privileges have been accorded to citizens in democratically oriented countries. In North America, for example, the following norms relating to rights and privileges currently prevail:

1. Governance by law
2. Individual freedom (as much as may be permitted in the social setting)
3. Protection from injury
4. Equality of opportunity
5. Privacy
6. Individual welfare

Second, based on a review of the literature, the following five categories or dimensions are recommended for a code of ethics for coaches:

a. The professional's conduct as a sport coach

(The intent here is that the sport coach should in the performance of his/her duties, (1) hold paramount the safety, health, and welfare of the public, (2) perform services only in his/her areas of competence, (3) issue public statements only in an objective and truthful manner, (4) act in professional matters for each employer or athlete/client as faithful agent or trustee, and (5) avoid improper solicitation of professional employment.)

b. The professional's ethical obligations to athletes/clients

(The intent here is that the professional should be completely trustworthy and that he/she has the following obligations or responsibilities in his/her relationship with athletes/clients: To exhibit <u>candor, competence, diligence, discretion, honesty, and loyalty</u>)

c. The professional's ethical responsibility to employers/employing organizations

(The intent here is that the professional should understand and and respect his/her responsibility to both the athlete/client and third parties (e.g., superior) by exhibiting <u>fairness, truthfulness, and non-maleficience</u>)

d. The professional's ethical responsibility to colleagues/ peers and the profession

(The intent here is that the professional has certain obligations to the profession in regard to doing research; working for reform; providing social leadership; improving professional knowledge and skills; and preserving and enhancing the role of the profession so that society's respect will be maintained.

Under this category, also, the professional should never forget that he/she has an obligation help with the self-regulation of the profession (1) by encouraging desirable young people to enter the profession and (2) by complying with, and seeing to it that others comply as well, with the established responsibilities and obligations of the profession as explained in the profession's code of ethics)

e. The professional's ethical responsibility to society

(The intent here is that the professional has an ethical

responsibility to society and therefore will make his/her full services available to all who need help regardless of age, sex, physical limitation, ethnic origin, religion, or sexual orientation. Additionally, the sport coach will make every effort to see that he/she personally, as well as his/her colleagues, will live up to the canons and principles of the profession'a code of ethics)

Third, proceeding from a fivefold categorization of the basic make-up of the proposed code of ethics, the recommended progression to be followed in the eventual determination of specific rules and regulations moves to a secondary categorization within the heading of professional <u>obligations</u> or <u>responsibilities</u>. Included here are (1) <u>standards</u> (virtues or vices), (2) <u>principles</u> (where some latitude is possible), and (3) <u>rules</u> that must be adhered to strictly (see Table 1, p. 22 below).

<u>Note</u>: It should be understood that there always are choices to be made when an individual acts personally or professionally in situations that are less than clear-cut. Thus, if one category is that of <u>obligations</u> (i.e. you must do so-and-so), a second category of available norms may be designated as <u>permissions</u> (i.e. you have freedom of choice because any action may be debatable). In this latter case, professionals are permitted to do (1) what is not prohibited by law; (2) what is not considered unethical in the society, generally speaking; and (3) what is not considered to be unethical by the professional society to which one belongs.

Fourth, and finally then, the listing of eight standards (virtues) has been explained above in Categories Two and Three (i.e., candor, competence diligence, discretion, honesty, and loyalty under Category Two; and fairness, non-maleficence, and truthfulness under Category Three). The brief, hortatory, approved Ethical Creed has been placed after the Preamble below. It remains for the somewhat more detailed Code of Ethics itself to include (1) a listing of the major principles or canons under which the professional sport coach <u>should</u> act, and (2) to show how coaches' associations may begin the process of developing a listing of the specific rules of practice that must be adhered to in daily professional life. (See Table 1 for examples that explain diagrammatically how rules of practice can be derived in the immediate future.)

Preamble to the Creed and Code of Ethics

<u>Statement of Purpose for a National Sport Coaching Society</u>

The purpose of a NATIONAL SPORT COACHING SOCIETY shall be to promote, stimulate, and encourage professional development, along with study, research, scholarly writing in the area of sport coaching (<u>broadly interpreted</u>). This statement of purpose means that the members of this society are concerned about the <u>theoretical</u> and <u>applied</u> aspects of sport coaching theory and practice specifically related to sport at the amateur, semiprofessional, and professional levels as these enterprises are pursued by the various sectors of the world population.

In the furtherance of these aims and objectives, the NSCS shall endeavor to carry out the following functions: (a) support and cooperate with local regional, national, and international organizations having similar purposes; (b) organize and administer meetings to promote the purpose stated above; and (c) issue appropriate proceedings and journals as this becomes possible.

The society shall conduct its activities solely to promote the above-stated purpose, but this shall in no way be construed as an effort to bring about pecuniary profit for the society itself. The fundamental aim is to assist in all ways possible with the professionalization of the field of sport coaching.

What Is a Profession Today? The NSCS includes typically those people who are functioning in a professional and/or disciplinary way within the broad field known generally as competitive sport. Merely stating that a group of people working within a field of endeavor at the public, semi-public or private levels represents a profession is a beginning, of course, but there is obviously much more to be accomplished than that. It can be argued, however, that there is no generally acceptable definition for a profession today--i.e., it is impossible to characterize professions by a set of necessary and sufficient features possessed by all professions--and <u>only</u> by professions (Bayles, 1981, p. 7). Nevertheless, the following is a brief attempt to define what constitutes a profession in the last quarter of the 20th century:

> (a) A profession can be defined as an occupation which requires specific knowledge of some aspect of learning before a person is accepted as a <u>professional</u> person.

> (b) There are <u>subcategories</u> of professions as follows: administering, teaching, supervising, consulting, research, etc. Sport coaching would presumably represent some combination of teaching, administering, supervising, and consulting duties and responsibilities. However, some within the profession or closely related fields should undoubtedly have a responsibility for scholarly and research endeavor.

> (c) The following may be considered as three <u>necessary</u> features of an occupation that can also be designated as a profession: (i) a need for extensive training; (ii) a significant intellectual component that must be mastered; and (iii) a

recognition by society that the trained person can provide an important basic service.

(d) Additionally, there are some other features that are common to most professions as follows: (i) licensing by state/province or professional body, (ii) establishment of professional societies, (iii) considerable autonomy in work performance, and (iv) establishment of a creed or code of ethics. Note: One aspect of a comprehensive code of ethics is that the controlling body should establish an code of ethics discipline committee to which infractions of the ethical code may be reported for deliberation and possible disciplinary action.

What Is the Professional Status of Coaching? Keeping the above seven necessary and common features of most professions in mind, the following may be said about the professional status of members of the embryonic coaching profession:

a. That there is some recognition by society that a qualified professional in sport coaching (broadly interpreted) can provide a basic, important service.

b. That there is a developing intellectual component to be mastered, and therefore an extensive training is required before and after a person becomes qualified as a professional in this aspect of the field. (Keeping this feature in mind, some provision should be made for the recognition of those men and women who coach on a volunteer or part-time basis.)

c. That sport coaching at the public, semi-public, and private agency levels is moving very slowly toward professional status based on the following accomplishments:

    i. Establishment of professional society
    ii. Conferences and symposia held to improve the knowledge and competency of professionals
    iii. Publication of one or more scholarly journals
    iv. Considerable autonomy in work performance

d. That, to promote sound, long range development, a specific creed for the society and the profession should be developed, and that this should be followed by a subsequent expansion to a detailed ethical code as soon as possible.

e. That professional certification procedures at the state or provincial level and voluntary registration at the national and international levels be promoted by the professional society as soon as possible. Also, voluntary accreditation procedures for professional training programs would be an excellent accompanying development. Further, in the relatively near future, required licensing for all practitioners (both in states/provinces and within the education system in respective countries) would necessarily have to take place on a political-unit basis.

f. That, in the development of such registration/licensing procedures, every effort should be made to avoid narrow discrimination on the basis of "professional/disciplinary labels" and training (i.e., unwillingness to accept obviously comparable course experiences from another profession/discipline as part of certification requirements). What must be guaranteed, of course, is that an acceptable level of knowledge, competency, and skill be determined, and that all who practice professionally possess such ability on a continuing basis.

An Ethical Creed for a International Sport Coaching Society

Members of the International Sport Coaching Society live in societies with democratic forms of government. As practitioners and scholars within a broad profession, we honor the preservation and protection of fundamental human rights. We are committed to a high level of professional practice and service. Our professional conduct shall be based on the application of sound coaching theory developed through a broadly based humanities, social science, and natural science body of knowledge about the role of competitive sport and related physical activity in the lives of all people. Such professional knowledge and service shall be made available to athletes/clients of all ages and conditions, whether such people are classified as accelerated, normal, or special insofar as their status or condition is concerned.

As International Sport Coaching Society members pursuing our professional service and related disciplinary endeavor, we will make every effort to protect the welfare of those who seek our assistance. We will use our professional skills only for purposes which are consistent with the values, norms, and laws of our country. Although we, as professional practitioners, demand for ourselves maximum freedom of inquiry and communication consistent with societal values, we fully understand that such freedom requires us to be responsible, competent, and objective in the application of our skills. We should always show concern for the best interests of our athletes/clients, our colleagues, and the public at large.

A Proposed Code of Ethics for an International Sport Coaching Society

Canons or Principles

The following canons or principles, arranged according to category or dimension, shall be considered by the sport coach in the performance of professional duties:

Category I. The professional's conduct as a sport coach

A. **Propriety.** The sport coach should maintain high standards of personal conduct in the capacity or identity of the coaching profession. For example, the coach should strive always to be fair.

B. **Service Where Competent.** The sport coach should perform services only in his/her areas of competence.

C. **Public Statements.** The sport coach should issue public statements in an objective and truthful manner, and shall make every effort to explaining where statements are personal opinions.

D. **Solicitation of Employment.** The sport coach should seek employment only where a position is available and an obvious need for service exists.

E. **Individual Welfare.** The sport coach should hold paramount the safety, health, and welfare of the individual in the performance of professional duties.

F. **Competence and Professional Development.** The sport coach should strive to become and remain proficient in professional practice and the performance of professional functions.

G. **Integrity.** The sport coach should act in accordance with the highest standards of professional integrity.

Category II. The professional's ethical obligations to athletes/clients

H. **Primacy of Athletes'/Clients' Interests.** The sport coach's primary responsibility is to athletes/clients.

I. **Service as Agent or Trustee.** The sport coach, when acting in professional matters for employer or athlete/client, should be a faithful agent or trustee.

J. Rights and Prerogatives of Clients. The sport coach should, in considering the nature of the relationship with the student/client, make every effort to foster maximum self-determination on the part of the athletes/clients.

K. Confidentiality and Privacy. The sport coach should respect the privacy of athletes/clients and hold in confidence all information obtained in the course of professional service.

L. Fees. When setting fees for service in private or commercial settings, the sport coach should ensure that they are fair, reasonable, considerate, and commensurate with the service performed and with due respect to the clients' ability to pay.

Category III The professional's ethical responsibility
             to employers/employing organizations

M. Commitments to Employers/Employing Organizations. The sport coach should adhere to any and all commitments made to the employing organization. The relationship should be characterized by fairness, non-maleficience, and truthfulness.

Category IV The professional's ethical responsibility
             to colleagues/peers and to the profession

N. Respect, Fairness, and Courtesy. The sport coach should treat colleagues with respect, courtesy, fairness, and good faith.

O. Dealing with Colleagues' Athletes/Clients. The sport coach has the responsibility to relate to the athletes/clients of colleagues with full professional consideration.

P. Maintaining the Integrity of the Profession. The sport coach should uphold and advance the values and ethical standards, the knowledge, and the mission of the profession.

Q. Community Service. The sport coach should assist the profession in making information and services relating to desirable sport, physical activity, and health practices available to the general public.

R. Development of Knowledge. The sport coach should take responsibility for identifying, developing, and fully utilizing established knowledge for professional practice.

S. Approach to Scholarship and Research. The sport coach engaged in study and/or research should be guided by the accepted convention of scholarly inquiry.

<u>Category V</u> The professional's ethical responsibility to society

T. Promoting the General Welfare. The sport coach should promote the general welfare of society.

U. Service. The sport coach should regard as primary his/her professional service to others.

V. Reporting Code Infractions. The sport coach has an ethical responsibility to society in that minor and major code infractions by colleagues should be reported to the appropriate committee of the professional society.

ISCS's Code of Ethics Discipline System

The ISCS's Creed and Code of Ethics were developed to help its members strive to approximate the highest standards of their profession. A profession become recognized by the quality and quantity of service provided for the citizens of the jurisdiction in which it is established. It is therefore the responsibility of members of the profession to make certain that the ideals or standards expressed in the code of ethics, along with established principles and specific rules, are upheld. Any noted infringements or violations of the Code of Ethics shall be reported to the Society's Ethics Code Discipline Committee and shall be adjudicated by the disciplinary system described below.

1. Jurisdiction.

The Code of Ethics Discipline Committee of the Society shall receive charges, in writing, of alleged violations of the Code of Ethics and shall then make determinations about the validity of the charges. If the charges are found to be true, the Code of Ethics Discipline Committee shall determine the appropriate sanctions and/or discipline to be imposed.

2. Composition and Terms of Office.

Composition. The discipline system of the International Sport Coaching Society shall consist of the Code of Ethics Discipline Committee and the Executive Council of the Society. The Committee shall consist of six (6) members of the Society appointed by the President of the Society. Keeping the importance of geographical representation in mind, three members of the Committee shall be from the United States and three shall be from Canada. These six (6) members will be appointed by the President of the Society in 19-- (?). Each year thereafter, the President of the Society will appoint two (2) members to the committee. The composition of the Executive Council of the society is defined by the existing ISPC By-Laws.

Terms of Office. Each Code of Ethics Discipline Committee member will serve a staggered three-year (3) term so that two new members will be appointed each year. The initial appointments will be made to begin in July 19--as follows:

Two members for a three-year term
Two members for a two-year term
Two members for a one-year term

Vacancies may be filled at any time through appointments made by the NSCS President.

3. Procedure for Reporting Violations.

Alleged violations should be reported in writing, accompanied by a full set of supporting documents or data, to the Code of Ethics Discipline Committee. This may included such items as (1) evidence supporting racial or ethnic bias; (2) supported claims that a sport coach breached confidentiality; (3) proof of the illegal breaking of a contract; (4) evidence that a sport coach is incompetent; (5) proof that a plagiarized manuscript was submitted for publication; (6) evidence that a member accepted a place on a convention program and then gave no sufficient explanation of a failure to appear, etc.

4. Committee Procedures

The Code of Ethics Discipline Committee will attempt initially to understand the violation reported as completely as possible by written communication and (possibly) telephone conversation(s) with the person(s) reporting the violation to the committee. Next the alleged violator will be provided with copies of the documents sent to the committee and asked to respond in writing to the allegations. Typically, especially if the alleged violation is categorized as major, it may be necessary to schedule a private hearing during the next ISCS Conference.

5. Violations.

Two classes of Code of Ethics Violations are established: Minor and Major. Minor violations are those that are not classified as major violations. When it is determined after due process (explained below) that specific rules of practice have been abrogated, the extent of violation of such rules will be determined by the Committee.

6. Sanctions.

Members found guilty of Minor Violations will receive a letter of reprimand with copies sent to the member's superior. Members found guilty of Major Violations, or who are repeat offenders of Minor Violations, will receive the letter of reprimand described above and will be prohibited from participating in NSCS functions for a period of not less than two years or more than five years (depending upon the severity of the violation). Such prohibition will affect NSCS membership, presentations at ISCS conferences and programs, and publications made available by ISCS. In addition, names of those who are guilty of Major Violations or repeat offenses of Minor Violations will be published, along with their official affiliation, in any ISSC newsletter. Repeated Code of Ethics Violations can result in discipline for the member's entire professional life.

7. Appeals.

As indicated above, a member may appeal any discipline by the Code of Ethics Discipline Committee to the Executive Council of the Society. Upon review of the case, the decision of the Executive Committee shall be final.

The Sport Management Profession in the 21st Century

Earle F. Zeigler
Canada

Note: This was a presentation to the 17th Annual
Conference of the North American Society for Sport
Management, Canmore, Alberta, Canada, June 1, 2002.

Our thoughts turn to the "adventure of civilization" as Earth enters
moves into "The 21st Century" (C.E.). However, any such pondering has
certainly been colored by the way things have been going since September 11,
2001. Any reasonably enlightened person would be forced to admit that what
we like to call "developing" civilization is *truly* an adventure into which we
are being drawn inexorably! I base this opinion on the dictionary definition of
the term as either an "exciting experience" or a "bold undertaking" (*Encarta
World English Dictionary*, 1999, p. 23).

The "Adventure" of Civilization

In retrospect, the adventure of civilization began to make some
headway because of now-identifiable forms of early striving which embodied
elements of great creativity (e.g., the invention of the wheel, the harnessing of
fire). The subsequent development in technology, very slowly but steadily,
offered humans some surplus of material goods over and above that needed
for daily living. For example, the early harnessing of nature created the
irrigatio systems of Sumeria and Egypt, and these accomplishments led to
the establishment of the first cities. Here material surpluses were collected,
managed, and sometimes squandered; nevertheless, necessary early
accounting methods were created that were subsequently expanded in a way
that introduced writing to the human scene. As we now know, the
development of this form of communication in time helped humans expand
their self-consciousness and to evolve gradually and steadily in all aspects of
culture. For better or worse, however, the end result of this social and
material progress has created a mixed agenda characterized by good and evil
down to the present. The world's blanketing communications network has
now exceeded humankind's ability to cope with it.

Muller (1952) concluded, "the adventure of civilization is necessarily
inclusive" (p. 53). By that he meant that evil will probably always be with
humankind to some degree, but it is civilization that sets the standards and
accordingly works to eradicate at least the worst forms of such evil. Racial
prejudice, for example, must be overcome. For better or worse, there are now
more than six billion people on earth, and that number appears to be growing
faster than the national debt! These earth creatures are black-, yellow-,
brown-, or white-skinned, but fundamentally we now know from genetic

research that there is an "overwhelming oneness" in all humankind that we dare not forget in our overall planning (Huxley, 1957).

As various world evils are overcome, or at least held in check, scientific and accompanying technological development will be called upon increasingly to meet the demands of the exploding population. Gainful work and a reasonable amount of leisure will be required for further development. Unfortunately, the necessary leisure required for the many aspects of a broad, societal culture to develop fully, as well as for an individual to grow and develop similarly within it, has come slowly. The average person in the world is far from a full realization of such benefits. Why "the good life" for all has been so slow in arriving is not an easy question to answer. Of course, we might argue that times do change slowly, and that the possibility of increased leisure has really come quite rapidly--once humans began to achieve some control of their environment.

Naipaul or Huntington: "Universal Civilization or the Clash of Civilizations?

Naipaul (1990) had theorized that we are developing a "universal civilization" characterized by (1) the sharing of certain basic values, (2) what their societies have in common (e.g., cities and literacy, (3) certain of the attributes of Western civilization (e.g., market economies and political democracy), and (4) consumption patterns (e.g., fads) of Western civilization. Samuel Huntington (1998), the eminent political scientist, doesn't see this happening, however, although he does see some merit in these arguments. He grants that Western civilization is different than any other civilization that has ever existed because of its marked impact on the whole world since 1500. However, he doesn't know whether the West will be able to reverse the signs of decay already present and thus renew itself.

Sadly, there have been innumerable wars throughout history with very little if any let-up down to the present. Nothing is so devastating to a country's economy as war. Now, whether we like it or not, the world is gradually sliding into what Huntington has designated as "the clash of civilizations." Some people have seized upon his analysis as a justification for the United States to move still further in the War on Terrorism by the installation of what has euphemistically been called a "modernized regime" in Iraq. It is argued that this "accomplishment" would help toward the gradual achievement of worldwide democratic values along with global capitalism and so-called free markets.

The Misreading of Huntington's Thought. This misreading of Huntington's thought, however, needs to be corrected. As it stands, he asserts, "Western belief in the universality of Western culture suffers three problems. . . .It is false; it is immoral; and it is dangerous" (p. 310). He believes strongly that these religion-based cultures, such as the Islamic and the Chinese, should be permitted to find their own way in the 21st century. In fact, they will probably do so anyhow, no matter what the West does. Then individually (hopefully not together!), they will probably each become superpowers themselves. The "unknown quality" of their future goals will undoubtedly fuel the desires of those anxious for the United States to maintain overwhelming military superiority along with continually expanding technological capability.

While this is going on, however, the United States needs to be more aware of its own internal difficulties. It has never solved its "inner-city problem," along with increases in antisocial behavior generally (i.e., crime, drugs, and violence). Certainly the decay of the traditional family has long-term implications as well. Huntington refers further to a "general weakening of the work ethic and rise of a cult of personal indulgence (p. 304). Still further, there is a definite decline in learning and intellectual activity as indicated by lower levels of academic achievement creating a need for course grade "aggrandizement" (i.e., the gentleman's "C" is "history"). Finally, there has been a marked lessening of "social capital" (the amount of "volunteering" including personal trust in others to meet individual needs).

Schlesinger's Analysis of America. These conflicting postulations by Huntington and Naipaul are stated here merely to warn that the present "missionary culture" of the United States is, in many ways, not really a true culture anyhow. So states Arthur Schlesinger, Jr. (1998), the distinguished historian. He points out that in recent years the U.S.A. has gradually acquired an ever-increasing multi-ethnicity. In his The disuniting of America, he decries the present schisms occurring in the United States. He is most concerned that the melting pot concept formerly so prominent in the States is becoming a "Tower of Babel" concept--just like Canada!

He understands, however, that "Canadians have never developed a strong sense of what it is to be a Canadian" by virtue of their dual heritage (p. 17). Huntington explains further that an attempt to export democratic and capitalistic values vigorously to the world's other cultures may be exactly the wrong approach. He believes that they may well be looking mainly for stability in their own traditions and identity. (Japan, for example, has shown the world that it's possible to become "rich and modern" without giving up their illiberal "core identity.") Struggle as all cultures do for renewal when internal decay sets in, no civilization has proven that it is invincible indefinitely. This is exactly why Muller characterized history as somehow being imbued with a "tragic sense."

The "Tragic Sense" of Life (Muller)

This "tragic sense' that history has displayed consistently was described by Herbert Muller (1952), in his magnificent treatise titled The uses of the past . Muller disagrees with the philosopher Hobbes (1588-1679), however, who stated in his De homine that very early humans existed in an individual state of nature in which life was anarchic and basically "solitary, poor, nasty, brutish, and short." Muller argued in rebuttal that life "might have been poor and short, but that it was never solitary or simply brutish" (p. 6).

Accordingly, Muller's approach to history was in the spirit of the great tragic poets, a spirit of reverence and/or irony. It is based on the assumption that the tragic sense of life is not only the profoundest, but also the most pertinent for an understanding of both past and present (p. viii).

Muller believed that the drama of human history has been characterized up to now by high tragedy in the Aristotelian sense. As he stated, "all the mighty civilizations have fallen because of tragic flaws; as we are enthralled by any golden age we must always add that it did not last, it did not do" (p. viii). This brings to mind that conceivably the 20th century of the modern era may turn out to have been the "Golden Age" of the United States. As unrealistic as this may sound because I am talking about what today is the most powerful nation in the history of life on Earth, there are also many misgivings developing about the blind optimism concerning history's malleability and compatibility in keeping with American ideals.

"The future as history." More than a generation ago, Heilbroner (1960) arrived at this position similarly. He explained in his "future as history" concept that America's belief in a personal "deity of history" may be shortlived in the 21st century. As he stated this, he emphasized the need to search for a greatly improved "common denominator of values" (p. 170) in the face of technological, political, and economic forces that are "bringing about a closing of our historic future." As the world turns today in 2002, you may laugh at this prediction. Yet, looking at the situation from a starkly different perspective even earlier, Arnold Toynbee (1947) came to a quite similar conclusion in his monumental A study of history from still another standpoint. He theorized that humankind must return to the one true God from whom it has gradually but steadily fallen away. You can challenge him on this opinion, as I (an agnostic) most assuredly do. Yet, no matter--the ways things are going at present--we on the Earth had best try to use our heads as intelligently and wisely as possible. As we get on with striving to make the world as effective, efficient, and humane as possible, we need to make life as replete with Good, as opposed to Evil, as we possibly can. With this plea for an abundance of righteousness, you may no longer be wondering where this analysis is heading. Let us turn now to what I have termed "the plight" of sport management.

The "Plight" of Sport Management

At this point, having placed the "adventure of civilization" in some perspective, I will now shift my focus to sport and related physical activity.

Here is a societal institution that became an ever-more powerful social force in the 20th century. In this study I am attempting to analyze philosophically and sociologically what I have called reluctantly the "plight" of sport management. Basically, I am arguing that society is governed by strong social forces or institutions. Among those social institutions are (1) the values (and accompanying norms devised) , (2) the type of political state in vogue, (3) the prevailing economic system, (4) the religious beliefs or system present, etc. To these longstanding institutions I have added the influence of such other forces as education, science and technological advancement, concern for peace, and now sport itself. (Zeigler, 1989, Part II) Of these, the values, and the accompanying norms that are developed, form the strongest social institution of all.

Crossing the Postmodern Divide. Whether we all recognize it or not, similar to all other professions today, the burgeoning sport management profession is presently striving to cross what has been termed the postmodern divide. An epoch in civilization approaches closure when many of the fundamental convictions of its advocates are challenged by a substantive minority of the populace. It can be argued that indeed the world is moving into a new epoch as the proponents of postmodernism have been affirming over recent decades. Within such a milieu there are strong indications that sport management is going to have great difficulty crossing this chasm, this so-called, postmodern divide.

A diverse group of postmodern scholars argues that many in democracies, undergirded by the various rights being propounded (e.g., individual freedom, privacy), have come to believe that now they too require-- and deserve!--a supportive "liberal consensus" within their respective societies. Conservative, essentialist elements prevail at present and are functioning strongly in many Western political systems. With their more authoritative orientation in mind, conservatives believe that the deeper foundation justifying this claim of a need for a more liberal consensus has never been fully rationalized. However, postmodernists now form a substantive minority that supports a more humanistic, pragmatic, liberal consensus in which highly competitive sport is viewed as an increasingly negative influence on society. If this statement is true--there are strong indications that the present sport management profession--as known today-- will have difficulty crossing this post-modern divide that has been postulated.

Characterizations of Competitive Sport

Having stated that "sport" has become a strong social force or institution, it is true also that there has been some ambiguity about what such a simple word means. In an earlier study I recall uncovering that the word "sport" was used in 13 different ways as a noun. Somehow this number has increased to 14 in the most recent Encarta World English Dictionary

(1999) (p. 1730). In essence, what we are describing here is an athletic activity requiring skill or physical prowess. It is typically of a competitive nature as in racing, wrestling, baseball, tennis, or cricket. For the people involved, sport is often serious, and participants may even advance to a stage where competitive sport becomes a semi-professional or a professional career choice. For a multitude of others, however, sport is seen more as a diversion, as recreational in nature, and as a pleasant pastime.

A Social Institution Without a Theory. Viewed collectively, I am now arguing that at present the "totality" of sport appears to have become a strong social institution--but one that is without a well-defined theory. This fact is being recognized increasingly. Yet, at this point the general public, including most politicians, seems to believe that "the more competitive sport we have, the merrier!" I believe, however, that we in the sport management profession need right now to answer such questions as (1) what purposes competitive sport has served in the past, (2) what functions it is fulfilling now, (3) where it seems to be heading, and (4) how it should be employed to serve all humankind.

How Sport Serves Society . In response to these questions, without very careful delineation at this point, I believe that sport as presently operative can be subsumed in a non-inclusive list as possibly serving in the following ways:

1. As an organized religion (for those with or without another similar competing affiliation)
2. As an exercise medium (often a sporadic one)
3. As a life-enhancer or "arouser" (puts excitement in life)
4. As a trade or profession (depending upon one's approach to it)
5. As an avocation, perhaps as a "leisure-filler" (at either a passive, vicarious, or active level)
6. As a training ground for war (used throughout history for this purpose)
7. As a "socializing activity" (an activity where one can meet and enjoy friends)
8. As an educational means (i.e., the development of positive character traits, however described)

As I review the list developed above, I find it most interesting that I didn't list "sport as a developer of positive character traits" until last! I wonder why. . .
.

My listing could undoubtedly be larger. I could have used such terms as (1) sport "the destroyer," (2) sport "the redeemer," (3) sport "the social institution being tempted by science and technology," (4) sport "the social phenomenon by which heroes and villains are created," or, finally, (5) sport "the social institution that has survived within an era characterized by a vacuum of belief for many." But I must stop. I believe this listing is sufficient to make the necessary point in the present discussion.

I am hoping that you agree that the sport manager truly needs to understand what competitive sport has become in society, as well as why many of its promoters are confronted with a dilemma. I assert this since I believe that sport too--as all other social institutions--is inevitably being confronted by the postmodern divide. In crossing this frontier, many troubling and difficult decisions, often ethical in nature, will have to be made as the professor of sport management seeks to prepare prospective professionals who will guide sport into becoming a responsible social institution. The fundamental question facing the profession is: "What kind of sport do we want to promote to help shape what sort of world in the 21st century?"

Is Sport Fulfilling Its Presumed Educational and Recreational Roles Adequately?

What implications does all of this have for sport as it enters the 21st century? I believe that there are strong indications that sport's presumed educational and recreational roles in the "adventure" of civilization are not being fulfilled adequately. Frankly, the way commercialized, over-emphasized sport has been operated, it can be added to the list of symptoms of American internal decay enumerated above (e.g., drugs, violence, decline of intellectual interest, dishonesty, greed). If true, this inadequacy inevitably throws a burden on sport management as a profession to do something about it. Sport, along with all of humankind, is facing the postmodern divide.

Reviewing this claim in some detail. Depauw (Quest, 1997) argues that society should demonstrate more concern for those who have traditionally been marginalized in society by the sport establishment (i.e., those excluded because of sex or "physicality"). She speaks of "The (In)Visibility of (Dis)Ability" in our culture. Depauw's position is backed substantively by what Blinde and McCallister (1999) call "The Intersection of Gender and Disability Dynamics."

A second point of contention about sport's contribution relates to the actual "sport experience." The way much sport has been conducted, we have every right to ask, "Does sport build character or 'characters'?" Kavussannu & Roberts (*Journal of Sport and Exercise Psychology*, 2001) recently showed that, even though "sport participation is widely regarded as an important opportunity for character development," it is also true that sport "occurs in a context that values ego orientation (e.g. winning IS the most important thing)."

Sport's Contribution Today. What is competitive sport's contribution today? If we were to delve into this matter seriously, we might be surprised--or perhaps not. We may well learn that sport is contributing significantly in the development of what are regarded as the social values--that is, the values of teamwork, loyalty, self-sacrifice, and perseverance consonant with prevailing corporate capitalism in democracy and in other political systems as well. Conversely, however, we will also discover that there is now a great deal of evidence that sport may be developing an ideal that opposes the fundamental moral virtues of honesty, fairness, and responsibility in the innumerable competitive experiences provided (Lumpkin, Stoll, and Beller, 1999).

Significant to this discussion are the results of investigations carried out by Hahm, Stoll, Beller, Rudd, and others in recent years. The Hahm-Beller Choice Inventory (HBVCI) has now been administered to athletes at different levels in a variety of venues. It demonstrates conclusively that athletes will not support what is considered "the moral ideal" in competition. As Stoll and Beller (1998) see it, for example, an athlete with moral character demonstrates the moral character traits of honesty, fair play, respect, and responsibility whether an official is present to enforce the rules or not. This finding was further substantiated by Preist, Krause, and Beach (1999) who reported that their findings in the four-year changes in college athlete's ethical value choices were consistent with other investigations. They showed decreases in "sportsmanship orientation" and an increase in "professional" attitudes associated with sport.

On the other hand, even though dictionaries define social character similarly, sport practitioners, including participants, coaches, parents, and officials, have come to believe that character is defined properly by such values as self-sacrifice, teamwork, loyalty, and perseverance. The common expression in competitive sport is: "He/she showed character"--meaning "He/she 'hung in there' to the bitter end!" [or whatever]. Rudd (1999) confirmed that coaches explained character as "work ethic and commitment." This coincides with what sport sociologists have found. Sage (1998. p. 614) explained that "Mottoes and slogans such as 'sports builds character' must be seen in the light of their ideological issues" In other words, competitive sport is structured by the nature of the society in which it occurs. This would appear to mean that over-commercialization, drug-taking, cheating, bribe-taking by officials, violence, etc. at all levels of sport are simply reflections of the culture in which we live. So much for sport's presumed relationship with moral character development.

At this point, we can't help but recall that the ancient Olympic Games became so excessive with its ills that they were abolished. They were begun again only by the spark provided in the late 19th century byde Coubertin's "noble amateur ideal." The way things are going today, it is not unthinkable that the steadily increasing excesses of the present Olympic Games

Movement could well bring about their demise again. However, they are only symptomatic of a larger problem confronting an American culture. Despite its claims to be "the last best hope on earth," American culture appears to be facing what Berman (2000) calls "spiritual death" (p. 52). He makes this claim because of "its crumbling school systems and widespread functional illiteracy, violent crime and gross economic inequality, and apathy and cynicism."

This discussion about whether's sport's presumed educational and recreational roles have justification in fact could go on indefinitely. So many negative incidents have occurred that one hardly knows where to turn to avoid further negative examples. On the one hand we read the almost unbelievably high standards set in the Code of Conduct developed by the Coaches Council of the National Association for Sport and Physical Education (NASPE) (2001); yet, conversely we learn that today athletes' concern for the presence of moral values in sport declines over the course of a university career (Priest, Krause, and Beach, 1999).

Sedentary Living Has Caught Up With Us. With this as a backdrop, we learn further that Americans, for example, are increasingly facing the cost and consequences of sedentary living (Booth & Chakravarthy, 2002). Additionally, Malina (2001) tells us that there is a need to track people's physical activity across their lifespans. Finally, Corbin and Pangrazi (2001) explain that we haven't yet been able to devise and accept a uniform definition of wellness for all people. The one thought that emerges from these various assessments is as follows: We give every evidence of wanting our "sport spectaculars" for the few much more than we want all people of all ages and all conditions to have meaningful sport and exercise involvements throughout their lives.

Having made this statement, I report further that Tibbetts (2002) in Canada, for example, described a most recent Environics survey that explained that "65% of Canadians would like more government money spent on local arenas, playgrounds, and swimming pools, as well as on sports for women, the poor, the disabled, and aboriginals." At the same time, Dr. Ayotte, director of the only International Olympic Committee-accredited testing laboratory in Canada, explains that young athletes believe you must take drugs to compete successfully. "People have no faith in hard work and food now," she says, to achieve success in sport (Long, 2001).

Official Sport's Response to the Prevailing Situation

And where do we find what we often call "sport officialdom" responding to this situation? Answers to this question are just about everywhere as we think, for example, of the various types of scandals tied to both the summer and winter Olympic Games. For example, the Vancouver Province (2000) reported that the former "drug czar" of the U.S. Olympic

Team, Dr. Wade Exum, has charged that half ot the team used performance-enhancing drugs to prepare for the 1996 Games. After making this statement, the response was rapid: he was forced to resign! He is currently suing the United States Olympic Committee for racial discrimination and harassment.

Viewed in a different perspective, as reported by David Wallis (2002), Dr. Vince Zuaro, a longtime rules interpreter for Olympic wrestling, said recently: "Sports are so political. If you think what happened with Enron is political, [try] Olympic officiating. . . .Every time there's judging involved, there's going to be a payoff." Further, writing about the credibility of the International Olympic Committee, Feschuk (2002) stated in an article titled "Night of the Olympic Dead": "The IOC has for so long been inflicting upon itself such severe ethical trauma that its survival can only be explained by the fact that it has passed over into the undead. Its lifeless members shuffle across the globe in a zombie-like stupor, one hand extended to receive gratuities, the other held up in exaggerated outrage to deny any accusations of corruption."

Dick Pound's Reward for Distinguished Service. Closing out reference to the Olympic Games Movement, recall the case of Dick Pound, the Canadian lawyer from Montreal, who had faithfully and loyally striven most successfully to bolster the Games' finances in recent decades. He had also taken on the assignment of monitoring the situation with drugs and doping, as well as the bribery scandal associated with the Games held in Salt Lake City. In the race to succeed retiring President Samaranch, Pound unbelievably finished in third place immediately behind a man caught in a bribery scandal just a short time earlier. Just punish "the messenger". . . .

Finally, in the realm of international sport, Dr. Hans B. Skaset (2002), a Norwegian professor, is set to make a prediction at a conference on drugs in sport scheduled for November, 2002. He will predict as keynote speaker that "Top international sport will cut itself free from its historical values and norms. After working with a clear moral basis for many years, sport by 2008-2010 will continue to be accepted as a leading genre within popular culture--but not, as it was formerly, a model for health, fairness, and honorable conduct. . . ."

Switching venues, you don't see the hockey promoters doing anything to really curb the neandertal antics of professional hockey players. Or considering professional sport generally, note the view of sport sociologist, Steven Ortiz, who has found in his study that "there clearly seems to be a 'fast-food sex' mentality among professional athletes" (Cryderman, 2001)

In addition, in the realm of higher education, Canadian universities are gradually moving toward the athletic-scholarship approach that certain universities in the East and Midwest sections of Canada have been following for years illegally (Naylor, 2002)! In September, 2001, a Halifax, Nova Scotia team (the St. Mary Huskies) beat Mount Allison's, New Brunswick's football team by a score of 105-0. In this article, one of a series sponsored by The Globe and Mail (Toronto), various aspects of this disturbing development were considered. Interestingly, this is just "penny-ante" compared to the financial practices of various upper-division university conferences in the United States .

How to Reclaim Sport (Weiner). In writing about how society's obsession with sport has "ruined the game," Jay Weiner (2000) of the Minneapolis Star-Tribune asks the question: "How far back must we go to remember that sports matter?" Recalling the time when "sports had meaning," and "sports were accessible," he recommends that society can only "reclaim sports from the corporate entertainment behemoth" if it does the following:

1. Deprofessionalize college and high school sports,
2. Allow some form of public ownership of professional sports teams,
3. Make sports affordable again, and
4. Be conscious of the message sport is sending.

To summarize, the sport industry has quite simply conducted itself in keeping with the prevailing political environment and the ethos of the general public. It has not understood and consequently not accepted the contention that there is an urgent need for sport to serve as a beneficient social institution with an underlying theory looking to humankind's betterment (an "IF 'this,' THEN 'that' will result" type of approach). Thus, it could be argued that society does indeed believe that competitive sport is doing what it is intended to do--i.e., provide both non-moral and moral values to those involved. The non-moral values could be listed as recognition, money, and a certain type of power, whereas the moral values could be of a nature designed to help the team achieve victory--dedication, loyalty, self-sacrifice. If this assessment is accurate, the following question must be asked: What then does the prevailing ethos in sport competition do to help boys and girls, and men and women , to learn honesty fair play, justice, responsibility, and beneficence (i.e., doing good)?

There are continuing strong indications that the sport industry is "charging ahead" driven by the prevailing capitalistic, "global village" image of the future. Increasingly in competitive sport, capitalistic theory is embraced ever more strongly, an approach in which winning is overemphasized with resulting higher profits through increased gate receipts. This same sport industry is aided and abetted by a society in which the majority do not recognize sufficiently the need for sport to serve as a social institution that truly results in individual and social good. Thus, on the one hand there are scholars who argue that democratic states, under girded by the various human rights legislated (e.g., equal opportunity), need a supportive "liberal consensus" to maintain a social system that is fair to all. Yet, conservative, essentialist elements functioning in the same social system do not see this need for a more humanistic, pragmatic consensus about the steadily mounting evidence showing a need for ALL people to be active physically throughout their lives.

It is argued here, therefore, that commercialized sport will have great difficulty "crossing the post-modern divide." Zeigler (*Quest*, 1996) points out that almost every approach to "the good life" stresses a need for an individual's relationship to developmental physical activity such as sport and fitness. Should not we in NASSM be assessing this social institution of sport to determine to what extent the way we present sport to our students is resulting in their becoming imbued with a desire to promote the concept of "sport for all" tp foster overall human betterment?

Functioning With an Indeterminate, Muddled Theory. Once again, before considering future societal scenarios that our culture is facing, I repeat my argument that today sport is functioning vigorously with an indeterminate, muddled theory that implies that sport competition builds both "moral" and "social" character traits consonant with democracy and capitalism. I am arguing further that crossing the post-modern divide means basically that we in NASSM as sport and physical activity management educators should see through the false front and chicanery of the developing economic and technological facade of the global hegemony. Face it: Sport is simply being used as a powerful institution in this "Brave New World" of the 21st century.

Future Societal Scenarios (Anderson)

Walter Truett Anderson (1997), president of the American Division of the World Academy of Art and Science, has sketched four different scenarios as postulations for the future of earthlings in this ongoing adventure of civilization. In this essay "Futures of the Self," taken from *The future of the self: Inventing the postmodern person* (Tarcher/Putnam, 1997), Anderson argues convincingly that current trends are adding up to a turn-of-the-century identity crisis for humankind. The creation of the present "modern self," he explains, began with Plato, Aristotle, and with the rights of humans in Roman legal codes.

The developing conception of self bogged down in the Middle Ages, but fortunately was resurrected in the Renaissance Period described by many historians as the second half of The Middle Ages. Since then the human "self" has been advancing like a "house afire" as the Western world has gone through an almost unbelievable transformation. Without making this an historical treatise, I will say only that scientists like Galileo and Copernicus influenced philosophers such as Descartes and Locke to foresee a world in which the self was invested with human rights.

"One World, Many Universes." Anderson's "One World, Many Universes" version is the most likely to occur. This is a scenario characterized by high economic growth, steadily increasing technological progress, and globalization combined with high psychological development. Such psychological maturity , he predicts, will be possible for a certain segment of the world's population because "active life spans will be gradually lengthened through various advances in health maintenance and medicine" (pp. 251-253)

Nevertheless, a problem has developed with this dream of individual achievement of inalienable rights and privileges, one that looms large at the beginning of this new century. The modern self envisioned by Descartes, a rational, integrated self that Anderson likens to Captain Kirk at the command post of (the original)!) Starship Enterprise, appears to be having an identity crisis. The image of this bold leader (he or she!) taking us fearlessly into the great unknown has begun to fade as alternate scenarios for the future of life on Earth are envisioned. In a world where globalization and economic "progress" seemingly must be rejected because of catastrophic environmental concerns or "demands," the bold-future image could well "be replaced by a post-modern self; decentered, multidimensional, and changeable" (p. 50).

Captain Kirk, or "George W," as he "boldly goes where no man has gone before"--this time to rid the world of terrorists)--is facing a second crucial change. As they seek to shape the world of the 21st century, based on Anderson's analysis, there is another force--the systemic-change force mentioned above--that is shaping the future. This all-powerful force may well exceed the Earth's ability to cope. As gratifying as such factors as "globalization along with economic growth" and "psychological development" may seem to the folks in a coming "One-World, Many Universes" scenario, there is a flip side to this prognosis. This image, Anderson identifies, as "The Dysfunctional Family" scenario. All of these benefits of so-called progress are highly expensive and available now only to relatively few of the six billion plus people on earth. Anderson foresees this as "a world of modern people happily doing their thing; of modern people still obsessed with progress, economic gain, and organizational bigness; and of postmodern people being trampled and getting angry" [italics added] (p. 51). And, I might add further, as people get angrier, present-day terrorism in North America could seem like child's play.

What Kind of A World Do You Want for Your Descendants?

What I am asking here, my colleagues, is whether members of THE one North American professional society for sport management are cognizant of, and approve of, the situation as it has developed. Are we simply "going along with the crowd" while taking the path of least resistance? Can we do anything to improve the situation by implementing an approach with our students that could help to make the situation more wholesome?. More precisely, the question is, whether the North American Society for Sport Management can, and indeed should , re-orient itself to play a significant role in helping sport and physical activity become a social institution exerting a positive influence in the "adventure" of civilization.

To do this, we as professionals should determine what sort of a world we and our descendants should be living in. If you consider yourself an environmentalist, for example, the future looks bleak to you at present. If you are business oriented, however, continued economic and technologic growth could well be the answer to all upcoming problems. Finally, if you see yourself as something of a "New Ager," you can only hope for some sort of mass spiritual transformation to take place.

Finally, as I see it, the members of NASSM are at the moment, individual and collectively, typically conforming blindly to the power structure as it uses our medium of education and recreation--i.e., sport--for its selfish purposes. As one aging person who encountered corruption and sleaze in the intercollegiate athletic structure of several major universities in the United States, I retreated to a Canadian university where the term "scholar-athlete" still implied roughly what it says. However, I now see serious problems developing in Canadian inter-university sport as well.

Two Approaches to Consider. What can this diatribe possibly mean to the members of the North American Society for Sport Management? As I see it, we have several choices before us. One choice is to do nothing. By that I mean that we continue in the same vein as we are doing presently. This would require no great effort, of course. We can simply go along with the prevailing ethos of a society that is using sport to help in the promotion of social, as opposed to moral, character traits. In the process, "business as usual" will be supported one way or the other--by hook or by crook.

A second approach, one that I recommend strongly, is that we live up to the dictates of our constitution. Permit me to remind you what Article II (Purpose) of the Society's constitution calls for. After stating that we should "promote, stimulate, and encourage study, research, scholarly writing, and professional development in the area of sport management broadly interpreted " [the italics are not mine]. It continues by explaining that "this statement of purpose means that the members of this Society are concerned about the theoretical and applied aspects of management theory and practice specifically related to sport, exercise, dance, and play as these enterprises are pursued by all sectors of the population "

Still further, our constitution states that "in the furtherance of these aims and objectives, the Society shall endeavor to carry out the following functions: (a) support and cooperate with local, regional, national, and international organizations having similar purposes. (b) organize and administer meetings to promote the purpose stated above, and (c) issue appropriate proceedings and journals." I don't believe it is necessary to press this point any further. At present the farthest thing from our "collective mind" would be to show steady, deliberative concern about the theoretical and applied aspects of management theory and practice as related to exercise, dance, and play.

What we are showing deliberate concern about to a great extent--and doing it quite nicely--is about the theoretical and applied aspects of commercialized sport management (i.e., management quite narrowly interpreted). This in itself is good, we might say. However, this is simply not enough for a professional society such as ours. And, to repeat, this is especially true if ones reads our constitution. What we are doing, I suggest, is devoting ourselves to the type of sport that in the final analysis means least to our society and ignoring that which could mean the most. We should be seeking the answers to such questions as (1) what is sport's prevailing drift, (2) what are the advantages and disadvantages of sport involvement for life, and (3) what is sport's residual impact on society?

Even though I was personally involved in sport competitively throughout high school and college, and then coached university football, wrestling, and/or swimming over a period of 15 years, I have personally been conducting an informal boycott of the NFL, NBA, and NFL, and of all commercialized university sport for years. Frankly, it disgusts me, because it is basically non-educational and subversive to the higher purposes of democracy. I confess that I still watch golf and tennis on tv, but the rest of it is for the birds.

Further, I'm convinced that the commercialized Olympic Movement with its drugs, officiating, free-loading officials and bribery problems--not to mention its millionaire basketball and hockey players--will eventually suffer the same fate as the ancient Games did in 576 B.C.E. unless radical change takes place soon. The late Baron de Coubertin and Avery Brundage must indeed be "whirling in their graves" at a rate to soon exceed the sound barrier!

Concluding Statement

You may think that I am being unduly pessimistic and have reached the "old-curmudgeon" stage. This may be partially true, but I urge you, the members of NASSM, to adhere--in both your research and in your professional actions--to your stated and approved purpose more carefully than you are doing at present. I urge you further to seek the answer to two fundamental questions, The response to the first question might well cause action to be taken in the near future to answer question #2. These questions are: (1) in what ways can we accurately assess the present status of sport to learn if it is--or is not--fulfilling its role as a presumably beneficient social institution? and (2)--depending on the answer to #1, of course--will you then have the motivation and professional zeal to do your utmost to help sport achieve what could well be its rightful place in society? I believe sport and related physical activity--broadly interpreted--can indeed be a worthwhile social institution contributing to the wellbeing and health of people of all ages and conditions? As they say, "don't be part of the problem, be part of the solution!"

References

Anderson, W.T. (1997). The future of the self: Inventing the postmodern person. NY: Tarcher/Putnam.

Berman, M. (2001) The twilight of American culture, NY: W.W. Norton.

Blinde, E.m. & McCallister, S.G. (1999). Women, disability, and sport and physical fitness activity: The intersection of gender and disability dynamics. Research Quarterly for Sport and Exercise, 70, 3, 303-312.

Booth, F.W., & Chakravarthy, M.V. (2002). Cost and consequnces of sedentary living: New battleground for an old enemy. Research Digest (PCPFS), 3, 16, 1-8.

Cryderman, K. (2001). Sport's culture of adultery. The Vancouver Sun (Canada), August 21, C5.

Depauw, K.P. (1997). The (in)visibility of disability: Cultural contexts and "sporting bodies," Quest, 49, 416-430

Encarta World English Dictionary, The. (1999). NY: St. Martin's Press.

Feschuk, S. (2002). Night of the Olympic dead. National Post (Canada), Feb. 16, B10.

Hahm, C.H., Beller, J.M., & Stoll, S.K. (1989). The Hahm-Beller Values Choice Inventory. Moscow, Idaho: Center for Ethics, The University of Idaho.

Huntington, S.P. (1998). The Clash of Civilizations (and the Remaking of World Order. NY: Touchstone.

Huxley, J. (1957). New wine for new bottles. NY: Harper & Row.

Kavussanu, M. & Roberts, G.C. (2001). Moral functioning in sport: An achievement goal perspective. Journal of Sport and Exercise Psychology, 23, 37-54

Long, W. (2001. Athletes losing faith in hard work. The Vancouver Sun (Canada), Jan. 31. E5.

Lumpkin, A., Stoll, S.K., & Beller, J.M. (1999). Sport ethics: Applications for fair play (2nd ed.). St. Louis: McGraw-Hill.

Malina, R.M. (2001). Tracking of physical activity across the lifespan. Research Digest (PCPFS), 3-14, 1-8.

Muller, Herbert J. (1952) The uses of the past. NY: Mentor.

Naipaul, V.S. (Oct 30, 1990). "Our Universal Civilization." The 1990 Winston Lecture, The Manhattan Institute, New York Review of Books, p. 20.

National Association for Sport and Physical Education. (2001). The coaches code of conduct. Strategies, Nov.-Dec., 11.

Naylor, D. (2002), In pursuit of level playing fields. The Globe and Mail (Canada), March 9, S1.

Priest, R.F., Krause, J.V., & Beach, J. (1999). Four-year changes in college athletes' ethical value choices in sports situations. Research Quarterly for Exercise and Sport, 70, 1, 170-178.

Province, The (Vancouver, Canada) (2000). Drug allegations rock sports world. July 3, A2.

Rudd, A., Stoll, S.K., & Beller, J.M. (1999). Measuring moral and social character among a group of Division 1A college athletes, non-athletes, and ROTC military students. Research Quarterly for Exercise and Sport, 70 (Suppl. 1), 127.

Schlesinger, A.M. (1998). (Rev. & Enl.).The disuniting of America. NY: W.W. Norton.

Skaset, H.B., Email correspondence. May 14, 2002.

Tibbetts, J. (2002). Spend more on popular sports, Canadians say, National Post (Canada), A8, April 15.

Toynbee, A. J. (1947). A study of history. NY: Oxford University Press.

Wallis, D. (2002). Annals of Olympics filled with dubious decisions. National Post (Canada), Feb. 16, B2.

Weiner, J. (Jan.-Feb. 2000). Why our obsession has ruined the game; and how we can save it.Sports centered. Utne Reader, 97, 48-50.

Zeigler, E.F. (1989). An introduction to sport and physical education philosophy. Carmel, IN: Benchmark.

Selection #16
The 21st Century:
What Do We Do Now That We're Here?

Earle F. Zeigler
Canada

> Look not mournfully to the past--it comes not
> back again; wisely improve the present--it is
> thine; go forth to meet the shadowy future
> without fear, and with a manly heart.
> --Longfellow

If the title of this presentation, "The 21st Century: What Do We Do Now That We're Here?". sounds a bit pretentious, I really didn't intend it to be so. I will state at the outset that I make no claim to omniscience on this subject. The words of Longfellow above, it seems to me, are among the best I have seen for general guidance (with apologies for his unwitting chauvinism in his final words). We have made our mistakes in the past; we have a fairly good idea of where we are at the present; and we must move into the future strongly and boldly, but with great care and concern.

I plan to spell out what I consider the necessary steps for us to take as a field (and potential) profession as we "sculpt the future." Then I will conclude with some thoughts on "the task ahead." First, however, what I propose to say here will be offered in a somewhat different perspective or slant: it will be somewhat more general socially, and also more normatively philosophical. I am very matter of fact and very specific as to how our field and profession had been "modified." This occurred to a certain extent because of the impact of various social forces (e.g., economics), but also because of our many sins of omission and commission. In what follows I don't propose to repeat myself--although the occasional similar thought or phrase might slip in when an example is drawn.

If I were not worried about the future generally, and about the future of our own field specifically, I don't believe that I would have undertaken this task. (I have presumably been officially retired since 1985!) However, I want to make it clear that I don't for one minute buy the thought expressed by Sir Arthur Wing Pinero in his *The Second Mrs. Tanqueray* to the effect that "the future is only the past again, entered through another gate." I am much more inclined to the sentiment expressed by Henrik Ibsen in a letter to Georg Brandes in which he stated, "I hold that man is in the right who is most closely in league with the future." Indeed, but there's the rub, I suppose: Just how does one "get in league with the future"? The answer to this question is probably--"With some difficulty." Nevertheless, I think we would all agree that the achievement of such understanding is our task alone; no one else is going to do it *for* us.

Forecasting the Future

"Getting in league with the future" may come true, I presume, by making a sincere, solid effort to understand what "futurology" is all about. I turned first for some guidance to *Visions of the Future* (Melnick, 1984), a publication of the well-known Hudson Institute. Initially, we are told that there are three ways of "looking at the future": (1) the *possible* future, (2) the *probable* future, and (3) the *preferable* future (p. 4). The next step is to decide which of the three ways to consider first to apply these findings in our lives. Initially, then, it is the *possible* future of the profession of what I call physical activity education and educational sport that I consider first.

As you might imagine, the *possible* future includes everything that *could* happen. Thus, perceptions of the future can be formed by us either individually and collectively. The *probable* future refers to occurrences that are likely to happen, and here the range of alternatives should be considered. Finally, the *preferable* future relates to an approach whereby people first make choices that indicate how they would like things to happen. Underlying any thought, there are certain basic assumptions or premises:

(1) that the future hasn't been predetermined by some force or power,

2) that the future cannot be accurately predicted because we don't understand the process of change fully, and

(3) that the future will undoubtedly be influenced by choices that people make, but won't necessarily turn out the way they want it to be (Amara, 1981).

As we all appreciate, people have been predicting the future for thousands of years, undoubtedly with a limited degree of success. Considerable headway has been made, of course, since the time when animal entrails were examined to provide insight about the future (i.e., one of the techniques of so-called divination). Nowadays, for example, methods of prediction include forecasting by the use of trends and statistics. One most recent approach (Megatrends, 1982) along this line has been of great interest to me because I have been using a variation of this technique for more than 40 years, one that originated with John S. Brubacher (1947). It is termed a "a persistent problems approach". I have used it to help analyze my own field (see Zeigler, 1964, 1968, 1977a, 1977b, 1984, 1988, 1989, 1990, 1992, 1994a, 1994b, 2003, 2005).

John Naisbitt and The Naisbitt Group (Megatrends 1982 and subsequent publications) believe that "the most reliable way to anticipate the future is by understanding the present" (p. 2). Thus, they monitor occurrences all over the world through a technique of descriptive method known as *content analysis*. They actually monitor the amount of space given to various topics in newspapers, an approach they deem valid because "the news-reporting process is forced choice in a closed system" (p. 4).

Melnick and associates (1984) discussed a further aspect of futurology–the question of "levels of certainty." They explain that the late, great scholar, Herman Kahn, often used the term "Scotch Verdict" when he was concerned about the level of certainty available prior to making a decision. He borrowed this idea from the Scottish system of justice in which a person charged with the commission of a crime can be found "guilty," "not guilty," or "not been proven guilty." This "not been proven guilty" (or "Scotch") verdict implies there is enough evidence to demonstrate that the person charged is guilty, but that insufficient evidence has been presented to end *all reasonable doubt* about the matter. Thus, a continuum has been developed at one end of which we can state we are 100% sure that such-and-such is *not* true. Accordingly, at the other end of the continuum we can state we are 100% sure that such-and-such is the case (pp. 6-7). Obviously, in between these two extremes are gradations of the level of certainty. From here this idea has been carried over to the realm of future forecasting.

Next we are exhorted to consider the "Great Transition" that humankind has been experiencing, how there has been a pre-industrial stage, an industrial stage and, finally, a post-industrial stage that seems to have arrived in North America first. Each of the stages has its characteristics that we recognize. For example, in the pre-industrial era there was slow population growth, people lived simply with very little money, and the forces of nature made life very difficult. When the industrial stage or so-called modernization entered the picture, population growth was rapid, wealth increased enormously, and people became increasingly less vulnerable to the destructive forces of nature. The assumption here is that comprehension of the transition that is occurring now can give us some insight as to what the future might hold. We cannot be "100% sure", but at least we might be able to achieve a "Scotch Verdict" (p. 47). If North America is that part of the world that is the most advanced economically and technologically, and as a result will complete the Great Transition by becoming a post-industrial culture, then we must be aware of what this will mean to our society. Melnick believes that we have probably already entered a "super-industrial period" of the Industrial Stage in which "projects will be very large scale, services will be readily available, efficient and sophisticated, people will have vastly increased leisure time, and many new technologies will be created" (pp. 35-37).

It is important that we understand what is happening as we move further forward into what presumably is the final or third stage of the Great Transition. First, it should be made clear that the level of certainty here about predictions is at Kahn's "Scotch Verdict" point on the continuum. The world has never faced this situation before; so, we do not know exactly how to date the beginning of such a stage. Nevertheless, it seems to be taking place right now (i.e., with the super-industrial period starting after World War II). As predicted, those developments mentioned above (e.g., services readily available) appear to be continuing. It is postulated that population growth is slower than it was 20 years ago; yet it is true that people are living longer. Next, it is estimated that a greater interdependence among nations and the steady development of new technologies will contribute to a steadily improving economic climate for underdeveloped nations. Finally, the forecast is that advances in science and accompanying technology will bring almost innumerable technologies to the fore that will affect life styles immeasurably all over the world.

This discussion could continue almost indefinitely, but the important points to be made here are emerging rapidly. First, we need a different way of looking at the subject of natural resources. In this interdependent world, this "global village" if you will, natural resources are more than just the sum of raw materials. They include also the application of technology, the organizational bureaucracy to cope with the materials, and the resultant usefulness of the resource that creates supply and demand (p. 74). The point seems to be that the total resource picture (as explained here) is reasonably optimistic *if correct decisions are made* about raw materials, energy, food production, and use of the environment. These are admittedly rather large "IFS" (pp. 73-97).

Finally, in this "forecasting the future" section, the need to understand global problems of two types is stressed. One group is called "mostly understandable problems," *and they are solvable*. Here reference is made to:

> (1) population growth,
> (2) natural resource issues,
> (3) acceptable environmental health, (
> 4) shift in society's economic base to service
> occupations, and
> (5) effect of advanced technology.

However, it is the second group classified as "mostly uncertain problems," that could bring on disaster! First, the Great Transition is affecting the entire world, and the eventual outcome of this new type of cultural change is uncertain. Thus, we must be ready for these developments

346

attitudinally. Second, in this period of changing values and attitudes, people in the various countries and cultures have much to learn and they will have to make great adjustments as well. Third, there is the danger that society will, possibly unwittingly-, stumble into some irreversible environmental catastrophe (e.g., upper-atmosphere ozone depletion). Fourth, the whole problem of weapons, wars, and terrorism, and whether the world will be able to stave off all-out nuclear warfare. Fifth, and finally, whether bad luck and bad management will somehow block the entire world from undergoing the Great Transition successfully, obviously a great argument for the development of management art and science (pp. 124-129).

What Should We Avoid in the 21st Century?

Before recommending what we, in the field of physical activity education and educational sport under girded by the scholarly contributions of kinesiology or exercise science, *should do* as we move along in the 21st century, we should undoubtedly give brief consideration to the question of *what to avoid* along this path. First, there is evidence to suggest that we should maintain flexibility in our philosophical approach. This will be difficult for some who have worked out definite, explicit philosophic stances. For those who are struggling along with *an implicit sense of life* (as defined by Rand, 1960), however, having philosophic flexibility may be even more difficult because they don't fully understand "where they are coming from"! We all know people for whom Alvin Toffler's concepts of "future shock" and "third wave world" have become a reality. Life has indeed become stressful for these individuals.

Second, I believe that we as individuals should avoid what may be called either "naive optimism" or "despairing pessimism" in the years ahead. What we should assume, I believe, is a philosophical stance that is named "positive meliorism", a position that assumes that we should strive consciously to bring about a steady improvement in the quality of our lives. This "what-to-avoid" item is related to the recommendation above concerning flexibility in philosophical approach, of course. We cannot forget, however, how easy it is to fall into the seemingly "attractive traps" of either blind pessimism or blind optimism.

Third, I believe the professional in physical activity education and educational sport should continue to strive for "just the right amount" of "freedom" in his or her life generally and in one's professional affairs as well. Freedom for the individual is a fundamental characteristic of a democratic state, but it should never be forgotten that such freedom as may prevail in all countries today had to be won "inch by inch." It is evidently in the nature of the human animal that there are always people in our midst who "know what is best for us," and who seem anxious to take our hard-won freedoms away. This seems to be true whether crises exist or not. Of course, the concept of 'individual freedom' can not be stretched to include anarchy. On the other hand, the freedom to *teach* what we will responsibly in physical activity education and educational sport, or conversely the freedom to *learn* what one will in such a process, should be guarded almost fanatically.

A fourth pitfall in this matter of avoidance along the way is the possibility of the development of undue influence of certain *negative* aspects inherent in the various social forces capable of influencing our culture and everything within it (including, of course, physical activity education and educational sport). Consider the phenomenon of nationalism and how an overemphasis in this direction can soon destroy a desirable world posture or even bring about unconscionable isolationism. Another example of a "negative" social force that is not understood generally is the clash between capitalistic economic theory and the environmental crisis that has developed. "Bigger" is not necessarily "better" in the final analysis.

Fifth, moving back to the realm of education, we must be careful that our field doesn't contribute to what has consistently been identified as a fundamental anti-intellectualism in the United States. On the other hand, "intelligence or intellectualism for its own sake" is far being the answer to our problems. As long ago as 1961, Brubacher asked for the "golden mean" between the cultivation of the intellect and the cultivation of a high degree of intelligence because it is need as "an instrument of survival" in the Deweyan sense (pp. 7-9).

Sixth, and finally, despite the cry for a "return to essentials" in the final quarter of the 20th century–and I am not for a moment suggesting that Johnny or Mary shouldn't know how to read and calculate mathematically– we should avoid imposing a narrow academic approach on students in a misguided effort to promote the pursuit of excellence. I am continually both amazed and discouraged by decisions concerning admission to professional programs in undergraduate physical activity education programs made *solely* on numerical grades, in essence a narrowly defined academic proficiency. Do not throw out academic proficiency testing, of course, but by all means broaden the evaluation made of candidates by assessing other dimensions of excellence they may have–i.e., the actual life competencies they have achieved! Here, in addition to ability in human motor performance, I include such aspects as "sensitivity and commitment to social responsibility, ability to adapt to new situations, characteristics of temperament and work habit under varying conditions of demand," and other such characteristics, traits, and competencies as recommended as long ago as 1970 by the Commission on Tests of the College Entrance Examination Board (*The New York Times*, Nov. 2, 1970)

What *Should* We Do in the 21st Century?

What should we do--perhaps what *must* we do--to ensure that the profession will move more decisively and rapidly in the direction of what

348

might be called <u>true</u> professional status? Granting that the various social forces will undoubtedly influence us, what can we do collectively in the years immediately ahead? These positive steps should be actions that will effect a workable consolidation of purposeful accomplishments on the part of those men and women who have a concern for the future of developmental physical activity as a valuable component of the entire life of a human. The following represent a number of categories joined with action principles that are related to the listing of "modifications" that have occurred in the past 30 years. We should seek a North American consensus on the steps spelled out below. Then we, as dedicated professionals, should take as rapid and strong action as we can muster through our professional associations in the United States and Canada. These recommended steps are as follows:

1. A Sharper Image. In the past the field of physical education has tried to be "all things to all people," and now does not know exactly what it does stand for. Now we should now sharpen our image and improve the quality of our efforts by focusing primarily on developmental physical activity–specifically, human motor performance in sport, exercise, and related expressive movement. As we sharpen our image, we should make a strong effort to include those who are working in the private agency and commercial sectors. This implies further that we will extend our efforts to promote the finest type of developmental physical activity for people of all ages in "normal, accelerated, or special" populations.

2. Our Profession's Name. All sorts of name changes have been implemented to explain either what people think we are doing or should be doing, or to camouflage the presumed "unsavory" connotation of the term "physical education" that evidently conjures up the notion of a "dumb jock" working with the lesser part of a tri-partite human body. Nevertheless, we should continue to focus primarily on developmental physical activity as defined immediately above while moving toward an acceptable working term for our profession. In so doing, we should keep in mind the profession's bifurcated nature in that it has both theoretical and practical (*or disciplinary and professional*) aspects. At the moment we are still called physical education and sport professionally and physical and health education in a significant number of elementary and secondary schools in Canada where the professional association just changed its name to Physical and Health Education Canada. A desirable name might be developmental physical activity, and we could delineate this by our inclusion of sport, exercise, and expressive movement.

3. A Tenable Body of Knowledge. Various social forces and professional concerns have placed us in a position where we don't know where or what our body of knowledge is, we will strongly support the idea of disciplinary definition and the continuing

development of a body of knowledge based on such a consensual definition. From this should come a merging of tenable scientific theory in keeping with societal values and computer technology so that we will gradually, steadily, and increasingly provide our members with the knowledge that they need to perform as top-flight professionals. As professional practitioners we simply must possess the requisite knowledge, competencies, and skills necessary to provide developmental physical activity services of a high quality to the public.

4. Our Own Professional Associations. There is insufficient support of our own professional associations for a variety of reasons. Thus, we need to develop voluntary and mandatory mechanisms that relate membership in professional organizations both directly and indirectly to stature within the field. We simply must commit ourselves to work tirelessly and continually to promote the welfare of professional practitioners who are serving the public in areas that we represent. Incidentally, it may be necessary to exert any available pressures to encourage people to give first priority to our own groups (as opposed to those of related disciplines and/or allied professions). The logic behind this dictum is that our own survival comes first for us!

5. Professional Licensing. Teachers-coaches in the schools, colleges, and universities are protected indefinitely by the shelter of the all-embracing teaching profession. However, we should now move rapidly and strongly to seek official recognition of our endeavors in public, semi-public, and private agency work and in commercial organizations relating to developmental physical activity through professional licensing at the state or provincial level. Further, we should encourage individuals to apply for voluntary registration as qualified practitioners at the federal level in both the United States and Canada.

6. Harmony Within The Profession. An unacceptable series of gaps and misunderstandings has developed among (1) those in our field concerned primarily with the bio-scientific aspects of human motor performance, (2) those concerned with the social-science and humanities aspects, (3) those concerned with the general education of all students, and (4) those concerned with the professional preparation of physical educators/coaches, all at the college or university level. Hence, we should strive for a greater balance and improved understanding among these essential entities within the profession.

7. Harmony Among The Allied Professions. The field of physical education spawned a number of allied professions down through the years of the 20th century. Now we should seek to comprehend what they claim that they do professionally, and where there may be a possible overlap with what we claim that we do. Where disagreements prevail, they should be ironed out to the greatest extent possible at the

national level within the Alliance (AAHPERD)and within Physical and Health Education Canada (the former CAHPERD).

8. The Relationship With Intercollegiate Athletics. For several reasons an ever-larger wedge has been driven between units of physical education and interscholastic and intercollegiate athletics in educational institutions where gate receipts are a strong and basic factor. Such a rift serves no good purpose and is counter to the best interests of both groups. Thus, we will work for greater understanding and harmony with those people who are primarily interested in the promotion of highly organized, often commercialized athletics. At the same time it is imperative that we do all in our power to maintain athletics in a sound educational perspective within our schools, colleges, and universities.

9. The Relationship with Intramurals and Recreational Sports. Intramurals and recreational sports is in a transitional state at present in that it has proved that it is "here to stay" at the college and university level. Nevertheless, intramurals hasn't really taken hold yet, generally speaking, at the high school level, despite the fact that it has a great deal to offer the large majority of students in what may truly be called recreational (educational?) sport.

Both philosophically and practically, intramurals and recreational sports ought to remain within the sphere of the physical education profession. It is impractical and inadvisable to attempt to subsume all non-curricular activities on campus under one department or division. Thus, departments and divisions of physical education and athletics ought to work for consensus on the idea that intramurals and recreational sports are co-curricular in nature and deserve regular funding as laboratory experience in the same manner that general education course experiences in physical education receive their funding for instructional purposes.

10. Guaranteeing Equal Opportunity. "Life, liberty, and the pursuit of happiness" are guaranteed to all in North American society. As members of a profession, we should move positively and strongly to see to it that equal opportunity is indeed provided to the greatest possible extent to women, to minority groups, and to special populations as they seek to improve the quality of their lives through the finest type of experience in the many activities of our field.

11. The Physical (Activity) Education Identity. In addition to the development of the allied professions (e.g., school health education) in the second quarter of the twentieth century, we witnessed the advent of a disciplinary thrust in the 1960s that was followed by a splintering of many of the field's "knowledge components" to form many different

sub disciplinary societies. These developments have undoubtedly weakened the overall field of physical education in both educational institutions and in the larger society. Thus, it is now more important than ever that we hold high the physical education identity as we continue to promote vigorously the professional and scholarly foundations opf our profession.

12. Applying the Competency Approach. The failures and inconsistencies of the established educational process have become increasingly apparent. Thus, we will as a profession explore the educational possibilities of a competency approach as it might apply to general education, to professional preparation, and to all aspects of our professional endeavor in public, semi-public, private, and commercial agency endeavors. This means that initially we will indicate clearly what state or quality we are asking students to achieve in the various theoretical and practical experiences outlined in the curriculum. Then we will see to it that they achieve sufficient knowledge and skill to fulfill the curricular requirements before they advance to the next stage of their development.

13. Managing the Enterprise. All professionals in the unique field of sport and physical education are managers--but to varying degrees. The "one course in administration" approach with no laboratory or internship experience of earlier times is simply not sufficient for the future. There is an urgent need to apply a competency approach in the preparation (as well as in the continuing education) of those who will serve as managers either within educational circles or elsewhere in the society.

14. Ethics and Morality in Physical Activity Education and Educational Sport. In the course of the development of the best professions, the various, embryonic professional groups have gradually become conscious of the need for a set of professional ethics–that is, a set of professional obligations that are established as norms for practitioners in good standing to follow. Our profession needs a well-defined creed, as well as a detailed code of ethics as we move ahead in our development. Such a move is important because, generally speaking, ethical confusion prevails in North American society. Such a sound code of ethics should be combined with steady improvement in the three essentials of a fine profession would relatively soon place us in a much firmer position to claim that we are indeed members of a fine profession. These three "essentials" are (1) an extensive period of training, (2) a significant intellectual component that must be mastered before the profession is practiced, and (3) a recognition by society that the trained person can provide a basic, important service to its citizens (Zeigler, 1984, 1992, 2002, 2007).

15. Reunifying the Profession's Integral Elements. There now appears to be reasonable agreement that what is now called physical (activity) education and (educational) sport is concerned primarily with developmental physical activity as manifested in human motor performance in sport, exercise, and related expressive movement. Thus, we will now work for the reunification of those elements of our profession that should be uniquely ours within our disciplinary definition.

16. Cross-Cultural Comparison and International   Understanding. We have done reasonably well in the area of international relations within the Western world due to the solid efforts of many dedicated people over a considerable period of time. However, we now need to redouble our efforts to make cross-cultural comparisons of physical education and educational sport while reaching out for international understanding and cooperation in both the so-called Western and Eastern blocs. Much greater understanding on the part of all of the concepts of 'communication,' 'diversity,' and 'cooperation' is required for the creation of a better life for all in a peaceful world. Our profession can contribute significantly toward this long range objective.

17. Permanency and Change. The "principal principles" espoused for physical education and sport by the late Arthur Steinhaus of George Williams College still apply most aptly to our professional endeavors. These are the overload principle, the principle of reversibility, the principle of integration and integrity, and the principle of the priority of man and woman). We should now emphasize that which is timeless in our work, while at the same time accepting the inevitability of certain societal change. (See, also, "Physical education's 13 principal principles" by E.F. Zeigler, 1994).

18. Improving the Quality of Life. Our field is unique within education and in society. Since fine living and professional success involve so much more than the important verbal and mathematical skills, we will emphasize strongly that education is a lifelong enterprise. Further, we will stress that *the quality of life can be improved significantly through the achievement of a higher degree of kinetic awareness and through heightened experiences in sport, exercise, and related expressive movement.*

19. Reasserting Our "Will to Win". The developments of the past 40 years have undoubtedly created an uneasiness and concern about the future of the profession. Doubts have been raised by some as to the field's "will to win" through the achievement of the highest type of professional status. We *pledge ourselves to make still greater*

efforts to become vibrant and stirring through absolute dedication and commitment in our professional endeavors. Ours is a high calling as we seek to improve the quality of life for all through the finest type developmental physical activity in sport, exercise, and related expressive movement.

The Professional Task Ahead

What, then, is the professional task ahead? First, we should truly understand why we have chosen this profession as we rededicate ourselves anew to the study and dissemination of knowledge, competencies, and skills in human motor performance in sport, exercise, and related expressive movement. Concurrently, of course, we need to determine exactly what it is that we are professing.

Second, as either professional practitioners or instructors involved in professional preparation, we should search for young people of high quality in all the attributes needed for success in the field. Then we should follow through to help them develop lifelong commitments so that our profession can achieve its democratically agreed-upon goals. We should also prepare young people to serve in the many alternative careers in sport, exercise, dance, and recreational play that are becoming increasingly available in our society.

Third, we must place *quality* as the first priority of our professional endeavors. Our personal involvement and specialization should include a high level of competency and skill under girded by solid knowledge about the profession. It can be argued that our professional task is as important as any in society. Thus, the present is no time for indecision, half-hearted commitment, imprecise knowledge, and general unwillingness to stand up and be counted in debate with colleagues within our field and in allied professions and related disciplines, not to mention the public.

Fourth, the obligation is ours. If we hope to reach our potential, we must sharpen our focus and improve the quality of our professional effort. Only in this way will we be able to guide the modification process that the profession is currently undergoing toward the achievement of our highest professional goals. This is the time, right now, to employ sport, exercise, dance, and play to make our reality more healthful, more pleasant, more vital, and more life enriching. By "living fully in one's body," behavioral science men and women will be adapting and shaping this phase of reality to their own ends.

Finally, such improvement will not come easily; it can only come through the efforts of professional people making quality decisions, through the motivation of people to change their sedentary lifestyles, and through our professional assistance in guiding people as they strive to fulfill such motivation in their movement patterns. When our black brothers and sisters speak about the concept of 'soul,' they mean placing a special quality into some aspect of life (e.g., soul music). Our missions in the years ahead is to place this special quality in all of our professional endeavor.

References and Bibliography

Amara, R. (1981). The futures field. *The Futurist*, February.

Brubacher, J.S. (1947). *A history of the problems of education.* New York: McGraw-Hill.

Brubacher, J.S. (1961). Higher education and the pursuit of excellence. *Marshall University Bulletin*, 3:3.

Melnick, R. (1984). *Visions of the future.* Croton-on-Hudson, NY: Hudson Institute.

Naisbitt, J. (1982). *Megatrends.* New York: Warner

New York Times, The. (1970). Report by Commission on Tests of the College Entrance Examination Board, Nov. 2

Rand, A. (1960*). The romantic manifesto.* New York: World Publishing.

Zeigler, E. F. (1951). *A History of Professional Preparation for Physical Education in the United States* . Eugene, OR: University of Oregon Microform Publications, 1951).

Zeigler, E. F. (1968). *Problems in the History and Philosophy of Physical Education and Sport* Englewood Cliffs, NJ: Prentice-Hall.

Zeigler, E. F. (1977). Relationships in Physical Education: A Viewpoint from History and Philosophy. In The Academy Papers (No. 11), Relationships in Physical Education (Ed. M. Gladys Scott). Washington, DC: AAHPERD, 14-23.

Zeigler, E. F. (Ed. & Au.).(1975). *History of Sport and Physical Education in the United States and Canada. Champaign, IL:* Stipes, 1975).

Zeigler, E. F. (1979). *Issues in North American Physical Education and Sport.* Washington, DC: AAHPERD, 1979.

Zeigler, E. F. (1986). *Assessing Sport and Physical Education: Diagnosis and Projection* Champaign, IL: Stipes.

Zeigler, E. F. (1991*). Sport and Physical Education: Past, Present, Future.* Champaign, IL: Stipes, 1991).

Zeigler, E. F. (2003). *Socio-Cultural Foundations of Physical Education and Educational Sport.* Aachen: Germany: Meyer & Meyer.

Zeigler, E. F. (2005). *History and Status of American Physical Education and Educational Sport.* Victoria, Canada: Trafford.

Zeigler, E. F. (2007). *Applied Ethics for Sport and Physical Activity Professionals.* Victoria, Canada: Trafford